Pediatric Stroke Rehabilitation

An Interprofessional and Collaborative Approach

Pediatric Stroke Rehabilitation

An Interprofessional and Collaborative Approach

Heather L. Atkinson, PT, DPT, NCS
Board Certified Neurologic Clinical Specialist
Physical Therapy Department
The Children's Hospital of Philadelphia
Philadelphia, Pennsylvania

Kim Nixon-Cave, PT, PhD, PCS
Board Certified Pediatric Clinical Specialist
Department of Physical Therapy
Thomas Jefferson University
College of Health Professions
Philadelphia, Pennsylvania

Sabrina E. Smith, MD, PhD
Division of Pediatric Neurology
Fellow of the Academy of Medical Educators
Kaiser Permanente Oakland Medical Center
Oakland, California

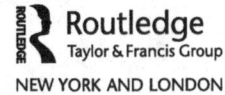

Routledge
Taylor & Francis Group

NEW YORK AND LONDON

Instructors: *Pediatric Stroke Rehabilitation: An Interprofessional and Collaborative Approach* includes ancillary materials specifically available for faculty use. Included are PowerPoint slides. Please visit www.routledge.com/9781617116186 to obtain access.

First published 2018 by SLACK Incorporated

Published 2024 by Routledge
605 Third Avenue, New York, NY 10158

and by Routledge
4 Park Square, Milton Park, Abingdon, Oxon OX14 4RN

Routledge is an imprint of the Taylor & Francis Group, an informa business

Library of Congress Cataloging-in-Publication Data

Names: Atkinson, Heather L., 1973- editor. | Nixon-Cave, Kim, editor. |
  Smith, Sabrina E., 1970- editor.
Title: Pediatric stroke rehabilitation : an interprofessional and
  collaborative approach / [edited by] Heather L. Atkinson, Kim Nixon-Cave,
  Sabrina E. Smith.
Description: Thorofare, NJ : SLACK Incorporated, [2018] | Includes
  bibliographical references and index.
Identifiers: LCCN 2017020333 (print) | ISBN 9781617116186
Subjects: | MESH: Stroke--therapy | Stroke Rehabilitation--methods | Child |
  Treatment Outcome
Classification: LCC RJ496.C45 (print) | NLM WL 356 |
  DDC 618.92/81--dc23
LC record available at https://lccn.loc.gov/2017020333

ISBN: 9781617116186 (hbk)
ISBN: 9781003525578 (ebk)

DOI: 10.4324/9781003525578

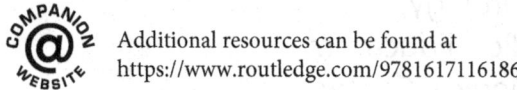
Additional resources can be found at
https://www.routledge.com/9781617116186

Dedication

This book is dedicated to the survivors of childhood stroke, their amazing families, and to the interprofessional teams who work in partnership to help the children and families achieve their goals.

Contents

Dedication v
About the Editors ix
Contributing Authors xi
Foreword by Rebecca Ichord, MD xiii
Introduction xv

Section I   **Pediatric Stroke: Medical Management and the Continuum of Care** 1
Chapter 1   Childhood Arterial Ischemic Stroke 3
       Adam Kirton, MD, MsC, FRCPC
Chapter 2   Perinatal Arterial Ischemic Stroke 21
       Sabrina E. Smith, MD, PhD
Chapter 3   Cerebral Sinovenous Thrombosis in Children 35
       Mubeen F. Rafay, MB.BS, FCPS, MSc
Chapter 4   Intracerebral Hemorrhage in Neonates and Children 59
       Shih-Shan Lang, MD and Gregory G. Heuer, MD, PhD
Chapter 5   The Provision of Rehabilitation Medicine Across the Continuum of Care in Pediatric Stroke 69
       Phillip R. Bryant, DO

Section II   **Optimizing Functional Outcomes After Pediatric Stroke.** 89
Chapter 6   Examination and Evaluation of Neuromotor Function in Children With Stroke 91
       Heather L. Atkinson, PT, DPT, NCS and Susan V. Duff, EdD, MPT, OTR/L, CHT
Chapter 7   Intervention for Functional Motor Skills in Children With Stroke 113
       Heather L. Atkinson, PT, DPT, NCS; Mardee Greenham, PhD;
       Anna Cooper, BOT, GC Paediatric OT; and Anne Gordon, PhD, MSc, BAppSc
Chapter 8   Communication and Feeding in Children With Stroke 135
       Amy Colin, MA, CCC-SLP and Elizabeth Yeh, MA, CCC-SLP
Chapter 9   Cognitive Changes and Potential in Children With Stroke 161
       Amanda Fuentes, PhD, C Psych and Robyn Westmacott, PhD, C Psych, ABPP
Chapter 10   Behavioral and Emotional Functioning in Children With Stroke 185
       Lauren Krivitzky, PhD, ABPP-CN and Danielle Bosenbark, PhD

Section III   **The Child's Environment: Family and Community** 205
       Introduction 206
       Kim Nixon-Cave, PT, PhD, PCS
Chapter 11   The Family and Child's Environment in Children With Stroke 211
       Lois J. Robbins, DSW, LSW and Kim Nixon-Cave, PT, PhD, PCS
Chapter 12   Educational Needs of a Child/Adolescent Following a Stroke 227
       Elisa Olson D'Achille, MEd and Juliana Bloom, PhD
Chapter 13   Prevention to Poststroke Rehabilitation: Lifelong Management, Advocacy, and Resources for Children With Stroke 247
       Kim Nixon-Cave, PT, PhD, PCS and Mary Kay Ballasiotes

Financial Disclosures 259
Index 261

About the Editors

Heather L. Atkinson, PT, DPT, NCS graduated from Arcadia University with a master of science in Physical Therapy and subsequently earned her Doctor of Physical Therapy degree from Temple University. She became a board-certified specialist in neurologic physical therapy in 2003. She has worked at the Children's Hospital of Philadelphia (CHOP) for over 20 years, including 10 years in the Pediatric Stroke Program. Dr. Atkinson works to expand pediatric stroke rehabilitation research and has served as an investigator on clinical studies examining modified constraint-induced therapy as well as asymmetric gait training in children with hemiparesis due to stroke. Dr. Atkinson teaches about pediatric stroke at local academic universities and is passionate about empowering children and families to maximize their functional potential. Dr. Atkinson is also interested in cultivating clinical reasoning skills along the continuum of professional development and she serves as a leader in the post-professional pediatric physical therapy residency and fellowship programs at CHOP. Dr. Atkinson aspires to better integrate shared decision making into physical therapist practice and she is currently leading a quality improvement project on building shared decision-making strategies into clinical practice with the aim of improving the overall patient experience of care.

Kim Nixon-Cave, PT, PhD, PCS is physical therapist who specializes in pediatrics. Dr. Nixon-Cave is an associate professor at Thomas Jefferson University, in the role of program director for the entry-level doctor of physical therapy and post-professional education, residency and fellowship education. She practices as a clinician in the Thomas Jefferson University Hospital in pediatrics, primarily the neonatal intensive care unit. Before taking the position at Thomas Jefferson University, Dr. Nixon-Cave was the manager of the Physical Therapy Department in The Center of Rehabilitation Services at The Children's Hospital of Philadelphia (CHOP) as well as providing direct patient care. She developed a physical therapy Pediatric Residency and Neonatology Fellowship program while at CHOP. Dr. Nixon-Cave has held several faculty appointments, including Temple University, as associate professor, program director and interim chair; associate professor at University of the Sciences; and associate faculty at Arcadia University. She has served on national boards for the American Physical Therapy Association, including the American Board of Physical Therapy Specialties, and American Board of Physical Therapy Residency and Fellowship Education, with the responsibility of developing board certification and post-professional educational programs. She has also focused efforts on addressing the changing health care environment and its impact on delivery of physical therapy services nationally. Recognized by APTA as an Innovator for changes in physical therapy practice as it relates to health care reform, Dr. Nixon-Cave's clinical focus is developing evidence-based clinical programs and protocols for various patient populations with a specific interest in infants and young children. Quality Improvement Projects have focused on clinical practice, reimbursement, episodic care in inpatient and outpatient practice settings, and best practice guidelines.

Dr. Nixon-Cave is a trained qualitative researcher but participates in research studies that utilize different research approaches including quantitative, qualitative, and mix methodologies to explore and examine health disparities, clinical decision-making of physical therapists, the impact of culture and environment on overall development, and the experience of patients and families and their interaction with the health care system. Dr. Nixon-Cave recently completed a research project examining the current practice of board certified pediatric specialists in physical therapy resulting in a description of specialty practice for physical therapy pediatric certified specialists. Dr. Nixon-Cave has published papers on various topics related to her research area and specifically clinical reasoning and cultural competence in physical therapy.

Dr. Nixon-Cave graduated from the University of Pittsburgh earning her entry-level degree in physical therapy followed by an advanced masters of science degree in Neurologic physical therapy and a PhD in Education from Temple University.

Sabrina E. Smith, MD, PhD is a pediatric neurologist at Kaiser Permanente Oakland Medical Center in Oakland, California. Before moving to Kaiser Permanente, Dr. Smith was a member of the Pediatric Stroke Team at the Children's Hospital of Philadelphia for 7 years, providing inpatient consultation for newborns and children who experienced a stroke, and running a multidisciplinary outpatient clinic for children who experienced a stroke in the newborn period. Dr. Smith graduated Magna Cum Laude from Princeton University before receiving her MD and a PhD in neurophysiology from New York University School of Medicine. She then completed a residency in pediatrics at the University of California-San Francisco School of Medicine and a residency in pediatric neurology at the University of Pennsylvania School of Medicine and the Children's Hospital of Philadelphia. Dr. Smith completed a postdoctoral fellowship in cognitive neurology at the University of Pennsylvania School of Medicine where her research focused on the cognitive effects of stroke and other types of brain injury in children. Dr. Smith has published numerous papers on perinatal and childhood stroke and has given talks at national and international meetings.

Contributing Authors

Mary Kay Ballasiotes (Chapter 13)
Co-Founder/President
International Alliance for Pediatric Stroke

Juliana Bloom, PhD (Chapter 12)
The Levin Center
Atlanta, Georgia

Danielle Bosenbark, PhD (Chapter 10)
The Children's Hospital of Philadelphia
Philadelphia, Pennsylvania

Phillip R. Bryant, DO (Chapter 5)
Clinical Professor of Pediatrics
University of Pennsylvania
Perelman School of Medicine
The Children's Hospital of Philadelphia
Philadelphia, Pennsylvania

Amy Colin, MA, CCC-SLP (Chapter 8)
The Children's Hospital of Philadelphia
Philadelphia, Pennsylvania

Anna Cooper BOT, GC Paediatric OT (Chapter 7)
Murdoch Children's Research Institute
The University of Melbourne
Parkville, Victoria, Australia

Susan V. Duff, EdD, MPT, OTR/L, CHT (Chapter 6)
Chapman University
Crean College of Health and Behavioral Sciences
Department of Physical Therapy
Irvine, California
Shriners Hospital for Children
Rehabilitation Department
Occupational Therapy & Physical Therapy
Philadelphia, Pennsylvania

Amanda Fuentes, PhD, C Psych (Chapter 9)
Department of Psychology
York University
Toronto, Ontario, Canada

Anne Gordon, PhD, MSc, BAppSc (Chapter 7)
Evelina London Children's Hospital
Guy's and St. Thomas Hospital NHS Foundation
    Trust
Institute of Psychiatry, Psychology and Neuroscience
King's College
London, United Kingdom

Mardee Greenham, PhD (Chapter 7)
Clinical Sciences
Murdoch Childrens Research Institute
School of Psychological Sciences
University of Melbourne
Melbourne, Victoria, Australia

Gregory G. Heuer, MD, PhD (Chapter 4)
Division of Neurosurgery
The Children's Hospital of Philadelphia
University of Pennsylvania
Perelman School of Medicine
Department of Neurosurgery
Philadelphia, Pennsylvania

Adam Kirton, MD, MSc, FRCPC (Chapter 1)
University of Calgary
Calgary, Alberta, Canada

Lauren Krivitzky, PhD, ABPP-CN (Chapter 10)
The Children's Hospital of Philadelphia
Philadelphia, Pennsylvania

Shih-Shan Lang, MD (Chapter 4)
Division of Neurosurgery
The Children's Hospital of Philadelphia
University of Pennsylvania
Perelman School of Medicine
Department of Neurosurgery
Philadelphia, Pennsylvania

Elisa Olson D'Achille, MEd (Chapter 12)
Education Coordinator
Pediatric Stroke Program
The Children's Hospital of Philadelphia
Philadelphia, Pennsylvania

Mubeen F. Rafay, MB.BS, FCPS, MSc (Chapter 3)
Associate Professor, Clinical Scientist
Section of Pediatric Neurology
Children's Hospital Winnipeg
Department of Pediatric and Child Health
University of Manitoba
Children's Hospital Research Institute of Manitoba
Winnipeg, Manitoba, Canada

Lois J. Robbins, DSW, LSW (Chapter 11)
Social Worker
Pediatric Stroke Program
The Children's Hospital of Philadelphia
Philadelphia, Pennsylvania

Robyn Westmacott, PhD, C Psych, ABPP (Chapter 9)
Department of Psychology
The Hospital for Sick Children
Toronto, Ontario, Canada

Elizabeth Yeh, MA, CCC-SLP (Chapter 8)
The Children's Hospital of Philadelphia
Philadelphia, Pennsylvania

Foreword

Caring for children recovering from stroke is a journey of endless and inspired discovery. The authors of this book embarked on that journey, each in their own way, when they began their careers in health care. They then found themselves through mutual dedication, curiosity, and good fortune brought together to create teams of caregivers, bound by the same mission—to help children and their families heal and find a way back to a new "normal." Along the way, each member of this unique team taught and learned from every other member of the team. Each found new ways of understanding the needs of each child and family by seeing through one another's eyes. In this book, they share that journey, to open eyes and minds to the great good that comes from working and understanding together in a way that is greater than the sum of the parts.

The first section of the book reviews the medical fundamentals, covering all of the major subtypes of stroke: arterial ischemic stroke, cerebral venous thrombosis, and hemorrhagic stroke. Chapter 1 starts, as it should, at the beginning, with Dr. Kirton's thoughtful and comprehensive review of the fundamentals of childhood stroke: definitions, epidemiology, pathophysiology, and approach to diagnosis and treatment. In Chapter 2, Dr. Smith reviews perinatal stroke, with its unique neurobiology, and especially emphasizes the importance of understanding the complexity of outcomes, and thereby the special rehabilitative needs, of children following perinatal stroke. Dr. Rafay does the same for the less common, but often deadly, subtype of stroke involving thrombosis of the cerebral venous system. Drs. Lang and Heuer take the reader through the many variations and unique problems facing children with intracranial hemorrhage. Finally, the section closes with a discussion of rehabilitation from a medical perspective. Dr. Bryant provides an overview in Chapter 5 emphasizing the critical importance that rehabilitation plays throughout the continuum of care. Here the true nature and the great power of teamwork become clear.

The second section of the book further addresses the heart of the matter: rehabilitation. In Chapter 6, Drs. Atkinson and Duff provide a richly detailed summary of the approach to neuromotor evaluation from the perspective of physical and occupational therapists, each with an abundance of hands-on experience with children and families recovering from stroke at all ages. In Chapter 7, Dr. Atkinson, Dr. Greenham, Ms. Cooper, and, Dr. Gordon further expand on intervention strategies and maximizing functional potential for children with stroke. Ms. Colin and Ms. Yeh follow in Chapter 8 with a review of the approach to impairments in feeding, speech, and language function. This provides a natural segue to Drs. Fuentes and Westmacott's chapter on cognitive assessment, aptly referring to both the "changes and potential" in the cognitive domains that are affected by stroke in children. Drs. Krivitzky and Bosenbark explore the ever-challenging and ever-present domains of emotion and behavior in Chapter 10.

The final section of the book expands the understanding of the child's recovery to the family and the community, and importantly, to the school environment. This section includes a chapter on the family by Drs. Robbins and Nixon-Cave, as well as integrating rehabilitation into the education system by Ms. Olson D'Achille and Dr. Bloom. Last but not least is a review of the importance of lifelong management, advocacy, and resources. Individual efforts and knowledge are the foundation, but as so well expressed by Dr. Nixon-Cave and Ms. Ballasiotes, much work remains to be done to raise awareness in the general public and in key organizations about the problems and needs of children and families with stroke.

Rebecca Ichord, MD
Professor, Neurology & Pediatrics
Perelman School of Medicine
University of Pennsylvania
Director, Pediatric Stroke Program
Department of Neurology
Philadelphia, Pennsylvania

Introduction

Welcome to *Pediatric Stroke Rehabilitation: An Interprofessional and Collaborative Approach*. This text aims to provide a comprehensive overview of the rehabilitative management of childhood stroke. Pediatric stroke is an important health issue, with an incidence of 0.6 to 13/100,000 children and 24 to 28/100,000 neonates.[1-5] Of these, at least 30% to 60% have persisting physical disability, 20% to 40% have persisting cognitive or neuropsychological disability, and 16% to 37% have behavioral problems.[5] These problems often result in an ongoing need to seek specialized treatment from health care professionals or special services in school.

Although there is a great deal of information regarding the treatment and rehabilitation of adults who have suffered a stroke, very little is available for children. This poses a unique problem to both the health care and school communities, as many providers struggle to seek information that will help meet the child's needs. Although many care providers will simply adapt techniques or knowledge learned from the adult population, there is a recognition that children are not "small adults" and have special and complex needs specific to them. These unique differences span every developmental area and include medical management, physical recovery, cognition, and language, as well as learning and emotional needs.

Interprofessional collaboration is critical in the recovery of pediatric stroke, and we believe that we can all be better care providers if we learn more from our colleagues in other disciplines and integrate that knowledge into our own areas of expertise. In this text we have assembled a diverse and expert panel of contributors from various places around the globe and have chapters representing perspectives from neurology, neurosurgery, physiatry, physical therapy, occupational therapy, speech language pathology, neuropsychology, education, and social work. Readers are encouraged to expand their understanding of pediatric stroke by exploring chapters outside their own disciplines and to consider ways to integrate interprofessional collaboration into practice.

We consider the family to be an integral member of the team, the one team member who traverses all areas of care and domains. Family-centered care is emphasized throughout the text, as health care providers can and should continually strive to improve collaboration with families. The text includes personal vignettes written by family members of children who have had a stroke. We hope that these important perspectives on living with the experience of childhood stroke will allow the reader to engage the material with a deeper understanding of the effect that stroke can have on the lives of families. Although this text is intended for health care providers, we recognize that some families may wish to use this text as a reference to help advocate for their child. Family focus boxes are included in several chapters, which help summarize the chapter content and can assist families with wading through unfamiliar concepts and terminology, as well as provide tools to help advocate for their child throughout his or her lifetime.

The book's overall structure emphasizes the *International Classification of Functioning, Disability and Health* (ICF) as put forth by the World Health Organization.[6] This classification enables a comprehensive and detailed understanding of an individual's experience of disability, including contextual aspects such as environmental barriers and facilitators, as well as personal factors that may have an impact on a person's functioning.[7] The ICF offers a meaningful construct through which to view the health and function of individuals, including those who have experienced a stroke. The *International Classification of Functioning, Disability and Health of Children and Youth* (ICF-CY) is a derivative of the ICF that underscores the developmental functioning of children and the environments in which they live.[8] The ICF-CY version of the ICF can assist providers, administrators, policy makers, and parents in documenting children and youth characteristics that are important for promoting growth, health, and development.[8] For readers unfamiliar with the ICF-CY, this framework shifts the emphasis away from negative connotations of disability and instead focuses on the abilities and participation of the individual child.[8] It provides health care and school professionals a comprehensive view of the whole person so that partnerships can truly be collaborative and meaningful for the person with the health condition. The ICF-CY has two main parts, each with two components. Part 1 focuses on physiological functioning of the body systems and how impairments of body structure and function affect the individual's ability to participate in tasks or perform actions to engage in life activities.[6] Part 2 focuses on the contextual aspects in the individual's environment and considers the environmental and personal factors that "make up the physical, social and attitudinal environment in which people live and conduct their lives."[6]

These perspectives are dynamically interconnected and influence each other, and the framework suggests that an individual's function and disability are an outcome of the interaction between the heath condition and the contextual factors. From a practical standpoint, the ICF-CY can afford the health care professional and education provider the ability to not only better collaborate with the individual, but also to prioritize areas for rehabilitation and recovery that are developmentally meaningful and important to the person. By using the ICF-CY, health care and school professionals can ensure that all aspects of the individual and his or her environment are holistically considered.

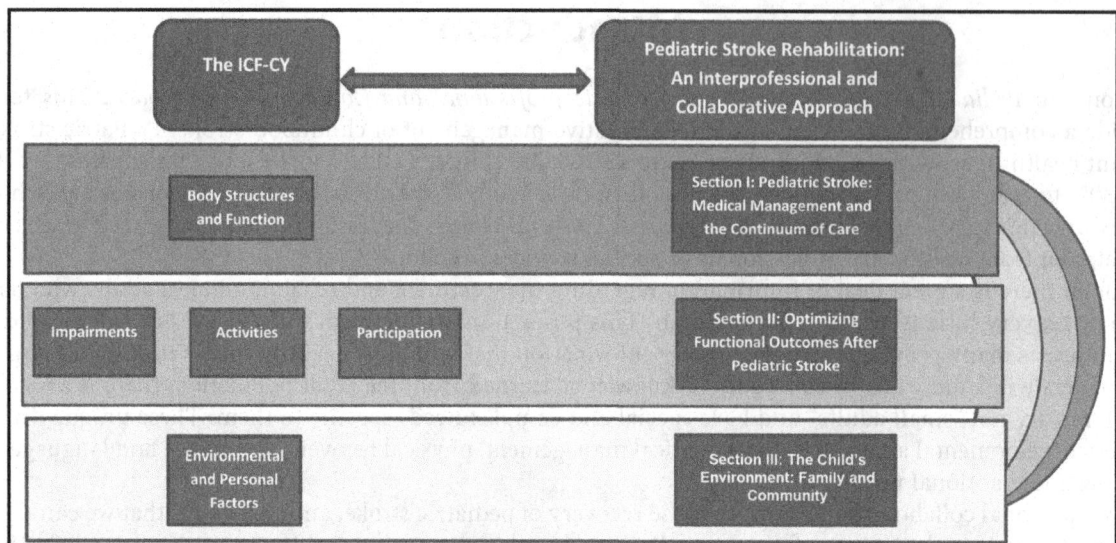

Figure I-1. This illustration depicts how the organization of the text mirrors the 3 levels of the ICF-CY.

Figure I-1 illustrates how the organization of the book shadows the three levels of the ICF-CY. Similar to the interplay between the various levels of the ICF-CY, the chapters and sections of this book integrate together to offer the reader a deeper and more complete understanding of the various aspects of childhood stroke. By learning more about the different attributes of the child, each care provider can deepen his or her own personal understanding of childhood stroke and work to provide more holistic and family-centered care.

Section I of the text, "Pediatric Stroke: Medical Management and the Continuum of Care," provides an overview of the first level of the ICF-CY (the child's health condition related to body structures and function). Chapters will review various types of childhood stroke and discuss rehabilitation medicine across the continuum of care. Section II, "Optimizing Functional Outcomes After Pediatric Stroke," highlights the second level of the ICF-CY (impairments, abilities, participation). This section will detail a child's neuromotor function, cognition, language, and behavioral functioning after stroke and discuss how clinicians can optimize long-term outcomes. Section III, "The Child's Environment: Family and Community" features the third level of the ICF-CY, which emphasizes the child's personal and environmental context and discusses the biopsychosocial model of health. Section III also includes helpful resources for health care providers, school professionals, and families. Just as the ICF-CY eloquently connects internal and external influences on an individual's functioning, disability, and health, this text seeks to connect these varied perspectives with the hope of creating a holistic, meaningful, and family-centered approach to the rehabilitation of children with stroke.

The future of rehabilitation for children with stroke is bright. Advances in scientific research over the past decade have catapulted stroke rehabilitation to a model of recovery, and clinical applications are multiplying. Technological advances in imaging techniques are allowing investigators to better understand the link between intervention and cortical reorganization, and collaboration between clinicians and scientists is inspiring the development of innovative therapies and devices that may help improve outcomes. Although a detailed discussion of neuroplasticity is beyond the scope of this book, many chapters highlight the difference between children and adults with stroke and provide therapeutic strategies to emphasize recovery.

Whereas in an ideal world, all children with stroke would have access to a pediatric stroke center of excellence with a highly functioning interprofessional team to manage their changing needs over their lifetime, we know this is not always available or realistic. We challenge the reader to become a steward for children and families with stroke, to help them seek out and develop an interprofessional team that will collaborate with the family, as well as with each other. As knowledge in the medical care and rehabilitation for children with stroke continues to evolve, family-centered care and collaboration among the interprofessional team will continue to be an essential driver in optimizing lifelong outcomes for children with stroke.

References

1. Fullerton HJ. Risk of stroke in children: ethnic and gender disparities. *Neurology.* 2003;61(2):189-194.
2. Giroud M, Lemesle M, Gouyon JB, Nivelon JL, Milan C, Dumas R. Cerebrovascular disease in children under 16 years of age in the city of Dijon, France: a study of incidence and clinical features from 1985 to 1993. *J Clin Epidemiol.* 1995;48(11):1343-1348.
3. Lee J, Croen LA, Backstrand KH, et al. Maternal and infant characteristics associated with perinatal arterial stroke in the infant. *JAMA.* 2005;293(6):723-729.
4. Lynch JK, Hirtz DG, deVeber G, Nelson KB. Report of the National Institute of Neurological Disorders and Stroke workshop on perinatal and childhood stroke. *Pediatrics.* 2002;109(1):116-123.
5. Hartel C, Schilling S, Sperner J, Thyen U. The clinical outcomes of neonatal and childhood stroke: review of the literature and implications for future research. *Eur J Neurol.* 2004;11(7):431-438.
6. World Health Organization. *ICF: The International Classification of Functioning, Disability and Health.* Geneva, Switzerland: World Health Organization; 2001.
7. Schneidert M, Hurst R, Miller J, Üstun B. The role of environment in the International Classification of Functioning, Disability and Health (ICF). *Disability Rehabil.* 2003;25(11-12):588-595. doi:10.1080/0963828031000137090.
8. World Health Organization. *ICF-CY, International Classification of Functioning, Disability, and Health.* Geneva, Switzerland: World Health Organization; 2007.

I

Pediatric Stroke
Medical Management and the Continuum of Care

1

Childhood Arterial Ischemic Stroke

Adam Kirton, MD, MsC, FRCPC

Stroke causes permanent brain injury, resulting in disability for many children affected by this condition. Stroke is often not considered in children, resulting in long delays in diagnosis. There are many different causes, most of which are not well understood. These reasons combine to make acute treatment very difficult and of limited efficacy. Most survivors incur long-term neurological deficits, creating a marked need for rehabilitation. The aim here is to provide a thorough, clinically relevant, evidence-based review of cerebrovascular disease in infants and children.

TERMINOLOGY: WHAT IS CHILDHOOD STROKE?

Stroke is the sudden occlusion or rupture of cerebral arteries or veins resulting in brain damage. Ischemic varieties are either arterial ischemic stroke (AIS) or cerebral sinovenous thrombosis (CSVT; see Chapter 3). AIS typically involves thromboembolic occlusion with focal infarction within an arterial territory. In CSVT, thrombosis of the cerebral veins or dural venous sinuses may or may not result in brain infarction. Hemorrhagic strokes involve vascular rupture and are classified by intracranial location (see Chapter 4). Overlap between ischemic and hemorrhagic strokes can occur, including hemorrhagic transformation of ischemic infarcts. Childhood strokes occur between 28 days of life and adulthood, distinguishing them from perinatal strokes, which are quite different and discussed in Chapter 2. Fundamental biological differences

between children and adults create specific differences in all elements of pediatric stroke. Principles and evidence from adult stroke are relevant but must be interpreted in a pediatric context.

EPIDEMIOLOGY: HOW COMMON IS STROKE IN CHILDREN?

Incidence rates for pediatric stroke are increasingly well defined and may be escalating.[1] This may relate to improved availability and specificity of diagnostic imaging, increased survival in high-risk conditions (see later), and heightened awareness. Studies of stroke rates are challenged by differences in definitions, data sources, and other variables. Combined rates for ischemic and hemorrhagic stroke in children have been relatively consistent across studies. Rates are approximately 2 to 5/100,000 children per year,[2-4] more than brain tumors or demyelinating disease in children, with stroke affecting more boys than girls. Rates more than double this have been suggested.[5] The relative balance of ischemic vs hemorrhagic stroke has been inconsistent across studies, but the rates are not likely similar.[2,3,5]

Limited hospital administrative data suggest stroke is among the top 10 causes of death in children.[6] The burden of childhood stroke is exacerbated by the high proportion of survivors with adverse outcomes and neurological morbidity that lasts decades. Economic costs of childhood stroke are substantial[7] and comparable to adult stroke when duration of morbidity is considered.

Atkinson HL, Nixon-Cave K, Smith SE, eds.
Pediatric Stroke Rehabilitation: An Interprofessional and Collaborative Approach (pp 3-20). © 2018 Taylor & Francis Group.

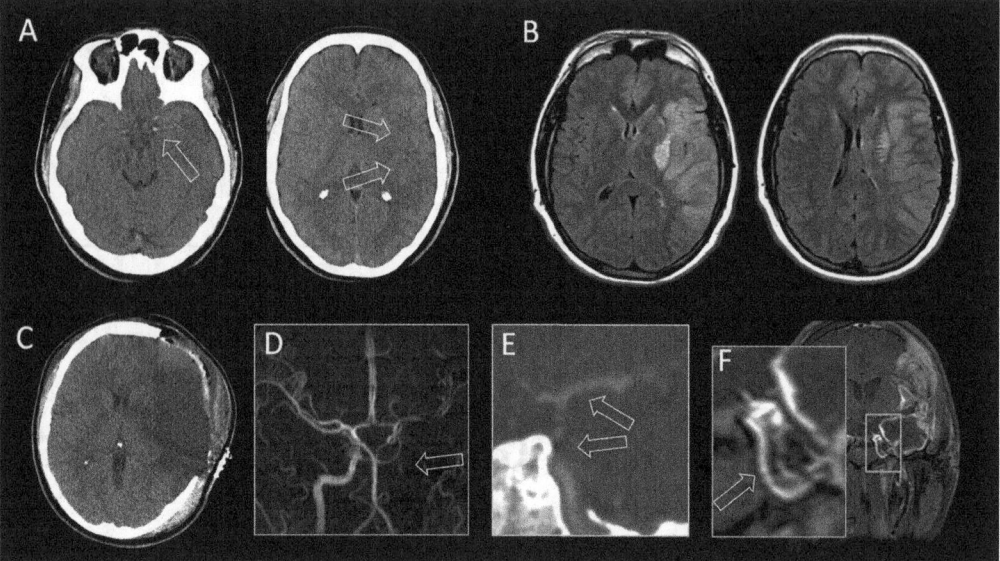

Figure 1-1. Acute imaging of a 15-year-old boy with childhood AIS. (A) Within an hour of the acute onset of inability to speak, a CT scan was done in the emergency room that showed a hyperdense (bright) middle cerebral artery and hypodensity (dark) in the left frontal and temporal lobes. (B) An MRI scan the next day confirmed large areas of acute infarction (bright) in the left middle cerebral artery territory. (C) Within 24 hours, swelling led to malignant cerebral edema requiring emergent hemicraniectomy—the left skull has been removed on a repeat CT scan. Imaging of the arteries shows severe narrowing on (D) MRI angiography, (E) CT angiography, and (F) enhancement of the internal carotid and middle cerebral arteries consistent with focal cerebral arteriopathy.

PATHOPHYSIOLOGY: HOW DOES ARTERIAL ISCHEMIC STROKE OCCUR IN CHILDREN?

Arterial Circulation

Arterial blood is delivered to the brain by the anterior (internal carotid, middle and anterior cerebral arteries) and posterior (vertebral, basilar, and posterior cerebral arteries) circulations. The posterior circulation supplies the brainstem, cerebellum, thalamus, and occipital lobes, whereas the anterior circulation does most of the rest. Communicating arteries link these systems at the circle of Willis. Small perforating arteries from these major vessels supply deep brain regions such as the basal ganglia and thalamus. Anastomoses across all these territories can provide collateral blood flow, affecting size and location of stroke. Clinical features of arterial stroke are dictated by which vessel is blocked. Occlusion of large arteries like the middle cerebral artery (MCA) typically results in peripheral, wedge-shaped lesions of cortex, white matter, and deep structures (Figure 1-1). Small artery strokes often involve perforating arteries to deep structures like the basal ganglia where deficits can also be devastating. The proportion of large- vs small-artery AIS is approximately equal in children. Pattern recognition aids in diagnosis, elucidation of underlying cause, and prognostication of outcome.

Mechanisms of Thromboembolism

AIS typically involves thrombotic occlusion of a cerebral artery. Thrombi may develop locally from regional disease (eg, vasculitis) or travel from an embolic source (eg, cardiac disease). The coagulation and platelet hemostatic systems generate thrombi. In slow-flow situations like cardiac dysfunction, the coagulation system predominates, generating fibrin-rich thrombi. In higher-flow, diseased arteries, platelet-rich thrombi may become more important. This relationship is complex and influenced by many factors, and most thrombi probably involve some combination of both systems. Important developmental differences in hemostasis are also likely important.[8,9] Recent studies suggest endothelial dysfunction also plays a role in childhood AIS.[10] Though less common, nonthrombotic cerebral embolization can occur, including infectious material in endocarditis, fat embolism, cardiac myxomas, and inert materials during intravascular procedures.

Mechanisms of Brain Injury

Multiple factors determine the extent of brain injury in AIS, including depth and duration of ischemia, the size and location of infarction, concurrent disease processes, such as seizures or infection, and the developmental stage of the child. Cerebral perfusion is a function of mean arterial pressure, intracranial pressure, and vascular resistance. Adult cerebral blood flow (CBF) is ~50 mL/100 g brain tissue/minute, whereas neonates and young children are ~40 and

130, respectively.[11-12] CBF represents 10% to 20% of cardiac output in infants and adults but > 50% in young children.[12] Autoregulation maintains steady perfusion across a wide range of pressures by altering arterial resistance in response to changes in pressure and metabolic substrates.

Such compromise in cerebral blood flow results in a central core of permanently damaged brain surrounded by a compromised, but potentially salvageable, penumbra. Regional ischemia causes hypoxia and energy depletion. Acidosis and lactate production may worsen injury. Ischemic neuronal cell death may occur via acute necrosis or more gradual apoptosis over days. Cellular mechanisms include glutamate excess, calcium-mediated toxicity, nitric oxide and free-radical generation, and neuroinflammatory components. Pharmacological interventions aimed at these mechanisms have been unsuccessful, with none focused on pediatric injuries. However, factors that worsen the imbalance between blood supply and metabolic demand in the penumbra are the primary target of immediate management to minimize injury. These include seizures, hyperthermia, blood pressure, and glucose imbalance.

CLINICAL PRESENTATION: HOW IS PEDIATRIC STROKE DIAGNOSED?

Sudden onset of a focal neurological deficit is a stroke until proven otherwise. Acute hemiparesis is most common where the differential diagnosis includes migraine, seizure Todd paralysis, demyelination, and others.[13,14] A differential diagnosis of stroke mimics is summarized in Table 1-1. Any focal deficit can occur, including hemianopsia, diplopia, gaze disorders, dysphasia or dysarthria, vertigo, nystagmus, ataxia, and hemisensory disturbances. Seizures are a more common presenting sign in children.[15,16] Diffuse, nonlocalizing presentations are also common such as headache and behavioral changes.[14,16] Stroke signs and symptoms are typically maximal at onset but may fluctuate.[17] A transient ischemic attack (TIA) is a brief episode of neurological dysfunction caused by focal brain ischemia, with clinical symptoms typically lasting less than one hour, and without MRI evidence of acute infarction. Many children with TIA have stroke risk factors, should be considered at risk, and promptly investigated.

Awareness and a high degree of clinical suspicion are required for the timely diagnosis of stroke in children. Most diagnoses are delayed, with the average being > 24 hours from symptom onset.[18-20] Children with acute neurological problems are typically brought quickly to medical attention with subsequent delays often in the hospital.[19] Poor recognition may relate to underawareness of primary care professionals, complex symptomology and signs, distracting features, limited examinations in smaller children, and a broad differential diagnosis.[14] Symptom screening tools

developed for adult stroke may be applicable in children.[21] Prompt diagnosis is essential in order to initiate early neuroprotective and prevention treatments.

Detailed history and examination are combined with imaging and ancillary studies to achieve timely diagnosis. History should focus on specific symptomology and exact time of onset (when was the child last seen well). Information about recent infection or trauma, including chiropractic neck manipulation, should be sought. Important medical history includes cardiac disease, chronic conditions, radiation of the head or neck, migraine history, immunization status (varicella), and medication use (oral contraceptives, chemotherapy, illicit drugs). Family history of thrombosis, young stroke or heart attack (< 50 years), use of anticoagulants, migraine, or neurological disease may be relevant. The examination focuses on the presenting complaints in the context of age and state of the child. The Pediatric National Institutes of Health Stroke Scale (PedNIHSS) is a validated, age-adjusted measure that can quickly estimate stroke severity.[22] Additional examination includes detailed cardiovascular evaluation with blood pressure, pulses, and bruit auscultation. Hypertension co-occurs in fibromuscular dysplasia and moyamoya disease.[23]

DIAGNOSIS: NEUROIMAGING

Stroke diagnosis is made by combining clinical reasoning with neuroimaging. Modern imaging provides tools that are both efficient and accurate when used properly, optimizing diagnosis and often elucidating probable mechanisms to guide management.

Computed tomography (CT) of the head is the most common initial imaging study in childhood AIS. Advantages include widespread and ready availability, short scan times without sedation, high negative predictive values for important exclusions (eg, hemorrhage), and excellent arterial imaging options. Done early, CT of the head is insensitive to childhood AIS, particularly smaller lesions or those in the posterior fossa.[19] AIS findings on CT typically feature focal hypodensity within an arterial territory. Possible additional findings such as a hyperdense artery sign suggesting thrombus, hemorrhagic transformation, or evolving cerebral edema are clinically relevant. Contrast-enhanced CT angiography can image major craniocervical arteries with sensitivity to suggest many arteriopathic diagnoses (see Figure 1-1E). Age-related complications of radiation exposure are low compared to acute stroke risks but should be considered in children.[24]

MRI is often the ideal imaging study in childhood cerebrovascular disease[25] (see Figure 1-1). The need for sedation in young children and longer scan times may be outweighed by increased utility. MRI sensitivity and specificity are greater than with CT. Diffusion-weighted imaging (DWI) has revolutionized acute stroke diagnosis

TABLE 1-1. DIFFERENTIAL DIAGNOSIS OF STROKE-LIKE EPISODES IN CHILDREN		
DISEASE	**CLINICAL DISTINCTION FROM STROKE**	**IMAGING DISTINCTION FROM STROKE**
Migraine	Evolving or "marching" symptoms, short duration, complete resolution, headache, personal or family history of migraine	Usually normal Migrainous infarction is rare
Seizure	Positive symptoms > negative symptoms; Todd paralysis may follow and is transient Altered level of consciousness	May identify source of focal seizures
Infection	Fever, encephalopathy, gradual onset, meningismus	Markers of encephalitis/cerebritis, typically diffuse and bilateral AIS and CSVT occur in bacterial meningitis
Demyelination (Acute disseminated encephalomyelitis [ADEM], multiple sclerosis [MS])	Gradual onset, multifocal symptoms, encephalopathy Past history of DM events (optic neuritis, transverse myelitis)	Multifocal lesions, typical appearance (eg, patchy in ADEM, ovoid in MS), typical locations (eg, pericallosal in MS), less likely to show restricted diffusion
Hypoglycemia	Risk factor (eg, insulin therapy), related to meals, additional neuroglycopenic symptoms	Bilateral, symmetrical May see restricted diffusion Posterior dominant pattern (neonates)
Watershed hypoxic ischemic encephalopath	Risk factor (eg, hypotension, sepsis), bilateral deficits	Bilateral, symmetrical restricted diffusion in arterial border zones
Inborn errors of metabolism (mitochondrial encephalomyo-pathy, lactic acidosis, and stroke-like episodes, mito)	Pre-existing delays/regression, multisystem disease, abnormal biochemical profiles	Possible restricted diffusion but often bilateral, not within arterial territories MR spectroscopy (eg, high lactate)
Hypertensive encephalopathy (posterior reversible encephalopathy syndrome)	Documented hypertension, bilateral visual symptoms, encephalopathy	Posterior dominant, bilateral, patchy lesions involving gray and white matter, usually no restricted diffusion
Vestibulopathy	Symptoms limited to vertigo Positional Nystagmus	Normal
Acute cerebellar ataxia	Gradual onset, bilateral, symmetric ataxia, postviral	Normal or diffusely swollen cerebellum
Channelopathies (alternating hemiplegia of childhood [AHC], episodic ataxia, familial hemiplegic migraine)	Syndromic cluster of recurring symptoms Switching sides Headaches Family history	Usually normal Need MRA to exclude moyamoya in AHC

with high sensitivity and specificity for acute focal ischemia within less than an hour. Bright DWI with a dark apparent diffusion coefficient map (restricted diffusion) in an arterial territory is diagnostic of AIS.[26,27] Changes in DWI signal over days and weeks may help time stroke occurrence. Blood-sensitive sequences can help recognize specific etiologies and hemorrhagic transformation. Magnetic resonance assessments of brain perfusion,[28] autoregulation,[29] pathway injury (diffusion tensor imaging), functional effects (functional MRI), and arterial wall imaging[30] all carry substantial potential for applications in childhood stroke.

Magnetic resonance angiography (MRA) can image major cerebral and cervical arteries and should be included in pediatric stroke MR protocols (see Figure 1-1D).[31-33] MRA can suggest embolic occlusions or characterize and follow cerebral arteriopathies.[34] MR parenchymal sequences also inform vascular status, including *Ivy sign* on fluid attenuation inversion recovery suggestive of impaired perfusion or cervical fat-saturation sequences to demonstrate dissection. Both time-of-flight and contrast-enhanced MRA provide relative alternatives.

Conventional angiography (CA) injects intra-arterial contrast via femoral puncture and is the gold standard for imaging cerebral arteries.[35] In a minority of childhood AIS cases, the noninvasive CT and MR modalities described earlier may not be adequate for diagnosis. Distinctive findings include double lumen or intimal flap signs of dissection, the banding or striae of focal cerebral arteriopathy, and small vessel diseases.[36] Moyamoya often requires CA for characterization and surgical planning.[37] CA should be considered in children with suspected but unconfirmed arteriopathy and possibly in otherwise unexplained AIS. The risk of CA in children is low with complication rates lower than adults at <0.5%.[38]

RISK FACTORS AND ASSOCIATIONS: WHAT CAUSES CHILDHOOD ARTERIAL ISCHEMIC STROKE?

Many conditions have been associated with childhood AIS. Of those considered "risk factors, only a select few carry strong evidence and biological plausibility suggesting a definitive causative role. For many others, evidence is limited, and pathophysiological mechanisms are incompletely understood. Prompt consideration and thorough evaluation of all factors is typically required for optimal management. Depending on evidence criteria, one possible risk factor is found in >80% of cases,[39-42] with the remainder being idiopathic. Most children are previously healthy.[41] The leading adult stroke risk factors for atherosclerosis are uncommon in children. A classification of possible childhood AIS etiologies is shown in Table 1-2. Three categories predominate: arteriopathy, cardiac, and prothrombotic and hematological disorders.

Arteriopathies

Diseases of the cerebral arteries are the leading cause of childhood AIS, found in >50%.[39,41,43-47] Arteriopathies also carry the highest rates of recurrence and are associated with poor outcome.[43,48] The importance of arteriopathy emphasizes the essential role of arterial imaging. Multiple classifications have been proposed based on imaging features, evolution over time, and presumed pathophysiology[49] with limited consensus across stroke experts. New classification schemes are being validated.[50] Three leading arteriopathies in childhood AIS are (1) a syndrome of focal, unilateral arteriopathy with possible inflammatory or infectious mechanisms; (2) dissection; and (3) moyamoya. Many other less common arteriopathies are listed in Table 1-2.

Focal or Transient Cerebral Arteriopathy: Inflammation?

An arteriopathy commonly seen in healthy school-aged children features irregular stenosis with banding or striae at the internal carotid artery (ICA)/MCA/anterior cerebral artery (ACA) trifurcation on one side. AIS within lenticulostriate and/or major MCA branches results. The arteriopathy may progress over days, but typically stabilizes or resolves over months. A typical case is shown in Figure 1-1. Early descriptions of this syndrome called it transient cerebral arteriopathy (TCA),[45,51] and many cases are self-limited with gradual resolution over months; though a minority may progress,[49] suggesting a different disorder.[50] Other terms offer varying conviction of the underlying mechanism, including nonspecific focal cerebral arteriopathy (FCA)[44] or implication of an inflammatory mechanism.[51] The term *nonprogressive childhood primary angiitis of the central nervous system* (CNS) has implied an isolated vasculitis (cPACNS).[52] Although parainfectious or inflammatory mechanisms predominate, they are speculative, and alternatives such as intracranial dissection are considered.[53]

More direct infectious pathophysiology has been suggested for similar cerebral arteriopathies. Postvaricella angiopathy (PVA) mimics the syndrome earlier, with the addition of varicella infection in the preceding year.[54] A comparable arteriopathy is described in adults with ophthalmic zoster.[55] Reactivation of trigeminal ganglion varicella may be responsible. Diagnostic testing to prove varicella is challenging,[56] but rare pathological cases have demonstrated arterial wall varicella virus. Varicella vaccination is not associated with childhood stroke and may lead to PVA decreasing.[57]

TABLE 1-2. POTENTIAL RISK FACTORS FOR CHILDHOOD ARTERIAL ISCHEMIC STROKE		
CATEGORY	**COMMON/HIGHLY PROBABLE**	**UNCOMMON/POSSIBLE/UNCERTAIN**
Arteriopathy	**Inflammatory/Parainfectious** Childhood primary angiitis of CNS (cPACNS) (nonprogressive or progressive; large vessel or small vessel) TCA FCA PVA **Infectious** Bacterial meningitis HIV **Dissection** Internal carotid artery Vertebral artery Intracranial arteries Moyamoya disease (idiopathic) Moyamoya syndrome Neurofibromatosis 1, trisomy 21	Secondary CNS vasculitis Systemic lupus erythematosus, polyarteritis nodosa, inflammatory bowel disease Takayasu arteritis **Infectious** Mycoplasma, toxoplasmosis, RMSF, Lyme disease, cryptococcus, chlamydia, Japanese encephalitis, coxsackie B4 and A9, influenza A, enterovirus, parvovirus B19, Post-radiation vasculopathy Reversible segmental cerebral vasospasm (Call-Flemming syndrome) **Genetic** COL4A1 Connective tissue disease (Marfan, Ehlers-Danlos) Pseudoxanthoma elasticum **Congenital** PHACE syndrome, progeria, Alagille, dwarfism (MOPDII), fibromuscular dysplasias
Cardiac	**Complex congenital heart disease** Cardiac surgery (eg, Fontan) Cardiac catheterization **Bacterial endocarditis** Atrial septal aneurysm Atrial septal defect Patent foramen ovale Venous thrombosis + right-to-left shunt	Cardiomyopathy, myocarditis Aortic coarctation Severe ventricular dysfunction Atrial myxoma Valvular disease (eg, rheumatic fever) Arrhythmia (atrial fibrillation) Extracorporeal membrane oxygenation Cerebral angiography Embolism (air, fat, amniotic fluid)
Prothrombotic	Factor V Leiden Prothrombin gene 20210A Elevated lipoprotein (a) Protein C deficiency Lupus anticoagulant Anticardiolipin antibodies	Methylene tetrahydrofolate reductase (MTHFR), hyperhomocysteinemia Protein S deficiency Antithrombin III deficiency Factor VII/IX/XI Plasminogen deficiency Dysfibrinogenemia Sticky platelet syndrome Pregnancy, puerperium

(continued)

TABLE 1-2 (CONTINUED). POTENTIAL RISK FACTORS FOR CHILDHOOD ARTERIAL ISCHEMIC STROKE		
CATEGORY	COMMON/HIGHLY PROBABLE	UNCOMMON/POSSIBLE/UNCERTAIN
Hematological	Sickle cell disease Iron-deficiency anemia	Leukemia Thalassemias Thrombocytosis Polycythemia Hemolytic uremic syndrome Immune thrombocytopenic purpura Thrombotic thrombocytopenic purpura
Medications/Drugs	Oral contraceptives Chemotherapy (L-asparaginase)	Cocaine, methamphetamine, ecstasy Ergots, triptans
Other	Migraine **Inborn Errors of Metabolism** Fabry disease, homocystinuria, mitochondrial	**Metabolic Syndrome** Hypertension, diabetes, insulin resistance, dyslipidemia, atherosclerosis Cigarette smoking, secondhand smoke

Evidence of any recent viral infection is well associated with childhood AIS[41,58] and FCA/TCA arteriopathy.[44] The Vascular Effects of Infection in Pediatric Stroke study should improve understanding of this relationship.[59] Specific infections associated with childhood AIS include definitive examples like bacterial meningitis, which causes both perforating and large-vessel diseases.[60] Severe examples include tuberculous meningitis[61] and HIV.[62] Other anecdotal associations include mycoplasma, toxoplasmosis, Rocky Mountain spotted fever (RMSF), Lyme disease, cryptococcus, Japanese encephalitis, coxsackie B4 and A9, influenza A, enterovirus, parvovirus B19, and chlamydia.[63]

Vasculitis or noninfectious arterial inflammation also causes childhood AIS. Diagnostic criteria and classifications are well described,[52] with most being cPACNS rather than associated with systemic vasculitis.[52] A unilateral, transient, large vessel variety indistinguishable from the FCA/TCA syndrome noted earlier is termed *nonprogressive large/medium (angiography-positive) cPACNS*. A progressive version with bilateral involvement may also occur. Small vessel or angiography-negative cPACNS features progressive, multifocal disease presenting with more insidious symptoms of headaches and behavioral changes. MRI is heterogeneous with few specific features.[64] CA is indicated but often normal, leading to brain biopsy for definitive pathological diagnosis.[34,52,64] Small vessel vasculitis may rarely be secondary to systemic vasculitides and connective tissue disorders like Kawasaki disease, Henoch-Schohnlein purpura, polyarteritis nodosa, Wegener granulomatosis, systemic lupus erythematosus, Behcet syndrome, and others.[65] Other forms of arteriopathy leading to stroke include extracranial and systemic arteriopathies like Takayasu arteritis,[66] nondissection cervical arteriopathies,[67] and pediatric forms of fibromuscular dysplasia.[23]

Recognition of arteriopathy invariably raises consideration of infectious and inflammatory mechanisms, with diagnostic and treatment implications. Testing should consider infectious studies (lumbar puncture and serology, virology, polymerase chain reaction) and screening for inflammatory biomarkers (erythrocyte sedimentation rate, C-reactive protein) or vasculitis (antinuclear antibodies, extractable nuclear antigens, complement). Such testing is both insensitive and nonspecific, and negative results do not constitute exclusion of inflammation. In cPACNS, laboratory tests are often normal or nonspecific. Small vessel cPACNS often has mild cerebrospinal fluid findings but brain biopsy is typically required for diagnosis.[68] Unique inflammatory biomarkers of focal cerebral arteriopathy require further study.[69]

Dissection and Physical Injury

Dissection occurs when arterial integrity is compromised, usually resulting in a subintimal hematoma. Craniocervical dissections cause AIS by the hematoma or thrombosis occluding the artery at the dissection site or artery-to-artery thromboembolism.[70] Any artery can dissect but high-risk locations include proximal and skull base sections of the ICA and the vertebral arteries at C1 to C2. Intracranial dissections may be more common in children[71] and can mimic FCA/TCA,[53] imparting a risk of subarachnoid hemorrhage.[71] Dissection is responsible for 1% to 20% of AIS in children.[71,72] Risk factors include obvious regional trauma, whereas subtle injuries like neck manipulation, extreme exertion, or contact sports are more difficult to determine.[72,73] Many pediatric dissections appear to be spontaneous, suggesting inherent differences in arterial structure supported by connective tissue studies in adults. Systemic arteriopathies like fibromuscular dysplasia are also associated with childhood dissection.[23]

Clinical presentations in dissection include new head or neck pain, often beginning a week or more before neurological symptoms. Horner syndrome or cervical bruits may be found on exam. Recurrence rates are likely 20% or higher[43,71-73] and may be greater than in adults. Medical management of dissection is controversial and without randomized trials. Pediatric guidelines recommend consideration of anticoagulation.[74,75] In contrast, a recent adult dissection meta-analysis found no difference between anticoagulation and antiplatelet strategies.[76] Both approaches appear safe. Activity restrictions postdissection are not well studied, although pediatric stroke experts generally advise against high-impact activities.[77]

Head and neck trauma within 3 months without dissection has been independently associated with AIS.[58] Additional arterial injuries associated with AIS include postradiation vasculopathy, ACA or PCA compression syndromes related to increased intracranial pressure, and mechanical trauma such as extracorporeal membrane oxygenation.

Moyamoya

Moyamoya is the progressive occlusion of the distal ICAs accompanied by abnormal collateral formation that produces a "puff of smoke" on CA.[37] Variants affecting the posterior circulation on only one side occur. Moyamoya disease was an idiopathic variety more common in Asia, but genetic causes such as RNF213 are now recognized.[78] Moyamoya syndrome is associated with conditions including sickle cell disease (SCD), neurofibromatosis type 1, Down syndrome, postradiation vasculopathy, fibromuscular dysplasia, and others.[23,37,79]

In addition to typical stroke signs and symptoms, unique presentations include hyperventilation-induced TIA, alternating hemiplegia, and slow cognitive decline. Stroke can be secondary to hypoperfusion or thrombotic occlusion. Recurrent, subclinical injuries may accumulate over time.[80] Risk of hemorrhagic stroke increases over time, often arising from collateral vessels. Hypertension is common, suggesting either a compensatory mechanism or associated renal arteriopathy.[23] Onset in infancy may predict a more rapid progression.[81] MRI may show typical AIS, watershed infarcts, collateral flow voids, or impaired perfusion such as the Ivy sign.[82] MRA can be diagnostic of moyamoya, but artifactual ICA flow voids can mimic the disease on time-of-flight studies, and CT angiography may be required. CA is required to define extent of disease and plan surgery.

Moyamoya treatment typically includes antiplatelet therapy with aspirin. Carbonic anhydrase inhibitors for vasodilation carry a risk of vascular "steal" and stroke. Hypertension must be cautiously treated to avoid hypoperfusion. Revascularization surgery is highly effective.[37] Direct procedures connecting extracranial and intracranial vessels are successful but limited in small children. Indirect surgeries approximate extracranial arterial branches with ischemic cortical areas, allowing neoangiogenesis to supply at-risk areas over months. Examples include encephalodural synangiosis and encephaloduralmyo synangiosis. Perioperative stroke risk is approximately 5% to 10%.[83] Serial vascular imaging can monitor surgical success. One study of 143 children undergoing pial synangiosis described 5-year symptom-free survival rates of >90%[84] with similar success rates in direct procedures.[85]

Cardiac

Heart disease accompanies 10% to 25% of childhood AIS.[39,41,42,86] Most AIS occur secondary to cardiogenic thromboembolism from differences in flow, structure, and function. Surgery, catheterization, and support devices further increase risk. AIS across multiple arterial territories suggests a cardiac origin. An international childhood AIS study found cardiac disorders in 204/667 (30%) with congenital defects in 60%, but also acquired diseases such as cardiomyopathy, valve disease, and arrhythmia.[86] Silent, preoperative strokes are common in congenital heart disease.[87] Risk of symptomatic stroke with cardiac surgery in children is 1:200.[88] Certain procedures are high risk such as Fontan (3% to 19%)[89] and balloon atrial septostomy.[90] Cardiac catheterization risk is 1:600 to 700.[91] One-third of children with stroke and congenital heart disease suffer recurrence.[92]

Patent foramen ovale (PFO) is a controversial risk factor for stroke.[93] Paradoxical embolization across a right-to-left intracardiac shunt requires higher pressures and venous clot in addition to the passageway found in 20% to 25% of children. Associations between PFO and young adult cryptogenic stroke but not stroke recurrence suggest most PFOs are incidental. Atrial septal aneurysm or thrombophilia may increase PFO stroke risk.[94] PFO closure trials in cryptogenic stroke found no effect on stroke recurrence.[95] Acquired cardiac conditions causing AIS in children include infective endocarditis, often resulting in mycotic aneurysm. Fever, constitutional symptoms, murmur, and skin and eye findings should raise suspicion. Multifocal microbleeds are common on susceptibility-weighted MRI, but long-term significance is unknown. Infective and metabolic cardiomyopathies, valve disease, arrhythmias, and atrial myxoma all cause childhood AIS. Ventricular assist devices have increased survival in children, but stroke rates approach 30%.[96]

Children with AIS typically require immediate cardiac evaluation, including examination, electrocardiogram, and echocardiography. Young children likely do not incur the added benefit of transesophageal echocardiography seen in adult stroke. Guidelines recommend anticoagulation therapy over antiplatelet agents in suspected cardiogenic childhood AIS,[74,75] typically with low-molecular-weight heparin (LMWH). Duration of anticoagulation depends on multiple factors and is informed by new guidelines for secondary stroke prevention in congenital heart disease.[97]

Prothrombotic and Hematological Disorders

Thrombophilias are associated with childhood AIS but rarely as a sole cause, and their precise role is complex.[98-100] Coagulation abnormalities are identified in 20% to 50% of children with AIS.[99,101] A meta-analysis found the following strengths of association (summary odds ratio/95% confidence intervals) with first childhood AIS: protein C deficiency (11.0/5.13 to 23.59), antiphospholipid antibodies or lupus anticoagulant (6.95 /3.67 to 13.14), and lipoprotein (a) (6.53/4.46 to 9.55).[102] Associations with factor V Leiden and prothrombin gene 20210A mutations were modest. MTHFR mutations are common, and significance in childhood AIS is unclear.[103] Thrombophilias also increase recurrence risk.[92,100,104,105] Platelet dysfunction has not been well studied. Testing for a prothrombotic condition should be considered in children with AIS, particularly those with idiopathic strokes, chronic high-risk conditions, or positive family history.[92] Testing is best completed in the absence of thrombosis and anticoagulants. Proven laboratory methods and experienced thrombosis experts are required for accurate interpretation of results.

SCD increases AIS risk 400-fold in children, and 25% will incur cerebrovascular complications. These include both large and small vessel diseases with AIS, moyamoya, and hemorrhage.[106] Ischemic strokes predominate, but hemorrhage risks increase with age.[107] Large vessel disease affects major arteries often in a moyamoya pattern, although extracranial carotid disease also occurs.[108] Small end artery disease leads to accumulation of white matter damage. Mechanisms probably include vascular occlusion, abnormal flow, endothelial injury, low hemoglobin, genetics, and hypertension. Transcranial Doppler screens for large vessel disease in SCD with MCA velocities >200 cm/s predicting stroke risk.[109,110] Annual screening from early childhood may be complemented by MR/MRA in those with stroke, new symptoms, or moyamoya.[111] In children with elevated velocities, regular transfusions reduce stroke risk by 90%.[110] Risk increases when transfusions are stopped[112] or the child is switched to hydroxyurea.[113] The effect of transfusions on small vessel disease is under investigation.[114] Transfusions are standard of care but with significant morbidity.[74,75] The role for antiplatelet agents, hydroxyurea, and nocturnal oxygen are not defined. Transplant therapies are increasingly available in SCD,[115] although cerebrovascular benefits in children are not known.

Iron-deficiency anemia is an independent, treatable risk factor for AIS[116] and may be present in up to 40% of cases.[41] Mechanisms are not well defined. An acute imaging study comparing SCD to other anemic children found high stroke rates in the non-SCD population.[117] Children with dietary risks, low hemoglobin, and microcytosis should have iron studies done and prompt treatment.

Many other conditions have been associated with childhood AIS (Table 1-2). Migraine rates are higher in young stroke patients,[118] but migrainous infarction is rare.[119] Reversible cerebral vasoconstriction syndrome may occur in children.[120,121] Medications and drug use may increase AIS risk, particularly oral contraceptives.[122] Treatable metabolic diseases include homocystinuria and Fabry disease.[123] The modifiable lifestyle factors of adult stroke such as diabetes, hypertension, dyslipidemia, smoking, and obesity are uncommon but should be considered in children.[41]

TREATMENT

Acute stroke in a child is a medical emergency. Initial management requires measured clinical assessment and judicious use of select interventions to optimize outcomes. The PedNIHSS provides an efficient, valid measure of stroke severity.[22] Consensus-based guidelines for childhood stroke are available to guide management.[74,75] Adult stroke best practice guidelines provide additional information.[124] A chronological approach to acute treatment is summarized later. Long-term management and rehabilitation are included in the concluding outcomes section.

Emergent management of acute stroke in children rests first on principles of neuroprotection. These are supportive interventions to optimize survival of brain tissue at risk. Targets include optimizing cerebral blood flow while minimizing neuronal metabolic demand. Mean arterial and intracranial pressures are the primary determinants of cerebral blood flow. Maintaining systemic blood pressures is required for penumbral perfusion, and targets in the upper half of normal (50th to 95th percentile) may be reasonable. Initial interventions should include continuous intravenous normal saline and placing the head of the bed flat. Abnormal glucose worsens adult stroke outcome and should be monitored,[125] although insulin may carry additional complications.[126] Normal oxygenation and ventilation should be maintained with no proven role for supplemental oxygen. Hyperthermia should be treated with antipyretics, external cooling, and infection management. Seizures are common and may be subclinical, so monitoring with an electroencephalogram and anticonvulsant treatment are often required. Children typically require admission to a pediatric intensive care unit[127] and are ideally managed at a tertiary care pediatric center with cerebrovascular expertise.[128]

Thrombolytic and recanalization procedures commonly used in adult stroke lack evidence in children and are not supported by current guidelines. Given within 4.5 hours, intravenous tissue plasminogen activator (tPA) improves outcome across widely selected adult stroke patients with a low risk of intracranial hemorrhage. Safety and efficacy are unknown in children and complicated by differences in stroke mechanisms, coagulation systems, and others. According to adult criteria, ~10% of children are probably eligible for thrombolytics.[129] An international study of >650 children with AIS found intravenous or intra-arterial thrombolytic use in 2%.[130] A limited administrative study found rates are increasing and suggested complication rates comparable to adults.[131] The Thrombolysis in Pediatric Stroke study, a safety and dose-finding trial of intravenous tPA in childhood AIS, was stopped due to poor recruitment.[128] Interventional mechanical therapies continue to be evaluated in adult stroke,[132] but only anecdotal experience in children limits their application.[133]

Antithrombotic therapies are the primary urgent medical treatment consideration to prevent recurrence and promote recanalization in childhood AIS. There are two primary strategies: antiplatelet therapy with aspirin or anticoagulation with heparins. Antiplatelet agents are a reasonable first-line therapy for noncardiogenic childhood AIS[74,75] and the primary agent for long-term stroke prevention. Dosing is 1 to 5 mg/kg/day. Aspirin is safe in children,[134,135] with typically mild side effects of bruising, nosebleeds, and stomach upset. Reye syndrome has not been reported at these doses.[136] Clopidogrel is an alternative antiplatelet agent with pediatric safety data.[137]

Anticoagulation is often recommended for specific mechanisms, including cardiogenic stroke, high-grade stenosis, or severe thrombophilia. Aspirin may be preferred for arteriopathies. There are no randomized controlled trials. Initial antithrombotic therapy choices vary across guidelines and pediatric stroke specialists.[42,74,75,138,139] The two approaches are not mutually exclusive, may be combined, and often change over time. Initiating one antithrombotic agent is supported by high recurrence risk and solid safety data for all agents.[42,135] Initial anticoagulation is consistently used for cardiac and dissection etiologies[139] and supported by safety data[140] and guidelines.[74] Contraindications may include intracranial hemorrhage, uncontrolled hypertension, or systemic bleeding. Options include unfractionated heparin (UFH) or LMWH. Age-specific dosing guidelines for childhood AIS are published for both.[74] Risks include hemorrhage with both and thrombocytopenia with UFH. Monitoring is easier for LMWH with less frequent Xa levels. Parents can administer subcutaneous LMWH with good tolerability. Oral anticoagulation with warfarin is usually only for long-term anticoagulation such as congenital heart disease where new guidelines are available.[97] New oral anticoagulants have not been evaluated for childhood stroke prevention.

A role for steroids or immunomodulatory treatments in childhood AIS is controversial and not recommended by current guidelines. There are no definitive diagnostic tools to confirm inflammation in syndromes such as FCA, TCA, or cPACNS. However, given the very high risk of recurrence

and progression in these syndromes and adult evidence that steroids do not worsen stroke outcome, some would consider a short course of high-dose steroid therapy. With TCA stabilization by 3 months, prolonged courses would not be required.[52] Such immunomodulation may be beneficial in small vessel cPACNS.[141] Additional treatment issues to consider include aspiration prevention, feeding, and nutrition. The benefits of adult stroke units may prompt development of specialized pediatric stroke centers.[128]

Malignant cerebral edema is another urgent, life-threatening acute treatment issue. A higher brain:skull volume ratio in children increases the risk. High-risk lesions are recognizable at diagnosis, such as larger ICA/MCA and cerebellar strokes. Herniation can develop within 24 hours, although edema usually peaks at 48 to 72 hours. Close observation and early reaction to any clinical sign is required, including headache, drowsiness, and pupillary changes. Management includes supportive care, emergent imaging (CT), and reduction of intracranial pressure with sedation, paralysis, and osmotic therapy. Decompressive hemicraniectomy improves outcomes in adult stroke,[142] and smaller studies suggest benefit in children.[143,144]

OUTCOMES AND CHRONIC MANAGEMENT

Most childhood stroke survivors suffer lifelong neurological morbidity with moderate to severe deficits or epilepsy in >50%.[15,145,146] Mortality rate estimates vary but are likely 5% to 10%.[15,145] Multidisciplinary rehabilitation programs must address the physical, occupational, communication, cognitive and educational, behavioral and mental health, and psychosocial consequences with consideration of the individual child and family.[147] Emerging evidence from both adult stroke and congenital hemiparesis (cerebral palsy) literature and practice guidelines can inform childhood AIS rehabilitation.[124] The concept of *enhanced plasticity* improving outcomes in young patients with brain injury is a gross oversimplification. Many complex variables determine neurological outcomes, and age is only one that must be considered. However, improved understanding of developmental plasticity following early stroke is being translated into new strategies to promote recovery.[148-150]

Hemiparesis and other motor impairments are common, with disabling consequences in childhood AIS.[145,146] Neuroimaging may allow some prediction of motor outcomes at diagnosis.[151,152] Lesion location can predict motor deficits, such as MCA strokes resulting in upper more than lower extremity spastic paresis, although lower extremity and gait problems are common. Basal ganglia injury often results in late-emerging dyskinetic movement disorders, whereas cerebellar lesions lead to hemiataxia syndromes.[151,153]

Physical and occupational therapy are the backbone of motor recovery therapy, although specific childhood AIS evidence is limited.[154] Programs combining strength and aerobic conditioning, task-specific training, and an active lifestyle are encouraged. Constraint-induced movement therapy (CIMT) restrains the unaffected limb while therapy promotes functional learning on the hemiparetic side. Marked long-term CIMT effectiveness has been demonstrated in adult stroke, where 2-week programs can generate gains lasting 2 years or more.[155-159] Similar evidence is emerging in children with perinatal stroke and congenital hemiparesis.[160-165] Trials specific to childhood AIS are needed.[166,167] Alternative bimanual therapies may have similar efficacy to CIMT in children.[163] The ability of noninvasive neuromodulation with repetitive transcranial magnetic stimulation or transcranial direct current stimulation to enhance motor learning therapy in adult stroke is supported by substantial randomized trial evidence.[168] A small childhood AIS trial suggested favorable tolerability and possible benefit.[169] Peripheral electrical stimulation is supported by adult stroke rehabilitation guidelines but has not been tested in children. Emerging technologies in adult stroke rehabilitation such as robot-assisted rehabilitation[170] or virtual reality[171] may have potential in children.

Increased tone, including spasticity and dystonia, often limit function in children with AIS. Botulinum toxin may alleviate both forms of hypertonia and, used strategically, enhance function. Issues of tolerability, cost, and objective measures of functional improvement should be considered. Ankle–foot orthoses, hand splints, and other simple assistive devices may improve limb positioning to enhance function.[172] These topics are discussed in greater detail in Chapters 5 to 7. Growing children with neurological disability require regular assessment for musculoskeletal complications, including bone density, joint health, and scoliosis. Morbidity-targeted interventions should use objective, blinded pre- and postinterventional outcome measures focused on function and participation to judge efficacy and relative benefit. An experienced, multidisciplinary team approach is ideal, combining orthopedic and physical medicine physicians; occupational, physical and speech therapists; child psychologists; educational specialists; and others.

Perhaps the most complex adverse outcomes are the neuropsychological impairments commonly incurred by children with AIS. Decreases across a range of higher brain functions may limit academic success, future employability, and psychosocial health.[173-175] Collectively, global intellectual function is moderately impaired in children with AIS.[176,177] Predictors are not well defined, with only weak, inconsistent associations with age, volume, laterality, and location.[178-183] Language dysfunction frequently

occurs,[184,185] with cortical deficits usually associated with dominant hemisphere lesions.[174,186] Verbal learning and memory are often impaired with major implications for learning.[175,178,179] Attention deficit hyperactivity disorder rates are higher in childhood AIS and potentially treatable.[187-189] Emotional and behavioral disorders including depression, anxiety, and impaired social function may develop[187-189] and affect health-related quality of life and peer relationships.[190] These topics are explored in greater detail in Chapters 8 to 10. Strategic, formal neuropsychological testing is often required to fully characterize stroke-induced deficits and optimize educational planning. Particularly in young children who often "grow into their deficits" over time, serial measures may be required during development.[191,192]

Secondary stroke prevention is an important chronic management issue. Recurrence risks may be as high as 35%,[39,40,145,193] with larger population-based studies reporting 5-year rates of 20%.[43] Presence of arteriopathy is highly associated with recurrence risk[39,193] where rates increase to >65%.[43] Observational studies suggest recurrence rates are lower in children on antithrombotic therapy, but randomized trials do not exist.[193] Aspirin (1 to 5 mg/kg/day) is usually chosen and is recommended in published guidelines.[74,75,139] Certain conditions such as congenital heart disease may require long-term anticoagulation.[97] Additional prevention options include immunomodulation for vasculitis, transfusion therapy for SCD, revascularization surgery for moyamoya, avoidance of medications, and treatment of medical conditions like iron deficiency. Good general health practices to optimize arterial health should be encouraged, including balanced nutrition, regular exercise, avoidance of smoking, and screening for hypertension and dyslipidemia.[194]

Remote symptomatic epilepsy occurs in 15% to 20% of childhood AIS patients.[145,195-197] Seizures are usually focal, although secondary generalized events and epileptic encephalopathies also occur.[197-199] Factors that increase epilepsy risk may include cortical involvement,[145,196,200] younger age, and seizures at presentation.[201] Historical screening and electroencephalography are required. Treatments adhere to pediatric anticonvulsant best practices. Children with AIS who develop refractory epilepsy are often excellent epilepsy surgery candidates.[202,203] Headaches are reported in one third of children with AIS[145] and may be associated with certain diseases (eg, moyamoya), a primary headache disorder (eg, migraine), or psychological factors. Worsening headaches may suggest disease progression in cPACNS or moyamoya. Usual headache treatments are generally safe in children with AIS, although vasoconstricting triptans might be avoided.

Fundamental to treatment of childhood AIS is the psychological and social support of the child and their family. Such family-centered care optimizes opportunities to recognize and address the complex psychosocial challenges faced by most families. These topics are further explored in Chapter 11. Quality of life deteriorates in most families, and the reasons are many,[204] relating to neurological, psychosocial, and other factors.[173] Coping strategies are a recognized therapeutic target in adult stroke[205] but unstudied in children. Supportive care must consider the individual child's lifestyle, goals, and level of development and functioning while integrating into school and home environments.[147] Parental guilt may be modifiable through educational initiatives that could improve parental outcomes.[206] Families also need guidance to interpret the validity of the many unproven therapeutic options presented to them, both legitimate (eg, stem cells) and not.[207] International educational and supportive organizations focused on childhood AIS are expanding.

FAMILY FOCUS BOX

1. Pediatric arterial ischemic stroke affects 2 to 5/100,000 children/year. This type of stroke occurs when a blood clot in an artery or narrowing of an artery prevents part of the brain from receiving adequate blood flow, resulting in permanent injury. In children, common symptoms at the time of stroke include sudden onset of weakness affecting one or both sides of the body, difficulty speaking or understanding language, abnormal eye movements, impaired coordination, or trouble walking. Seizures affect some children at the time of AIS.

2. Brain MRI is the test that is most sensitive for detecting a stroke. Blood vessel abnormalities are the most common cause of AIS in children, so one or more tests will be done to look at the arteries that supply blood to the brain. The risk of stroke is higher in children with heart disease or a tendency to form blood clots easily, so blood tests and an echocardiogram (ultrasound of the heart) may be done to look for these problems. Medication to prevent blood clot formation is typically given to decrease the risk of subsequent stroke.

3. Children who experienced an AIS may have lasting weakness and stiffness (affecting the side of the body opposite the side of the stroke), difficulty speaking or understanding language, trouble with coordination and balance, learning difficulties, seizures, or attention deficit hyperactivity disorder.

4. Physical, occupational, speech and language, and/or feeding therapy may be recommended following a stroke. Some children will require special education or accommodations in school after a stroke. Some children will have lasting difficulties after a stroke, but other children will recover fully.

CASE STUDY

A 15-year-old boy was previously healthy. A high school football star, he was studying 3 languages and in 10th grade. His parents left him well at home at noon, but he did not answer the phone 2 hours later. They returned an hour later to find him unable to speak, confused, and vomiting. He was rushed to the local emergency room where immediate concerns included seizures and meningitis. A head CT scan was read as normal but in retrospect demonstrated loss of cortical signal in the left temporal lobe and a hyperdense left middle cerebral artery (see Figure 1-1A). After undergoing other tests, he was given seizure medicine and became increasingly drowsy, whereupon he was intubated and flown to the tertiary care pediatric center. The next morning, decreased movement of his right side was appreciated. MRI revealed an evolving AIS of the entire left middle cerebral artery territory (see Figure 1-1B). His sedation was stopped, but he had minimal improvement in consciousness and signs of brainstem dysfunction consistent with impending herniation secondary to malignant cerebral edema. An emergency decompressive hemicraniectomy was lifesaving (see Figure 1-1C). He was diagnosed with probable large vessel vasculitis based on imaging findings (see Figure 1-1D to 1-1F). He was treated with aspirin and high-dose steroids. He would spend several months in hospital rehabilitation with complications including severe hemiparesis, expressive dysphasia, seizures, depression, and others. At 3 years following the stroke, his motor deficits remain severe but he performs all his self-care and participates independently in high school and community activities. His expressive speech is still limited, but he recently made large gains after a trial of experimental brain stimulation and speech therapy. He and his family agree that they have regained their previous quality of life in nearly all areas, with optimism and highly meaningful goals for his future.

SUMMARY

AIS in children occurs when cerebral blood flow through one or more arteries is diminished or prevented by thromboembolic occlusion or arterial narrowing, resulting in infarction of brain tissue. AIS should be considered in children who develop an acute focal neurological deficit. Diagnosis is confirmed with neuroimaging, with brain MRI providing the greatest sensitivity. Arteriopathies, cardiac disease, and prothrombotic abnormalities are risk factors for AIS in children. Acute AIS is a medical emergency, and treatments to optimize cerebral perfusion while minimizing metabolic demand should be implemented. Antithrombotic therapy decreases risk of recurrent stroke. The majority of pediatric stroke survivors have lasting motor, cognitive, or behavioral impairments or develop epilepsy. Physical, occupational, and speech and language therapy, and educational support play important roles in long-term recovery.

REFERENCES

1. Kleindorfer D, Khoury J, Kissela B, et al. Temporal trends in the incidence and case fatality of stroke in children and adolescents. *J Child Neurol.* 2006;21(5):415-418.

2. Broderick J, Talbot GT, Prenger E, Leach A, Brott T. Stroke in children within a major metropolitan area: the surprising importance of intracerebral hemorrhage. *J Child Neurol.* 1993;8(3):250-255.

3. Fullerton HJ, Wu YW, Zhao S, Johnston SC. Risk of stroke in children: ethnic and gender disparities. *Neurology.* 2003;61(2):189-194.

4. Agrawal N, Johnston SC, Wu YW, Sidney S, Fullerton HJ. Imaging data reveal a higher pediatric stroke incidence than prior US estimates. *Stroke.* 2009;40(11):3415-3421.

5. Lynch JK, Hirtz DG, deVeber G, Nelson KB. Report of the National Institute of Neurological Disorders and Stroke workshop on perinatal and childhood stroke. *Pediatrics.* 2002;109(1):116-123.

6. Murphy SL. Deaths: final data for 1998. *Natl Vital Stat Rep.* 2000;48(11):1-105.

7. Lo W, Zamel K, Ponnappa K, et al. The cost of pediatric stroke care and rehabilitation. *Stroke.* 2008;39(1):161-165.

8. Andrew M, Paes B, Johnston M. Development of the hemostatic system in the neonate and young infant. *Am J Pediatr Hematol Oncol.* 1990;12:95-104.

9. Monagle P, Barnes C, Ignjatovic V, et al. Developmental haemostasis. Impact for clinical haemostasis laboratories. *Thromb Haemost.* 2006;95(2):362-372.

10. Eleftheriou D, Ganesan V, Hong Y, Klein NJ, Brogan PA. Endothelial injury in childhood stroke with cerebral arteriopathy: a cross-sectional study. *Neurology.* 2012;79(21):2089-2096.

11. Altman DI, Powers WJ, Perlman JM. Cerebral blood flow requirements for brain viability in newborn infants is lower than in adults. *Ann Neurol.* 1988;24:218-226.

12. Wintermark M, Lepori D, Cotting J, et al. Brain perfusion in children: evolution with age assessed by quantitative perfusion computed tomography. *Pediatrics.* 2004;113(6):1642-1652.

13. Shellhaas RA, Smith SE, O'Tool E, Licht DJ, Ichord RN. Mimics of childhood stroke: characteristics of a prospective cohort. *Pediatrics.* 2006;118(2):704-709.

14. Mackay MT, Chua ZK, Lee M, et al. Stroke and nonstroke brain attacks in children. *Neurology.* 2014;82(16):1434-1440.

15. Delsing BJ, Catsman-Berrevoets CE, Appel IM. Early prognostic indicators of outcome in ischemic childhood stroke. *Pediatr Neurol.* 2001;24(4):283-289.

16. Trescher WH. Ischemic stroke syndromes in childhood. *Pediatr Ann.* 1992;21(6):374-383.

17. Braun KP, Rafay MF, Uiterwaal CS, Pontigon AM, deVeber G. Mode of onset predicts etiological diagnosis of arterial ischemic stroke in children. *Stroke.* 2007;38(2):298-302.

18. Gabis LV, Yangala R, Lenn NJ. Time lag to diagnosis of stroke in children. *Pediatrics.* 2002;110(5):924-928.

19. Rafay MF, Pontigon AM, Chiang J, et al. Delay to diagnosis in acute pediatric arterial ischemic stroke. *Stroke.* 2009;40(1):58-64.

20. Srinivasan J, Miller SP, Phan TG, Mackay MT. Delayed recognition of initial stroke in children: need for increased awareness. *Pediatrics.* 2009;124(2):e227-e234.

21. Yock-Corrales A, Babl FE, Mosley IT, Mackay MT. Can the FAST and ROSIER adult stroke recognition tools be applied to confirmed childhood arterial ischemic stroke? *BMC Pediatr.* 2011;11:93.

22. Ichord RN, Bastian R, Abraham L, et al. Interrater reliability of the Pediatric National Institutes of Health Stroke Scale (PedNIHSS) in a multicenter study. *Stroke.* 2011;42(3):613-617.

23. Kirton A, Crone M, Benseler S, et al. Fibromuscular dysplasia and childhood stroke. *Brain.* 2013;136(Pt 6):1846-1856.

24. Brenner DJ, Hall EJ. Computed tomography: an increasing source of radiation exposure. *N Engl J Med.* 2007;357(22):2277-2284.

25. Muir KW, Buchan A, von Kummer R, Rother J, Baron JC. Imaging of acute stroke. *Lancet Neurol.* 2006;5(9):755-768.

26. Groenendaal F, van der Ground J, Witkamp TD, de Vries LS. Proton magnetic resonance spectroscopic imaging in neonatal stroke. *Neuropediatrics.* 1995;26:243-248.

27. Warach S, Baron JC. Neuroimaging. *Stroke.* 2004;35(2):351-353.

28. Kirkham FJ, Calamante F, Bynevelt M, et al. Perfusion magnetic resonance abnormalities in patients with sickle cell disease. *Ann Neurol.* 2001;49(4):477-485.

29. Mikulis DJ, Krolczyk G, Desal H, et al. Preoperative and postoperative mapping of cerebrovascular reactivity in moyamoya disease by using blood oxygen level-dependent magnetic resonance imaging. *J Neurosurg.* 2005;103(2):347-355.

30. Swartz RH, Bhuta SS, Farb RI, et al. Intracranial arterial wall imaging using high-resolution 3-tesla contrast-enhanced MRI. *Neurology.* 2009;72(7):627-634.

31. Husson B, Lasjaunias P. Radiological approach to disorders of arterial brain vessels associated with childhood arterial stroke: a comparison between MRA and contrast angiography. *Pediatr Radiol.* 2004;34(1):10-15.

32. Wiznitzer M, Masaryk TJ. Cerebrovascular abnormalities in pediatric stroke: assessment using parenchymal and angiographic magnetic resonance imaging. *Ann Neurol.* 1991;29:585-589.

33. Ganesan V, Savvy L, Chong WK, Kirkham FJ. Conventional cerebral angiography in children with ischemic stroke. *Pediatr Neurol.* 1999;20(1):38-42.

34. Aviv RI, Benseler SM, Silverman ED, et al. MR imaging and angiography of primary CNS vasculitis of childhood. *AJNR Am J Neuroradiol.* 2006;27(1):192-199.

35. Hill MD, Demchuk AM, Frayne R. Noninvasive imaging is improving but digital subtraction angiography remains the gold standard. *Neurology.* 2007;68(24):2057-20208.

36. Tan MA, deVeber G, Kirton A, Vidarsson L, MacGregor D, Shroff M. Low detection rate of craniocervical arterial dissection in children using time-of-flight magnetic resonance angiography: causes and strategies to improve diagnosis. *J Child Neurol.* 2009;24(10):1250-1257.

37. Scott RM, Smith ER. Moyamoya disease and moyamoya syndrome. *N Engl J Med.* 2009;360(12):1226-1237.

38. Burger IM, Murphy KJ, Jordan LC, Tamargo RJ, Gailloud P. Safety of cerebral digital subtraction angiography in children: complication rate analysis in 241 consecutive diagnostic angiograms. *Stroke.* 2006;37(10):2535-2559.

39. Chabrier S, Husson B, Lasjaunias P, Landrieu P, Tardieu M. Stroke in childhood: outcome and recurrence risk by mechanism in 59 patients. *J Child Neurol.* 2000;15(5):290-294.

40. Lanthier S, Carmant L, David M, Larbrisseau A, deVeber G. Stroke in children: the coexistence of multiple risk factors predicts poor outcome. *Neurology.* 2000;54(2):371-378.

41. Ganesan V, Prengler M, McShane MA, Wade AM, Kirkham FJ. Investigation of risk factors in children with arterial ischemic stroke. *Ann Neurol.* 2003;53(2):167-173.

42. deVeber G; Canadian Paediatric Ischemic Stroke Study Group. Canadian Paediatric Ischemic Stroke Registry: Analysis of children with arterial ischemic stroke. *Ann Neurol.* 2000;48(3):514.

43. Fullerton HJ, Wu YW, Sidney S, Johnston SC. Risk of recurrent childhood arterial ischemic stroke in a population-based cohort: the importance of cerebrovascular imaging. *Pediatrics.* 2007;119(3):495-501.

44. Amlie-Lefond C, Bernard TJ, Sebire G, et al. Predictors of cerebral arteriopathy in children with arterial ischemic stroke: results of the International Pediatric Stroke Study. *Circulation.* 2009;119(10):1417-1423.

45. Sebire G. Transient cerebral arteriopathy in childhood. *Lancet.* 2006;368(9529):8-10.

46. Braun KP, Bulder MM, Chabrier S, et al. The course and outcome of unilateral intracranial arteriopathy in 79 children with ischaemic stroke. *Brain.* 2009;132(Pt 2):544-557.

47. Mackay MT, Wiznitzer M, Benedict SL, Lee KJ, deVeber GA, Ganesan V. Arterial ischemic stroke risk factors: the international pediatric stroke study. *Ann Neurol.* 2011;69(1):130-140.

48. Goldenberg NA, Jenkins S, Jack J, et al. Arteriopathy, D-dimer, and risk of poor neurologic outcome in childhood-onset arterial ischemic stroke. *J Pediatr.* 2013;162(5):1041-1046.

49. Sebire G, Fullerton H, Riou E, deVeber G. Toward the definition of cerebral arteriopathies of childhood. *Curr Opin Pediatr.* 2004;16(6):617-622.

50. Bernard TJ, Manco-Johnson MJ, Lo W, et al. Towards a consensus-based classification of childhood arterial ischemic stroke. *Stroke.* 2012;43(2):371-377.

51. Chabrier S, Rodesch G, Lasjaunias P, Tardieu M, Landrieu P, Sebire G. Transient cerebral arteriopathy: a disorder recognized by serial angiograms in children with stroke. *J Child Neurol.* 1998;13(1):27-32.

52. Benseler S, Pohl D. Childhood central nervous system vasculitis. *Handb Clin Neurol.* 2013;112:1065-1078.

53. Dlamini N, Freeman JL, Mackay MT, et al. Intracranial dissection mimicking transient cerebral arteriopathy in childhood arterial ischemic stroke. *J Child Neurol.* 2011;26(9):1203-1206.

54. Askalan R, Laughlin S, Mayank S, et al. Chickenpox and stroke in childhood: a study of frequency and causation. *Stroke.* 2001;32(6):1257-1262.

55. Amlie-Lefond C, Kleinschmidt-DeMasters BK, Mahalingam R, Davis LE, Gilden DH. The vasculopathy of varicella-zoster virus encephalitis. *Ann Neurol.* 1995;37(6):784-790.

56. Gilden D, Cohrs RJ, Mahalingam R, Nagel MA. Varicella zoster virus vasculopathies: diverse clinical manifestations, laboratory features, pathogenesis, and treatment. *Lancet Neurol.* 2009;8(8):731-740.

57. Donahue JG, Kieke BA, Yih WK, et al. Varicella vaccination and ischemic stroke in children: is there an association? *Pediatrics.* 2009;123(2):e228-e234.

58. Hills NK, Johnston SC, Sidney S, Zielinski BA, Fullerton HJ. Recent trauma and acute infection as risk factors for childhood arterial ischemic stroke. *Ann Neurol.* 2012;72(6):850-858.

59. Fullerton HJ, Elkind MS, Barkovich AJ, et al. The vascular effects of infection in Pediatric Stroke (VIPS) Study. *J Child Neurol.* 2011;26(9):1101-1110.

60. Chang CJ, Chang WN, Huang LT, et al. Cerebral infarction in perinatal and childhood bacterial meningitis. *QJM.* 2003;96(10):755-762.

61. Springer P, Swanevelder S, van Toorn R, van Rensburg AJ, Schoeman J. Cerebral infarction and neurodevelopmental outcome in childhood tuberculous meningitis. *Eur J Paediatr Neurol.* 2009;13(4):343-349.

62. Patsalides AD, Wood LV, Atac GK, Sandifer E, Butman JA, Patronas NJ. Cerebrovascular disease in HIV-infected pediatric patients: neuroimaging findings. *AJR Am J Roentgenol.* 2002;179(4):999-1003.

63. Takeoka M, Takahashi T. Infectious and inflammatory disorders of the circulatory system and stroke in childhood. *Curr Opin Neurol.* 2002;15(2):159-164.

64. Benseler SM, deVeber G, Hawkins C, et al. Angiography-negative primary central nervous system vasculitis in children: a newly recognized inflammatory central nervous system disease. *Arthritis Rheum.* 2005;52(7):2159-2167.

65. Benseler S, Schneider R. Central nervous system vasculitis in children. *Curr Opin Rheumatol.* 2004;16(1):43-50.

66. Morales E, Pineda C, Martinez-Lavin M. Takayasu's arteritis in children. *J Rheumatol.* 1991;18(7):1081-1084.

67. Ganesan V, Cox TC, Gunny R. Abnormalities of cervical arteries in children with arterial ischemic stroke. *Neurology.* 2011;76(2):166-171.

68. Elbers J, Benseler SM. Central nervous system vasculitis in children. *Curr Opin Rheumatol.* 2008;20(1):47-54.

69. Mineyko A, Narendran A, Fritzler ML, Wei XC, Schmeling H, Kirton A. Inflammatory biomarkers of pediatric focal cerebral arteriopathy. *Neurology.* 2012;79(13):1406-1408.

70. Morel A, Naggara O, Touze E, et al. Mechanism of ischemic infarct in spontaneous cervical artery dissection. *Stroke.* 2012;43(5):1354-1361.

71. Fullerton HJ, Johnston SC, Smith WS. Arterial dissection and stroke in children. *Neurology.* 2001;57(7):1155-1160.

72. Chabrier S, Lasjaunias P, Husson B, Landrieu P, Tardieu M. Ischaemic stroke from dissection of the craniocervical arteries in childhood: report of 12 patients. *Eur J Paediatr Neurol.* 2003;7(1):39-42.

73. Rafay MF, Armstrong D, deVeber G, Domi T, Chan A, MacGregor DL. Craniocervical arterial dissection in children: clinical and radiographic presentation and outcome. *J Child Neurol.* 2006;21(1):8-16.

74. Monagle P, Chan AK, Goldenberg NA, et al. Antithrombotic therapy in neonates and children: Antithrombotic Therapy and Prevention of Thrombosis, 9th ed: American College of Chest Physicians Evidence-Based Clinical Practice Guidelines. *Chest.* 2012;141(2 Suppl):e737S-e801S.

75. Roach ES, Golomb MR, Adams R, et al. Management of stroke in infants and children: a scientific statement from a Special Writing Group of the American Heart Association Stroke Council and the Council on Cardiovascular Disease in the Young. *Stroke.* 2008;39(9):2644-2691.

76. Kennedy F, Lanfranconi S, Hicks C, et al. Antiplatelets vs anticoagulation for dissection: CADISS nonrandomized arm and meta-analysis. *Neurology.* 2012;79(7):686-689.

77. Bernard TJ, deVeber GA, Benke TA. Athletic participation after acute ischemic childhood stroke: a survey of pediatric stroke experts. *J Child Neurol.* 2007;22(8):1050-1053.

78. Kamada F, Aoki Y, Narisawa A, et al. A genome-wide association study identifies RNF213 as the first Moyamoya disease gene. *J Hum Genet.* 2011;56(1):34-40.

79. Jea A, Smith ER, Robertson R, Scott RM. Moyamoya syndrome associated with Down syndrome: outcome after surgical revascularization. *Pediatrics.* 2005;116(5):e694-e701.

80. Suzuki J, Kodama N. Moyamoya disease: a review. *Stroke.* 1983;14(1):104-109.

81. Kim SK, Seol HJ, Cho BK, Hwang YS, Lee DS, Wang KC. Moyamoya disease among young patients: its aggressive clinical course and the role of active surgical treatment. *Neurosurgery.* 2004;54(4):840-844.

82. Vuignier S, Ito M, Kurisu K, et al. Ivy sign, misery perfusion, and asymptomatic moyamoya disease: FLAIR imaging and (15) O-gas positron emission tomography. *Acta Neurochir (Wien).* 2013;155(11):2097-2104.

83. Fung LW, Thompson D, Ganesan V. Revascularisation surgery for paediatric moyamoya: a review of the literature. *Childs Nerv Syst.* 2005;21(5):358-364.

84. Scott RM, Smith JL, Robertson RL, Madsen JR, Soriano SG, Rockoff MA. Long-term outcome in children with moyamoya syndrome after cranial revascularization by pial synangiosis. *J Neurosurg.* 2004;100(2 Suppl):142-149.

85. Funaki T, Takahashi JC, Takagi Y, et al. Incidence of late cerebrovascular events after direct bypass among children with moyamoya disease: a descriptive longitudinal study at a single center. *Acta Neurochir (Wien).* 2014;156(3):551-559.

86. Dowling MM, Hynan LS, Lo W, et al. International Paediatric Stroke Study: stroke associated with cardiac disorders. *Int J Stroke.* 2013;8(Suppl A100):39-44.

87. Miller SP, McQuillen PS, Vigneron DB, et al. Preoperative brain injury in newborns with transposition of the great arteries. *Ann Thorac Surg.* 2004;77(5):1698-1706.

88. Domi T, Edgell DS, McCrindle BW, et al. Frequency, predictors, and neurologic outcomes of vaso-occlusive strokes associated with cardiac surgery in children. *Pediatrics.* 2008;122(6):1292-1298.

89. Monagle P, Karl TR. Thromboembolic problems after the Fontan operation. *Semin Thorac Cardiovasc Surg Pediatr Card Surg Annu.* 2002;5:36-47.

90. McQuillen PS, Hamrick SE, Perez MJ, et al. Balloon atrial septostomy is associated with preoperative stroke in neonates with transposition of the great arteries. *Circulation.* 2006;113(2):280-285.

91. Liu XY, Wong V, Leung M. Neurologic complications due to catheterization. *Pediatr Neurol.* 2001;24(4):270-275.

92. Rodan L, McCrindle BW, Manlhiot C, et al. Stroke recurrence in children with congenital heart disease. *Ann Neurol.* 2012;72(1):103-111.

93. Kizer JR, Devereux RB. Clinical practice. Patent foramen ovale in young adults with unexplained stroke. *N Engl J Med.* 2005;353(22):2361-2372.

94. Mas JL, Arquizan C, Lamy C, et al. Recurrent cerebrovascular events associated with patent foramen ovale, atrial septal aneurysm, or both. *N Engl J Med.* 2001;345(24):1740-1746.

95. Furlan AJ, Reisman M, Massaro J, et al. Closure or medical therapy for cryptogenic stroke with patent foramen ovale. *N Engl J Med.* 2012;366(11):991-999.

96. Fraser CD Jr, Jaquiss RD, Rosenthal DN, et al. Prospective trial of a pediatric ventricular assist device. *N Engl J Med.* 2012;367(6):532-541.

97. Giglia TM, Massicotte MP, Tweddell JS, et al. Prevention and treatment of thrombosis in pediatric and congenital heart disease: a scientific statement from the American Heart Association. *Circulation.* 2013;128(24):2622-2703.

98. Mackay MT, Monagle P. Perinatal and early childhood stroke and thrombophilia. *Pathology.* 2008;40(2):116-123.

99. Barnes C, deVeber G. Prothrombotic abnormalities in childhood ischaemic stroke. *Thromb Res.* 2006;118(1):67-74.

100. Strater R, Becker S, von Eckardstein A, et al. Prospective assessment of risk factors for recurrent stroke during childhood: a 5-year follow-up study. *Lancet.* 2002;360(9345):1540-1545.

101. deVeber G, Monagle P, Chan A, et al. Prothrombotic disorders in infants and children with cerebral thromboembolism. *Arch Neurol.* 1998;55(12):1539-1543.

102. Kenet G, Lutkhoff LK, Albisetti M, et al. Impact of thrombophilia on risk of arterial ischemic stroke or cerebral sinovenous thrombosis in neonates and children: a systematic review and meta-analysis of observational studies. *Circulation.* 2010;121(16):1838-1847.

103. Nowak-Goettl U, Strater R, Heinecke A, et al. Lipoprotein (a) and genetic polymorphisms of clotting factor V, prothrombin, and methylenetetrahydrofolate reductase are risk factors of spontaneous ischemic stroke in childhood. *Blood.* 1999;94(11):3678-3682.

104. Ganesan V, Prengler M, Wade A, Kirkham FJ. Clinical and radiological recurrence after childhood arterial ischemic stroke. *Circulation.* 2006;114(20):2170-2177.

105. Goldenberg NA, Bernard TJ, Hillhouse J, et al. Elevated lipoprotein (a), small apolipoprotein (a), and the risk of arterial ischemic stroke in North American children. *Haematologica.* 2013;98(5):802-807.

106. Pegelow CH. Stroke in children with sickle cell anaemia: aetiology and treatment. *Paediatr Drugs.* 2001;3(6):421-432.

107. Satoh S, Shibuya H, Matsushima Y, Suzuki S. Analysis of the angiographic findings in cases of childhood moyamoya disease. *Neuroradiology.* 1988;30(2):111-119.

108. Telfer PT, Evanson J, Butler P, et al. Cervical carotid artery disease in sickle cell anemia: clinical and radiological features. *Blood.* 2011;118(23):6192-6199.

109. Adams R, McKie V, Nichols F, et al. The use of transcranial ultrasonography to predict stroke in sickle cell disease. *N Engl J Med.* 1992;326:605-610.

110. Adams RJ, McKie VC, Hsu L, et al. Prevention of a first stroke by transfusions in children with sickle cell anemia and abnormal results on transcranial Doppler ultrasonography. *N Engl J Med.* 1998;339(1):5-11.

111. Zimmerman RA. MRI/MRA evaluation of sickle cell disease of the brain. *Pediatr Radiol.* 2005;35(3):249-257.

112. Adams RJ, Brambilla D. Discontinuing prophylactic transfusions used to prevent stroke in sickle cell disease. *N Engl J Med.* 2005;353(26):2769-2778.

113. Ware RE, Helms RW. Stroke with transfusions changing to hydroxyurea (SWiTCH). *Blood.* 2012;119(17):3925-3932.

114. Hulbert ML, McKinstry RC, Lacey JL, et al. Silent cerebral infarcts occur despite regular blood transfusion therapy after first strokes in children with sickle cell disease. *Blood.* 2011;117(3):772-779.

115. Walters MC, Patience M, Leisenring W, et al. Bone marrow transplantation for sickle cell disease. *N Engl J Med.* 1996;335(6):369-376.

116. Maguire JL, deVeber G, Parkin PC. Association between iron-deficiency anemia and stroke in young children. *Pediatrics.* 2007;120(5):1053-1057.

117. Dowling MM, Quinn CT, Plumb P, et al. Acute silent cerebral ischemia and infarction during acute anemia in children with and without sickle cell disease. *Blood.* 2012;120(19):3891-3897.

118. Rothrock JF. Migrainous stroke. *Cephalalgia.* 1993;13(4):231.

119. Feucht M, Brantner S, Scheidinger H. Migraine and stroke in childhood and adolescence. *Cephalagia.* 1995;15(1):26-30.

120. Kirton A, Diggle J, Hu W, Wirrell E. A pediatric case of reversible segmental cerebral vasoconstriction. *Can J Neurol Sci.* 2006;33(2):250-253.

121. Probert R, Saunders DE, Ganesan V. Reversible cerebral vasoconstriction syndrome: rare or underrecognized in children? *Dev Med Child Neurol.* 2013;55(4):385-389.

122. Gillum LA, Mamidipudi SK, Johnston SC. Ischemic stroke risk with oral contraceptives: a meta-analysis. *JAMA* 2000;284(1):72-78.
123. Bodensteiner JB, Hille MR, Riggs JE. Clinical features of vascular thrombosis following varicella. *Am J Dis Child.* 1992;146(1):100-102.
124. deVeber G, Kirton A, D'Anjou G, et al. Canadian best practice recommendations for stroke care 2010. *Canadian Stroke Network.* 2012;11(4):459-484.
125. Baird TA, Parsons MW, Phanh T, et al. Persistent poststroke hyperglycemia is independently associated with infarct expansion and worse clinical outcome. *Stroke.* 2003;34(9):2208-2214.
126. McCormick M, Hadley D, McLean JR, Macfarlane JA, Condon B, Muir KW. Randomized, controlled trial of insulin for acute poststroke hyperglycemia. *Ann Neurol.* 2010;67(5):570-578.
127. Fox CK, Johnston SC, Sidney S, Fullerton HJ. High critical care usage due to pediatric stroke: results of a population-based study. *Neurology.* 2012;79(5):420-427.
128. Bernard TJ, Rivkin MJ, Scholz K, et al. Emergence of the primary pediatric stroke center: impact of the thrombolysis in pediatric stroke trial. *Stroke.* 2014.
129. Lehman LL, Kleindorfer DO, Khoury JC, et al. Potential eligibility for recombinant tissue plasminogen activator therapy in children: a population-based study. *J Child Neurol.* 2011;26(9):1121-1125.
130. Amlie-Lefond C, deVeber G, Chan AK, et al. Use of alteplase in childhood arterial ischaemic stroke: a multicentre, observational, cohort study. *Lancet Neurol.* 2009;8(6):530-536.
131. Alshekhlee A, Geller T, Mehta S, Storkan M, Al KY, Cruz-Flores S. Thrombolysis for children with acute ischemic stroke: a perspective from the kids' inpatient database. *Pediatr Neurol.* 2013;49(5):313-318.
132. Broderick JP, Palesch YY, Demchuk AM, et al. Endovascular therapy after intravenous t-PA versus t-PA alone for stroke. *N Engl J Med.* 2013;368(10):893-903.
133. Amlie-Lefond C, Chan A, Ichord R, deVeber G; Members of IPSS. TPA in children with arterial ischemic stroke: cases from the IPSS compared with literature-based cases. *Thromb Hemostas.* 2007;5(Suppl 2):579.
134. Monagle P, Chan A, deVeber G, Massicotte P. *Andrew's Pediatric Thromboembolism and Stroke,* 3 ed. Valley Stream, NY: BC Decker; 2006.
135. Strater R, Kurnik K, Heller C, Schobess R, Luigs P, Nowak-Goettl U. Aspirin versus low-dose low-molecular-weight heparin: antithrombotic therapy in pediatric ischemic stroke patients: a prospective follow-up study. *Stroke.* 2001;32(11):2554-2558.
136. Schror K. Aspirin and Reye syndrome: a review of the evidence. *Paediatr Drugs.* 2007;9(3):195-204.
137. Soman T, Rafay MF, Hune S, Allen A, MacGregor D, deVeber G. The risks and safety of clopidogrel in pediatric arterial ischemic stroke. *Stroke.* 2006;37(4):1120-1122.
138. Fullerton H, deVeber G, IPSS investigators. Practice variability in the treatment of childhood acute ischemic stroke: results of the International Pediatric Stroke Study. *Stroke.* 2007;38(2):485.
139. Goldenberg NA, Bernard TJ, Fullerton HJ, Gordon A, deVeber G. Antithrombotic treatments, outcomes, and prognostic factors in acute childhood-onset arterial ischaemic stroke: a multicentre, observational, cohort study. *Lancet Neurol.* 2009;8(12):1120-1127.
140. Bernard TJ, Goldenberg NA, Tripputi M, Manco-Johnson MJ, Niederstadt T, Nowak-Goettl U. Anticoagulation in childhood-onset arterial ischemic stroke with non-moyamoya arteriopathy: findings from the Colorado and German (COAG) collaboration. *Stroke.* 2009;40(8):2869-2871.
141. Hutchinson C, Elbers J, Halliday W,, et al. Treatment of small vessel primary CNS vasculitis in children: an open-label cohort study. *Lancet Neurol.* 2010;9(11):1078-1084.
142. Vahedi K, Hofmeijer J, Juettler E,, et al. Early decompressive surgery in malignant infarction of the middle cerebral artery: a pooled analysis of three randomised controlled trials. *Lancet Neurol.* 2007;6(3):215-222.
143. Ramaswamy V, Mehta V, Bauman M, Richer L, Massicotte P, Yager JY. Decompressive hemicraniectomy in children with severe ischemic stroke and life-threatening cerebral edema. *J Child Neurol.* 2008;23(8):889-894.
144. Smith SE, Kirkham FJ, deVeber G,, et al. Outcome following decompressive craniectomy for malignant middle cerebral artery infarction in children. *Dev Med Child Neurol.* 2011;53(1):29-33.
145. deVeber G, MacGregor D, Curtis R, Mayank S. Neurologic outcome in survivors of childhood arterial ischemic stroke and sinovenous thrombosis. *J Child Neurol.* 2000;15(5):316-324.
146. Ganesan V, Hogan A, Shack N, Gordon A, Isaacs E, Kirkham FJ. Outcome after ischaemic stroke in childhood. *Dev Med Child Neurol.* 2000;42(7):455-461.
147. Paediatric Stroke Working Group. *Stroke in Childhood: Clinical Guidelines for Diagnosis, Management and Rehabilitation.* London, United Kingdom: Royal College of Physicians of London (UK); 2004.
148. Ward NS. Functional reorganization of the cerebral motor system after stroke. *Curr Opin Neurol.* 2004;17(6):725-730.
149. Teasell R, Bayona N, Salter K, Hellings C, Bitensky J. Progress in clinical neurosciences: stroke recovery and rehabilitation. *Can J Neurol Sci.* 2006;33(4):357-364.
150. Kirton A. Modeling developmental plasticity after perinatal stroke: defining central therapeutic targets in cerebral palsy. *Pediatr Neurol.* 2013;48(2):81-94.
151. Boardman JP, Ganesan V, Rutherford MA, Saunders DE, Mercuri E, Cowan F. Magnetic resonance image correlates of hemiparesis after neonatal and childhood middle cerebral artery stroke. *Pediatrics.* 2005;115(2):321-326.
152. Domi T, deVeber G, Shroff M, Kouzmitcheva E, MacGregor DL, Kirton A. Corticospinal tract pre-Wallerian degeneration: a novel outcome predictor for pediatric stroke on acute MRI. *Stroke.* 2009;40(3):780-787.
153. Kwak CH, Jankovic J. Tourettism and dystonia after subcortical stroke. *Mov Disord.* 2002;17(4):821-825.
154. Dobkin BH. Strategies for stroke rehabilitation. *Lancet Neurol.* 2004;3(9):528-536.
155. Taub E, Crago JE, Uswatte G. Constraint-induced movement therapy: a new approach to treatment in physical rehabilitation. *Rehab Psychol.* 1998;43(2):152-170.
156. Taub E, Uswatte G, Elbert T. New treatments in neurorehabilitation founded on basic research. *Nat Rev Neurosci.* 2002;3(3):228-236.
157. Wolf SL, Winstein CJ, Miller JP,, et al. Effect of constraint-induced movement therapy on upper extremity function 3 to 9 months after stroke: the EXCITE randomized clinical trial. *JAMA.* 2006;296(17):2095-2104.
158. Wolf SL, Winstein CJ, Miller JP,, et al. Retention of upper limb function in stroke survivors who have received constraint-induced movement therapy: the EXCITE randomised trial. *Lancet Neurol.* 2008;7(1):33-40.
159. Hakkennes S, Keating JL. Constraint-induced movement therapy following stroke: a systematic review of randomised controlled trials. *Aust J Physiother.* 2005;51(4):221-231.
160. Taub E, Ramey SL, DeLuca S, Echols K. Efficacy of constraint-induced movement therapy for children with cerebral palsy with asymmetric motor impairment. *Pediatrics.* 2004;113(2):305-312.
161. Taub E, Griffin A, Nick J, Gammons K, Uswatte G, Law CR. Pediatric CI therapy for stroke-induced hemiparesis in young children. *Dev Neurorehabil.* 2007;10(1):3-18.

162. Willis JK, Morello A, Davie A, Rice JC, Bennett JT. Forced use treatment of childhood hemiparesis. *Pediatrics*. 2002;110(1 Pt 1): 94-96.

163. Charles J, Gordon AM. Development of hand-arm bimanual intensive training (HABIT) for improving bimanual coordination in children with hemiplegic cerebral palsy. *Dev Med Child Neurol*. 2006;48(11):931-936.

164. Deluca SC, Echols K, Law CR, Ramey SL. Intensive pediatric constraint-induced therapy for children with cerebral palsy: randomized, controlled, crossover trial. *J Child Neurol*. 2006;21(11):931-938.

165. Sung IY, Ryu JS, Pyun SB, Yoo SD, Song WH, Park MJ. Efficacy of forced-use therapy in hemiplegic cerebral palsy. *Arch Phys Med Rehabil*. 2005;86(11):2195-2198.

166. Sakzewski L, Ziviani J, Boyd R. Systematic review and meta-analysis of therapeutic management of upper-limb dysfunction in children with congenital hemiplegia. *Pediatrics*. 2009;123(6):e1111-e1122.

167. Brady K, Garcia T. Constraint-induced movement therapy (CIMT): pediatric applications. *Dev Dis Res Rev*. 2009;15(2):102-111.

168. Hsu WY, Cheng CH, Liao KK, Lee IH, Lin YY. Effects of repetitive transcranial magnetic stimulation on motor functions in patients with stroke: a meta-analysis. *Stroke*. 2012;43(7):1849-1857.

169. Kirton A, Chen R, Friefeld S, Gunraj C, Pontigon AM, deVeber G. Contralesional repetitive transcranial magnetic stimulation for chronic hemiparesis in subcortical paediatric stroke: a randomised trial. *Lancet Neurol*. 2008;7(6):507-513.

170. Khadilkar A, Phillips K, Jean N, Lamothe C, Milne S, Sarnecka J. Ottawa panel evidence-based clinical practice guidelines for post-stroke rehabilitation. *Top Stroke Rehabil*. 2006;13(2):1-269.

171. Saposnik G, Levin M. Virtual reality in stroke rehabilitation: a meta-analysis and implications for clinicians. *Stroke*. 2011;42(5):1380-1386.

172. Lannin NA, Herbert RD. Is hand splinting effective for adults following stroke? A systematic review and methodologic critique of published research. *Clin Rehabil*. 2003;17(8):807-816.

173. Friefeld S, Yeboah O, Jones JE, deVeber G. Health-related quality of life and its relationship to neurological outcome in child survivors of stroke. *CNS Spectr*. 2004;9(6):465-475.

174. Nass RD, Trauner D. Social and affective impairments are important recovery after acquired stroke in childhood. *CNS Spectr*. 2004;9(6):420-434.

175. Studer M, Boltshauser E, Capone MA, et al. Factors affecting cognitive outcome in early pediatric stroke. *Neurology*. 2014;82(9):784-792.

176. Hetherington R, Tuff L, Anderson P, Miles B, deVeber G. Short-term intellectual outcome after arterial ischemic stroke and sinovenous thrombosis in childhood and infancy. *J Child Neurol*. 2005;20(7): 553-559.

177. McLinden A, Baird AD, Westmacott R, Anderson P, deVeber G. Early cognitive outcome after neonatal stroke. *J Child Neurol*. 2016;22(9):1111-1116.

178. Lansing AE, Max JE, Delis DC, et al. Verbal learning and memory after childhood stroke. *J Int Neuropsychol Soc*. 2004;10(5):742-752.

179. Max JE. Effect of side of lesion on neuropsychological performance in childhood stroke. *J Int Neuropsychol Soc*. 2004;10(5):698-708.

180. Ricci D, Mercuri E, Barnett A, et al. Cognitive outcome at early school age in term-born children with perinatally acquired middle cerebral artery territory infarction. *Stroke*. 2008;39(2):403-410.

181. Stiles J. Neural plasticity and cognitive development. *Dev Neuropsychol*. 2000;18(2):237-272.

182. Westmacott R, Barry V, MacGregor D, deVeber GA. Age at stroke and involvement of cortex modulate cognitive outcome in children with basal ganglia infarcts. Paper presented at: Annual Meeting of The Society for Pediatric Research; 2007. Toronto, Ontario, Canada.

183. Allman C, Scott RB. Neuropsychological sequelae following pediatric stroke: a nonlinear model of age at lesion effects. *Child Neuropsychol*. 2013;19(1):97-107.

184. Hertz-Pannier L, Chiron C, Jambaque I, et al. Late plasticity for language in a child's non-dominant hemisphere: a pre- and post-surgery fMRI study. *Brain*. 2002;125(Pt 2):361-372.

185. Van Dongen HR, Paquier PF, Raes J, Creten WL. An analysis of spontaneous conversational speech fluency in children with acquired aphasia. *Cortex*. 1994;30(4):619-633.

186. Chilosi AM, Cipriani PP, Bertuccelli B, Pfanner PL, Cioni PG. Early cognitive and communication development in children with focal brain lesions. *J Child Neurol*. 2001;16(5):309-316.

187. Max JE, Fox PT, Lancaster JL, et al. Putamen lesions and the development of attention-deficit/hyperactivity symptomatology. *J Am Acad Child Adolesc Psychiatry*. 2002;41(5):563-571.

188. Max JE, Mathews K, Manes FF, et al. Attention deficit hyperactivity disorder and neurocognitive correlates after childhood stroke. *J Int Neuropsychol Soc*. 2003;9(6):815-829.

189. Max JE, Robin DA, Taylor HG, et al. Attention function after childhood stroke. *J Int Neuropsychol Soc*. 2004;10(7):976-986.

190. Neuner B, von MS, Krumpel A, et al. Health-related quality of life in children and adolescents with stroke, self-reports, and parent/proxies reports: cross-sectional investigation. *Ann Neurol*. 2011;70(1):70-78.

191. Westmacott R, Barry V, MacGregor D, deVeber G. Intellectual function in preschool and school-aged children with a history of acute neonatal stroke. *Stroke*. 2007;38(2):581.

192. Westmacott R, MacGregor D, Askalan R, deVeber G. Late emergence of cognitive deficits after unilateral neonatal stroke. *Stroke*. 2009;40(6):2012-2019.

193. Lanthier S, Kirkham FJ, Mitchell LG, et al. Increased anticardiolipin antibody IgG titers do not predict recurrent stroke or TIA in children. *Neurology*. 2004;62(2):194-200.

194. Sultan SM, Schupf N, Dowling MM, deVeber GA, Kirton A, Elkind MS. Review of lipid and lipoprotein(a) abnormalities in childhood arterial ischemic stroke. *Int J Stroke*. 2014;9(1):79-87.

195. deVeber G, Andrew M; Canadian Pediatric Ischemic Stroke Study Group. Cerebral sinovenous thrombosis in children. *N Engl J Med*. 2001;345(6):417-423.

196. Yang JS, Yong DP, Hartlage P. Seizures associated with stroke in childhood. *Pediatr Neurol*. 1995;12:136-138.

197. Fitzgerald KC, Williams LS, Garg BP, Golomb MR. Epilepsy in children with delayed presentation of perinatal stroke. *J Child Neurol*. 2007;22(11):1274-1280.

198. Kirton A, deVeber G, Pontigon AM, MacGregor D, Shroff M. Presumed perinatal ischemic stroke: vascular classification predicts outcomes. *Ann Neurol*. 2008;63(4):436-443.

199. Soman TB, Moharir M, deVeber G, Weiss S. Infantile spasms as an adverse outcome of neonatal cortical sinovenous thrombosis. *J Child Neurol*. 2006;21(2):126-131.

200. Morais NM, Ranzan J, Riesgo RS. Predictors of epilepsy in children with cerebrovascular disease. *J Child Neurol*. 2013;28(11):1387-1391.

201. Hsu CJ, Weng WC, Peng SS, Lee WT. Early-onset seizures are correlated with late-onset seizures in children with arterial ischemic stroke. *Stroke.* 2014; 45(4):1161-1163.
202. Wyllie E, Lachhwani DK, Gupta A, et al. Successful surgery for epilepsy due to early brain lesions despite generalized EEG findings. *Neurology.* 2007;69(4):389-397.
203. Guzzetta F, Battaglia D, Di RC, Caldarelli M. Symptomatic epilepsy in children with poroencephalic cysts secondary to perinatal middle cerebral artery occlusion. *Childs Nerv Syst.* 2006;22(8):922-930.
204. Gordon AL, Ganesan V, Towell A, Kirkham FJ. Functional outcome following stroke in children. *J Child Neurol.* 2002;17(6):429-434.
205. Donnellan C, Hevey D, Hickey A, O'Neill D. Defining and quantifying coping strategies after stroke: a review. *J Neurol Neurosurg Psychiatry.* 2006;77(11):1208-1218.
206. Bemister T, Brooks B, Rothenmund S, Kirton A. Development, reliability and validity of the Alberta Perinatal Stroke Project (APSP) Parental Outcome Measure. *Ped Neurol.* 2014;51(1):43-52.
207. Rosenbaum P. Controversial treatment of spasticity: exploring alternative therapies for motor function in children with cerebral palsy. *J Child Neurol.* 2003;18(Suppl 1):S89-S94.

2

Perinatal Arterial Ischemic Stroke

Sabrina E. Smith, MD, PhD

During childhood, the neonatal period is the time when the risk of ischemic or hemorrhagic stroke is highest. The focus of this chapter is perinatal arterial ischemic stroke (PAIS), defined as "a cerebrovascular event occurring during fetal or neonatal life, before 28 days after birth, with pathological or radiological evidence of focal arterial infarction of brain."[1] Discussion of perinatal cerebral sinovenous thrombosis is included in Chapter 3, and discussion of intracerebral hemorrhage in neonates can be found in Chapter 4.

In recent population-based studies, the incidence of PAIS has been reported as 13 to 23/100,000 births/year in term and near-term infants.[2-4] Rates as high as 1/2300 births have been reported in smaller studies.[5] The incidence of PAIS is comparable to that of large vessel ischemic stroke in adults.[6] Not only is PAIS relatively common, but the clinical impact is significant. PAIS accounts for 30% of cases of congenital hemiparesis in term infants, making it the most common cause of hemiplegic cerebral palsy in this population.[7] In this chapter, the typical clinical presentation and risk factors of PAIS will be reviewed. Recommended evaluation will be discussed, and representative neuroimaging will be presented. Treatment and outcome will also be reviewed.

CLINICAL PRESENTATION

The majority of neonates with PAIS are diagnosed within the first 28 days of life with an acute stroke. In one population-based study that included children with an acute presentation as well as those with a delayed presentation, 58% came to attention during the neonatal period.[4] In an international registry, the vast majority (87%) were diagnosed within the first week of life.[8] Among term infants, clinical seizures are the most common presenting symptom, appearing in approximately 70%,[4,8] and 12% of neonatal seizures are due to PAIS.[9] Nonspecific symptoms such as abnormal tone, altered level of consciousness, and respiratory or feeding difficulties are also common. Focal neurological signs occur in the minority.[8] Stroke affects the left hemisphere more often than the right, and most perinatal strokes involve the middle cerebral artery (MCA) territory.[10]

Acute PAIS also occurs in preterm infants, though less is known about this subgroup. In one series, the majority (83%) came to clinical attention because of apnea or other respiratory difficulties, and only 30% presented with seizures.[11] In a population-based study that included term and preterm infants, acute stroke diagnosis was prompted by an incidental abnormality on routine surveillance head ultrasounds in all but one preterm infant. PAIS was then confirmed by additional neuroimaging.[4] As in term infants, preterm infants were more likely to have PAIS on the left side, and MCA location was most common.[12]

More than one-third of infants with PAIS do not have recognizable symptoms in the neonatal period, and diagnosis is made months to years later. Most often these children come to medical attention because of early hand preference indicating an emerging hemiparesis. In other cases, seizures or developmental delays prompt neuroimaging, which reveals a chronic arterial ischemic stroke.[4,13,14]

Atkinson HL, Nixon-Cave K, Smith SE, eds.
Pediatric Stroke Rehabilitation: An Interprofessional and Collaborative Approach (pp 21-33). © 2018 Taylor & Francis Group.

TABLE 2-1. RISK FACTORS FOR PERINATAL ARTERIAL ISCHEMIC STROKE

MATERNAL/PREPARTUM
Drug use (cocaine)
Gestational diabetes
History of infertility/ovarian stimulation
Intrauterine growth restriction
Placental abnormalities
Preeclampsia
Smoking during pregnancy
Thrombophilia
Twin–twin transfusion syndrome
INTRAPARTUM
Apgar score <7 at 5 minutes
Fetal heart rate abnormalities
Maternal fever/chorioamnionitis
Prolonged rupture of membranes
FETAL/NEONATAL
Congenital heart disease (CHD)
Early-onset sepsis/meningitis
Extracorporeal membrane oxygenation
Hypoglycemia
Thrombophilia

In these children the strokes are thought to have occurred in the perinatal period, but the precise timing is unknown because no symptoms were appreciated at the time of infarction, so these are considered presumed perinatal arterial ischemic strokes (PPAIS). In a Canadian study, parents first reported concerns at a median age of 5 months. Physicians did not become concerned until a median age of 7 months, and diagnosis was not confirmed until a median age of 12 months.[13] In utero timing of arterial ischemic stroke has also been confirmed on routine fetal ultrasound or magnetic resonance imaging (MRI), although the incidence is unknown.[15]

RISK FACTORS

Numerous maternal and fetal conditions have been associated with an increased risk of PAIS, although causation has not been confirmed. For a summary, see Table 2-1. Risk of stroke is increased when multiple risk factors are identified.[4] Maternal/prepartum conditions associated with PAIS include infertility, especially ovarian stimulation, preeclampsia, intrauterine growth restriction, twin–twin transfusion, and gestational diabetes.[2,4,12,16] Both maternal cocaine use and smoking during pregnancy have been associated with PAIS. In one case-control study from a neonatal intensive care unit, 17% of infants born to mothers with confirmed cocaine abuse had a cortical infarction.[17] In another case-control study nested within a whole population, maternal tobacco smoking during pregnancy was associated with increased risk of PAIS in multivariate analysis.[2]

Intrapartum conditions associated with PAIS include Apgar score <7 at 5 minutes, fetal heart rate abnormalities, maternal fever, chorioamnionitis, and prolonged rupture of membranes.[2,4,12,16,18] Several fetal characteristics have been associated with PAIS. CHD is a risk factor for PAIS, and in one study 72% of strokes in children with CHD were identified following a cardiac procedure.[19] Infants with cyanotic CHD who underwent palliative surgery with persistence of right-to-left shunting were at highest risk. In another study that performed postoperative imaging in a series of neonates and infants with CHD, half of strokes could be dated to the preoperative period based on imaging characteristics.[20] Extracorporeal membrane oxygenation has also been associated with increased risk of stroke in neonates with or without CHD.[21,22] Both sepsis and meningitis have been linked to PAIS. Proposed mechanisms include release of inflammatory cytokines, endothelial damage, and stimulation of a prothrombotic state.[10] Hypoglycemia has also been associated with PAIS in preterm and term infants.[12,18]

Neonates and pregnant women have a naturally prothrombotic state, which likely contributes to the high risk of stroke in the perinatal period. The risk of maternal ischemic stroke during pregnancy is 34 times greater in the 2 days before delivery and 1 day after delivery than earlier in the pregnancy or outside of pregnancy.[23] Inherited and acquired thrombophilia in the neonate, mother, or both have been associated with increased risk of stroke in the neonate,[24] and the presence of more than one prothrombotic risk factor may further increase risk.[25] Specific conditions that have been linked to PAIS are factor V Leiden gene mutation, prothrombin gene mutation,[26] elevated lipoprotein (a), protein C deficiency, anticardiolipin antibodies,[27] lupus anticoagulant, beta-2-glycoprotein antibodies, protein S deficiency, methylenetetrahydrofolate reductase C677T homozygosity,[28] elevated homocysteine, and antithrombin III deficiency.[29,30] Polycythemia has also been described in PAIS.[31] Not only have prothrombotic abnormalities been reported in neonates with acute PAIS, but they have also been described in infants with PPAIS.[14]

Although few studies of PAIS have included placental pathology, the placenta is thought to be a common source for thromboembolism in PAIS. In the normal fetal circulation, blood clots from the fetal side of the placenta or umbilical vein can bypass the lungs and liver and travel directly to the brain via the patent foramen ovale. Placental infarction, vessel thrombosis, decreased placental reserve, thromboinflammatory changes including chorioamnionitis, and evidence of a sudden catastrophic event have been described in the placenta in cases of PAIS.[28,32]

Diagnosis and Additional Evaluation

Diagnosis of PAIS requires neuroimaging. PAIS is diagnosed when abnormal signal is detected in a region of the brain that conforms to a known arterial vascular territory. Although arterial ischemic stroke (AIS) may be detected by head ultrasound or computed tomography (CT), MRI of the brain is the gold-standard study for detection of PAIS due to its greater sensitivity, especially in the acute period.[33] MRI also avoids the risk of radiation exposure inherent in CT scans. Abnormal signal can be seen on conventional T1 and T2 sequences, but these changes may be subtle initially.[34] The diffusion-weighted imaging (DWI) sequence and derived apparent diffusion coefficient (ADC) map on MRI are particularly sensitive to acute ischemic injury. These sequences reflect the movement of water molecules. With acute ischemic injury, water molecules move from the extracellular space to the intracellular space, causing cytotoxic edema. The resulting restricted diffusion of water molecules in the extracellular space appears as abnormal signal intensity on the DWI sequence and ADC map, and this can be detected within hours of AIS. In neonates, abnormal signal persists on the DWI sequence and ADC map for about 7 days after AIS, which allows the timing of the stroke to be estimated.[35] After this time, pseudonormalization of the DWI sequence and ADC map occurs, so conventional T1 and T2 sequences must be used for diagnosis of stroke if imaging is obtained 1 to 2 weeks after stroke onset. After 14 days, facilitated diffusion is seen on the DWI sequence, and abnormal signal persists on DWI, ADC, T1, and T2 sequences as the subacute infarction evolves to a chronic infarction.[34,36] Typical changes on T2, DWI, and ADC sequences in acute PAIS are found in Figure 2-1. Gradient echo imaging and susceptibility-weighted sequences are sensitive to acute and chronic blood products and may provide additional information about mechanism of injury or comorbid conditions. In infants with PPAIS in whom the diagnosis is made after the first month of life, imaging studies show chronic infarction in an arterial territory (Figure 2-2). Additional information about the pathophysiology of PAIS can be obtained from vascular imaging. Although vascular imaging in PAIS has not been studied in a systematic way, arterial occlusion may be seen on magnetic resonance angiography (MRA) of the head, and arterial dissection has been reported on MRA of the neck.[8,37]

Once a diagnosis of acute PAIS is confirmed on neuroimaging, evaluation for risk factors is recommended (Table 2-2). This should include evaluation for sepsis, blood tests to evaluate for a prothrombotic state, echocardiogram and electrocardiogram to assess for cardiac abnormalities that could predispose to stroke, and placental pathology (if available). The normal levels of protein C, protein S, and antithrombin III are age dependent and are lower in the neonatal period than in later childhood or adulthood. Therefore, lab values must be interpreted using age-adjusted normative values. Levels may also be transiently low in the setting of thrombosis, so a pediatric hematologist should be consulted if any of the prothrombotic labs are abnormal.

Given that the majority of infants with PAIS have seizures as the initial symptom of stroke, and seizures may be the only symptom of stroke in this age group, accurate identification of seizures is extremely important. Recognition of seizures should prompt neuroimaging with brain MRI, leading to a diagnosis of PAIS. Clinical seizures may be subtle in neonates, and funny movements may be misidentified as seizures, leading to errors in classification. Even experienced observers have difficulty distinguishing neonatal seizures from nonictal movements.[38] Furthermore, the majority of seizures in neonates are subclinical, meaning that the abnormal electrical activity in the brain is not accompanied by any change in movement or behavior. In one study of electroencephalogram (EEG) features in term infants with acute PAIS, 78% of the seizures were electrographic without clinical signs.[39] Therefore, an EEG is required to diagnose most seizures in neonates.

An EEG measures electrical activity in the brain through electrodes placed on the scalp. The sensitivity and specificity of seizure detection depend on the number of electrodes placed, the duration of the recording, and the presence of video. A routine conventional EEG provides a snapshot of brain activity over a 20- to 30-minute period. Although seizures may be detected during this time, a longer study is recommended in order to increase the likelihood of detecting them. The standard montage (electrode arrangement) for a routine clinical EEG utilizes 19 recording electrodes, although a neonatal montage consisting of 9 recording electrodes is sometimes used. The gold-standard study for seizure detection is continuous conventional EEG with video. Continuous EEG monitoring increases the likelihood of capturing the spells that are thought to be seizures, and video monitoring allows the EEG reader to determine if a change in behavior has an electrographic correlate on the EEG consistent with a seizure. Simultaneous video recording also helps the EEG reader determine if a change in electrical activity is due to a change in brain activity or if it

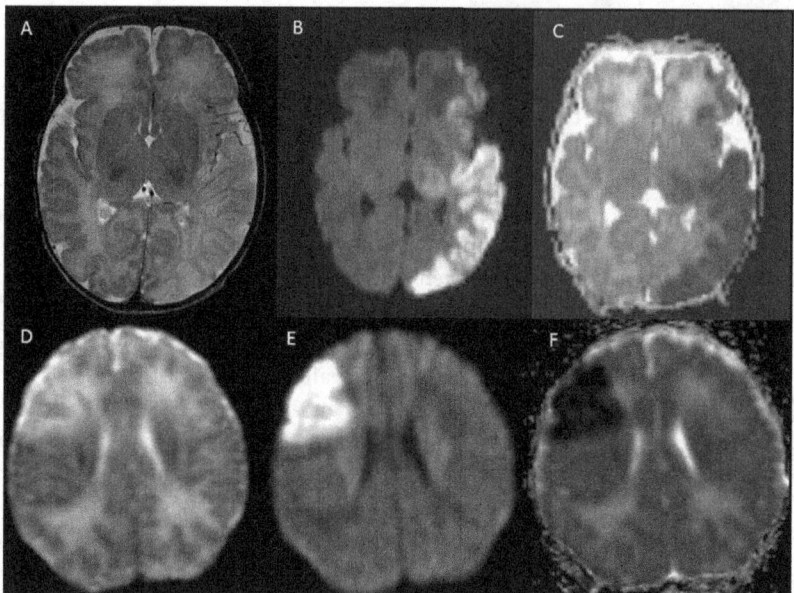

Figure 2-1. Representative axial images from brain MRI from 2 full-term neonates with acute perinatal AIS who presented with focal clonic seizures in the nursery. One neonate had acute left middle cerebral AIS (A-C), and the other neonate had acute right middle cerebral AIS. (A, D) T2-weighted imaging (B, E) Diffusion-weighted imaging (C, F) Apparent diffusion coefficient.

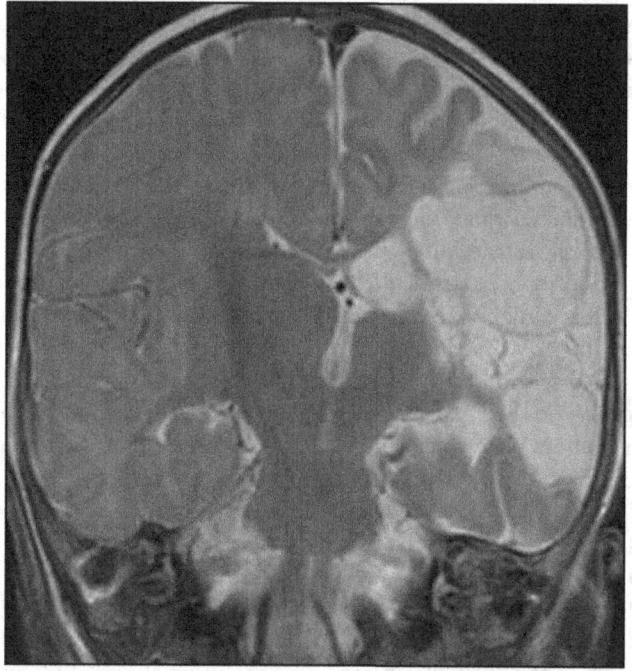

Figure 2-2. Representative coronal T2 image from brain MRI from a 4-month-old former full-term infant with early left hand preference and acquired microcephaly. Image demonstrates an area of chronic infarction in the territory of the left middle cerebral artery, consistent with presumed PAIS.

reflects electrical artifact from an external source (such as a nurse repositioning or patting the neonate). Although continuous video EEG monitoring allows for the most accurate detection of seizures, it requires specialized equipment and access to a trained EEG technologist to apply the electrodes and record the study, as well as a pediatric neurologist to interpret the study, making this cost prohibitive at many centers.

TABLE 2-2. SUGGESTED EVALUATION FOR NEONATES WITH ARTERIAL ISCHEMIC STROKE

NEUROIMAGING

- MRI brain including DWI and ADC
- MRA of head
- Consider MRA of neck

OTHER DIAGNOSTIC STUDIES

- Echocardiogram
- Electrocardiogram
- EEG, including continuous monitoring
- Consider venous ultrasound if right-to-left shunt is present

LABORATORY EVALUATION

- Glucose
- Complete blood count
- Blood cultures
- C-reactive protein

Thrombophilia

- Partial thromboplastin time	- Beta-2-glycoprotein antibodies
- International normalized ratio	- Lupus anticoagulant
- Protein C activity	- Lipoprotein (a)
- Protein S activity	- Homocysteine
- Antithrombin III activity	- Factor V Leiden gene mutation
- Anticardiolipin antibodies	- Prothrombin gene mutation

Cerebrospinal Fluid

- Cell count	- Protein
- Glucose	- Culture

MATERNAL STUDIES

- Placental pathology
- Consider evaluation for thrombophilia, as above

TREATMENT

In the acute period, treatment of PAIS is supportive. Cerebral perfusion can be optimized by maintaining adequate hydration. Efforts should be made to maintain normoglycemia, avoid hypoxemia and hyperthermia, and treat infections and seizures. Thrombolytic therapy with treatments such as tissue plasminogen activator is not recommended until information about safety and efficacy in neonates is available.[40] In adults this treatment has been approved for intravenous administration within 4.5 hours of stroke onset[41]; however, the precise time of stroke onset is rarely, if ever, known in neonates with acute PAIS, limiting

the potential use of this and other time-sensitive treatments. For example, therapeutic hypothermia appeared to be beneficial in a small number of neonates who were treated for neonatal encephalopathy and were later found to have PAIS.[42] In this study, none of the 5 infants with acute PAIS who received therapeutic hypothermia developed seizures compared to 7 of 10 infants with acute PAIS who did not receive therapeutic hypothermia and did have seizures. Unfortunately, the broader application of therapeutic hypothermia for acute PAIS is not likely to be feasible because this treatment must be instituted within 6 hours of injury to be effective. Neuroprotective treatments that exert beneficial effects for hours to days after stroke onset hold greater promise. For example, erythropoietin administration has been shown to preserve hemispheric volume in an animal model of neonatal stroke[43] and to be safe in neonates with PAIS.[44] Although no change in infarct volume or neurodevelopmental outcome was seen in the initial feasibility and safety study in humans, larger studies are planned to evaluate for efficacy.

In most cases of PAIS, secondary prevention with antithrombotic therapy is not required because the risk factors for stroke are unique to the perinatal period, making the chance of recurrent stroke low. In one series of children with PAIS, recurrent symptomatic arterial ischemic stroke occurred in just 4/215 during a median follow-up period of 3.5 years.[29] All of these children had risk factors for recurrent stroke, including moyamoya, CHD, and prothrombotic abnormalities. In selected cases of neonates with severe prothrombotic disorders, multiple systemic thrombi, or cardiac disease, treatment with anticoagulation or antiplatelet agents may be considered to decrease the risk of stroke recurrence.

Feeding difficulty is common in neonates with acute PAIS, so supplementation with nasogastric or orogastric tube feedings may be needed. Evaluation by a feeding therapist should be requested if feeding difficulties occur. A discussion of the evaluation of feeding in infants following stroke can be found in Chapter 8. Evaluation by an occupational or physical therapist during the acute hospitalization is also reasonable, although significant hemiparesis is not typically present in the neonatal period. Referral for ongoing outpatient therapy should occur at the time of hospital discharge. The duration and frequency of therapy should be guided by the infant's clinical status.

A detailed discussion of the evaluation of neuromotor function in infants and children following stroke can be found in Chapter 6, and a discussion of therapeutic interventions can be found in Chapter 7. Some of the most promising rehabilitation approaches, including constraint-induced movement therapy (CIMT), which leads to increased use of the hemiparetic arm by restraining the ipsilesional arm during functional tasks, and hand–arm bimanual training, which emphasizes bimanual tasks, have resulted in improved function in children with hemiplegic cerebral palsy.[45] These will be covered in Chapter 7. A recent randomized controlled trial of CIMT and repetitive transcranial magnetic stimulation (rTMS) for 2 weeks in children aged 6 to 19 years with hemiparesis due to perinatal stroke, the PLASTIC CHAMPS trial, confirmed that both treatments are well tolerated. Even more exciting, all treated children exhibited improved hand function 6 months after the intervention. The combination of CIMT and rTMS resulted in the greatest improvement, although significant improvement persisted at 6 months following treatment with either CIMT or rTMS.[46]

OUTCOME

The majority of children with PAIS develop persistent neurological deficits or epilepsy. In a review of cases of perinatal stroke published over a 30-year period, 40% were neurologically normal, 57% were neurologically or cognitively abnormal, and 3% had died.[10] In a population-based study of acute PAIS and PPAIS in term and preterm infants who were followed for at least 1 year (median follow-up of 41 months), 58% developed cerebral palsy, 39% developed epilepsy, 25% had a language delay, and 22% had behavioral abnormalities, including hyperactivity and poor attention.[47] All of these abnormalities were more common in children with PPAIS compared with those children who were diagnosed with stroke in the neonatal period. For example, 37% of children with acute stroke presentation in the first 28 days of life later developed cerebral palsy, whereas 82% of those with a delayed presentation (no symptoms in the neonatal period) were diagnosed with cerebral palsy. It is possible that the higher rate of deficits in children with a delayed presentation of PAIS reflects a detection bias because only children with deficits come to medical attention in that group, whereas children with acute symptoms of stroke in the neonatal period are identified before long-term deficits develop. Alternatively, differences in lesion location between these groups may account for the higher risk for motor deficits in children with presumed perinatal stroke (see later).

Motor and Sensory Deficits

Hemiparesis is the most common motor deficit to occur after PAIS, and stroke is the most common cause of hemiplegic cerebral palsy in children born at term.[48] Typically, a motor asymmetry first becomes apparent at 4 to 6 months when infants begin to reach for objects. A clear hand preference at this age raises strong concern for a structural lesion such as PAIS. Most children with PAIS walk independently even if hemiparesis is present, and the time to walking was not significantly delayed in children with unilateral injury.[49] However, in children with bilateral strokes, only two-thirds walked independently. Somatosensory deficits have not been studied much in children with PAIS, but proprioceptive deficits were noted frequently in a preliminary study using robots in children with PAIS.[50]

Several imaging features have been associated with an increased risk of motor deficit. In the population-based study by Lee et al[47] described earlier, predictors of hemiparesis included large stroke size, injury to Broca or Wernicke areas, internal capsule, or basal ganglia. Internal capsule injury was significantly more common in children with a

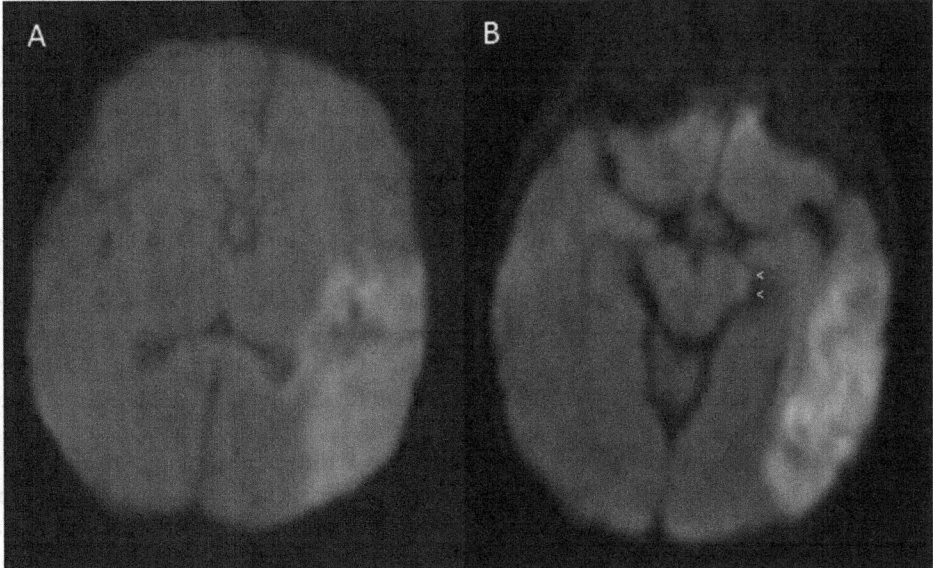

Figure 2-3. Representative axial DWI from a full-term neonate with acute perinatal left middle cerebral artery AIS who presented with focal clonic seizures in the nursery. (A) Area of cortical injury. (B) Area of cortical injury and area of restricted diffusion in the left cerebral peduncle (<). This indicates early Wallerian degeneration of the corticospinal tract and has been associated with increased risk of contralateral hemiparesis.

delayed diagnosis of stroke, occurring in 76% of children in that group, whereas internal capsule injury was seen in just 30% of children who were diagnosed with stroke in the neonatal period. Two single-center studies confirmed that a stroke involving motor cortex, internal capsule, and basal ganglia was highly associated with hemiparesis, with an odds ratio of 99 for the development of hemiparesis in the study by Boardman and colleagues.[51,52]

The presence of restricted diffusion in the descending corticospinal tract on acute neuroimaging predicts hemiparesis in infants with acute PAIS (Figure 2-3). In one study of term infants with acute PAIS, the presence of diffusion restriction at the level of the internal capsule was associated with a high likelihood of developing hemiparesis.[53] Moreover, follow-up MRI revealed Wallerian degeneration of the corticospinal tract when the acute study showed restricted diffusion. Another group of investigators sought to quantify the changes in the corticospinal tract on DWI that were associated with later hemiparesis. They found that the percentage of cerebral peduncle with abnormal DWI signal, as well as the length and the relative volume of descending corticospinal tract affected, was higher in children with poor motor outcome.[54] In another study diffusion tensor imaging, which allows for detailed analysis of white matter tracts, was performed at 3 months of age, and significant asymmetry in white matter integrity in the corticospinal tract had a positive predictive value of 100% for identifying unilateral motor deficits. This was in contrast to a positive predictive value of 86% for abnormal DWI signal in the ipsilesional cerebral peduncle on the acute scan obtained in the neonatal period.[55]

Cognitive and Behavioral Deficits

Cognitive and behavioral impairments are also common after PAIS. Following is an overview regarding the deficits that are typically seen. More information about the cognitive effects of PAIS can be found in Chapter 9 and the behavioral effects in Chapter 10. In the early years, children often show delays in motor and cognitive skills regardless of the hemisphere injured. In one study of infants with acute perinatal ischemic stroke who were assessed at 12 and 24 months with the Bayley Scales of Infant Development, the average Psychomotor Development Index was lower than the general population at 12 months, and both Mental and Psychomotor Development Indices were lower at 24 months.[56] In later childhood, average intelligence quotient (IQ) scores are generally lower than the population average though within the normal range following unilateral PAIS. In one study confined to children with unilateral perinatal ischemic stroke who were tested at school age, verbal IQ, performance IQ, and full-scale IQ scores fell within the lower end of the average range and were stable over time unless seizures were present. In children who experienced seizures outside the neonatal period, IQ scores primarily fell within the borderline range and were significantly lower compared to the children with stroke who had not experienced seizures after the first month of life. Performance on measures of academic achievement in children without seizures was in the low-average range for reading and spelling, whereas scores were in the average range for arithmetic. Performance was worse in all domains for children with seizures.[57] In another study of children with unilateral PAIS that excluded children with epilepsy, full-scale IQ, verbal IQ, and performance IQ fell within the normal range though were lower than the population mean.[58] In a small study of twin pairs who were discordant for PAIS in the MCA, IQ scores were significantly lower in the children with stroke. This suggests that when genetics and environment are comparable, an effect of PAIS on IQ can be detected. However, 3 of the 5 children with stroke had epilepsy, and 4 of the 5 had large strokes involving the complete MCA territory, so these factors likely contributed to the adverse cognitive outcomes.[59]

Although IQ is normal to low-normal in the majority of children following PAIS, detailed testing reveals more subtle deficits across most cognitive domains. Impaired function has been noted in language function, visuospatial processing, facial recognition, and emotional processing (for review, see Stiles et al[60]). Regarding language skills, mild delays in language acquisition are typical with good functional language by school age. However, impairments in language skills can be detected throughout childhood, especially on more complex tasks. In contrast to adults with stroke, language impairment occurs regardless of the specific hemisphere affected. As with global cognition, the presence of seizures adversely affects language function. Interestingly, in one study expressive language continued to improve in later childhood, suggesting that compensation continues for years after injury.[57] Functional neuroimaging studies have demonstrated more bilateral activation on language tasks following perinatal stroke compared with healthy controls and subjects who experienced stroke in later childhood or adulthood.[61]

Deficits in vision and visuospatial skills have been reported following PAIS, though these aspects of cognition have not been studied as much as language and global cognition.[50] In one small study of visual function at school age in children with PAIS, only 28% exhibited deficits. Two of 16 children had abnormal visual acuity, 2 had abnormal crowding acuity, 2 had weak stereopsis, and 2 had strabismus, with some children exhibiting impairment in more than one area. Only 2 children had a visual field deficit, and both of those children also had hemiparesis related to large MCA strokes involving the optic radiations.[62]

One important aspect of visuospatial attention is the ability to attend to both the big picture (global-level processing) and the details within a visual scene (local-level processing). In adults, the right temporal lobe is important for global-level processing, whereas the left temporal lobe is important for local-level processing. The effect of perinatal stroke on these skills shares some similarities, in that children with right hemisphere injury have more trouble reproducing the global organization of a complex figure than controls, and children with left hemisphere injury have more trouble reproducing the details within the figure. However, children with left hemisphere injury have trouble with both types of visuospatial processing when

compared to controls, even though local-level reproduction is relatively more affected.[60]

Another aspect of visuospatial attention is the ability to attend to information on both sides of the body. Visuospatial neglect, in which children attend less to visual stimuli in the contralesional hemifield in the absence of a primary visual defect, has been described in children following PAIS. This deficit has been noted following injury to cortical or subcortical areas, as well as the cerebellum, and neglect may occur following left or right brain injury (for review, see Smith & Chatterjee[63]). For example, when presented with a tray of toys, young children preferentially selected toys from ipsilesional space following perinatal brain injury to either hemisphere, consistent with mild neglect of the contralesional field.[64] In another study using 5 different tasks to assess for visuospatial neglect in children months to years following perinatal or childhood stroke, nearly half of the children showed neglect on at least one task. In contrast to adult studies in which neglect is more persistent and severe following right hemisphere injury, the presence of mild neglect did not differ between children with left or right brain injury.[65]

Visuospatial processing can also be separated into dorsal stream processes, which provide information about the location of an object in space (*where*), and ventral stream processes, which provide information about the identity of an object (*what*). In one study children with perinatal brain injury including PAIS exhibited deficits in both of these processes, though dorsal stream functions were only mildly impaired.[66] One common ventral stream process is face recognition, and in this study children with right hemisphere injury had impaired facial recognition, consistent with data from adults.

Deficits in global attentional processes have also been reported following perinatal stroke. In one study of children with either perinatal or childhood stroke, the majority had attention deficit hyperactivity disorder (ADHD) or ADHD traits. When lesion location was considered in the subset of subjects with smaller lesions, injury to the ventral putamen was more common in children with ADHD symptoms, though the association was not statistically significant.[67] Working memory and processing speed are also impaired following unilateral PAIS.[58]

Little has been published on outcome following PAIS in preterm infants. In one small study of 23 infants from a single center identified from neurology clinic records, patient referrals, and ICD-9 code searches, one child died in the neonatal intensive care unit and all of the surviving children had disabilities at follow-up. Specifically, 77% had cerebral palsy, 45% had epilepsy, and 77% had cognitive impairment. However, most of these children did not have isolated PAIS. Rather, the majority had multiple mechanisms of brain injury, including intraventricular hemorrhage in 55% and white matter injury in 55%, which likely contributed to the poor neurological outcome. Because this cohort was identified from neurology clinic charts and patient referrals, a referral bias also may have contributed to the presence of disability in all survivors. In another study of 31 preterm infants with PAIS identified from a prospectively studied hospital-based population, language problems were more common at 2 years of age compared to term infants.[68] In a recent imaging study of term and pre-term infants with large MCA ischemic stroke, the pattern of injury differed between and term and preterm infants. Specifically, 3/12 of the preterm infants had complete spar-ing of the cortex with underlying white matter injury, and 4/12 had partial cortical sparing, whereas only 1/28 full-term infants showed partial sparing of the cortex, and none of the term infants had complete sparing. This suggests that developmental differences in the vascular system likely exist when preterm infants are compared to term infants, resulting in a different pattern of injury.[69]

Epilepsy

Seizures are common at the time of acute PAIS. A smaller number of children with PAIS will go on to have recurrent seizures outside of the neonatal period. Some children may have a single seizure or seizures only with fever, whereas other children will have 2 or more unprovoked seizures, leading to a diagnosis of epilepsy and treatment with daily anticonvulsant medication. In one prospective study of 46 children with acute PAIS, just under 25% of children experienced a seizure outside of the neonatal period with a mean follow-up of 31.3 months.[70] The median age at the time of first seizure was 8 months. Of the 11 children who had a seizure, 3 had a single seizure with fever, and 2 had a single episode of unprovoked seizures. The other 6 children developed epilepsy. In this study, stroke size was significantly associated with the development of later seizures, with larger stroke size conferring more than a 6-fold higher risk of seizure outside of the neonatal period. When stroke size was dichotomized as small or large, only 11% of children with a small stroke had a seizure outside the neonatal period, whereas 45% of children with a large stroke had at least 1 seizure. In a population-based study of remote seizure following either acute or presumed perinatal AIS, 43% of children had one or more seizures with a median follow-up of 7.1 years, and 28% had active epilepsy at last follow-up.[71] When adjusted for duration of follow-up, the risk of remote seizure was 46% at 5 years and 54% at 10 years. In this study, a history of neonatal seizures was associated with 2 times greater risk of remote seizure and 2.6 times greater risk of active epilepsy. Of those with epilepsy, one-third were having monthly seizures despite treatment with anticonvulsant medication.

Health Status, Quality of Life, and Cost

As discussed, the majority of children with PAIS have long-term physical, cognitive, psychological, or medical conditions as a result of the stroke. Although most of the studies described thus far have focused on deficits noted by a health care provider or educator, less is known about how function is perceived by children and their families. In one recent study, children with perinatal and childhood stroke or hemorrhage and their parents rated the health status of the child using the Pediatric Quality of Life Inventory, a standardized instrument that asks how much of a prob-lem the child has had in a specific area for the last month. Almost half of the subjects had PAIS, with almost equal numbers presenting acutely or in a delayed fashion. Overall, children with stroke had worse reported health status than healthy controls. Factors associated with worse reported health status included degree of hemiparesis, epilepsy, and lower IQ, although children and parents did not always agree on how the stroke affected the child.[72]

Another line of research has evaluated how parents are affected by raising a child with PAIS. In one study both mothers and fathers reported more depressive symptoms and poorer marital satisfaction, quality of life, and family functioning when their children had moderate to severe deficits. Mothers expressed more guilt and higher levels of anxiety than fathers. However, the parents of children with PAIS who had normal neurological function or mild impairments reported feelings comparable to controls.[73] For further discussion on the impact of PAIS on the family, see Chapter 11.

In addition to the physical and emotional toll of PAIS, the financial cost is significant. In one study of PAIS and hemorrhagic stroke, the adjusted 5-year cost was $51,719. Although the majority of this cost was incurred during the initial hospitalizations, even in the fifth year after stroke the annual cost continued to exceed control costs by nearly $2000/year.[74] This study only looked at direct costs captured by the managed health plan. Given that the majority of children with PAIS have lasting motor and/or cognitive impairment, the direct costs of ongoing medical care and academic services, as well as indirect costs related to lost productivity, are likely high. Thus, PAIS results in a long-term financial burden to families and society.

FAMILY FOCUS BOX

1. Neonatal AIS affects 1/4000 infants. This type of stroke occurs when a blood clot in an artery prevents part of the brain from receiving adequate blood flow, resulting in permanent brain injury. In newborns, common symptoms at the time of stroke include seizures, lethargy, poor feeding, low muscle tone, and breathing difficulties. Some newborns have no symptoms at the time of the stroke, but may be diagnosed with a stroke at a later age when they develop symptoms that prompt imaging of the brain.

2. Brain MRI is the test that is most sensitive for detecting a stroke. The risk of stroke is higher in children with CHD or a tendency to form blood clots easily, so blood tests and an echocardiogram (ultrasound of the heart) may be done to look for these problems. Abnormalities of the placenta also increase stroke risk. However, in most newborns with stroke, a specific cause is not found. The risk of recurrent stroke is very low, so typically no medication is needed to prevent another stroke.

3. Children who experienced a stroke in the newborn period are at risk for motor, language, and cognitive delays; weakness and stiffness (affecting the side of the body opposite the side of the stroke); seizures; learning disabilities; and ADHD. However, average intelligence remains within the normal range, and most children walk independently following a stroke in the newborn period.

4. Physical, occupational, speech and therapy, feeding, and/or developmental therapy may be recommended following a stroke in the newborn period. Some children will require special education or accommodations in school; however, some children have no lasting difficulties from the stroke.

CASE STUDY

Baby Boy (BB) was born at 39 weeks to a 33-year-old woman with history of infertility. Conception occurred via intrauterine insemination. This was her first pregnancy and it was unremarkable. She developed a fever prior to delivery and was treated with antibiotics. BB was born via spontaneous vaginal delivery. Apgars were 7 and 9, and birth weight was 3.3 kg. At 24 hours of life, BB developed focal clonic movements of the right arm and leg. EEG confirmed that these were seizures, and he was treated with phenobarbital. MRI of the brain revealed an acute AIS in the left middle cerebral artery territory. Blood, urine, and cerebrospinal fluid (CSF) cultures did not reveal an organism, and CSF cell count, glucose, and protein were normal. Clinical seizures resolved, but BB continued to have electrographic seizures for another 24 hours, requiring additional doses of phenobarbital. Placental pathology demonstrated acute chorioamnionitis. Echocardiogram was normal. Prothrombotic laboratory tests were significant for a heterozygous mutation in the factor V Leiden gene. BB had a normal neurological exam in the nursery and was nursing well by day of life 5. He had no further seizures and was discharged home on phenobarbital on day of life 7.

EEG at 3 months-of-age showed no epileptiform discharges, and BB was tapered off phenobarbital without seizure recurrence. At 4 months-of-age, parents reported that BB was reaching with his left hand but not with his right, and he tended to keep his right arm flexed with his hand in a fisted posture. BB began receiving occupational and physical therapy through his local early intervention program. By 12 months-of-age, BB was diagnosed with right hemiplegic cerebral palsy. He began walking at 14 months. He had mild expressive and receptive speech delay and began receiving speech therapy services at age 2 years. He was discharged from speech therapy prior to kindergarten, and he entered a typical kindergarten class with ongoing school-based occupational therapy. In first grade, BB was noted to have significant difficulty paying attention in class, and he was diagnosed with ADHD.

SUMMARY

PAIS affects nearly 1 in 4000 term and near-term infants, making this condition as common as large vessel ischemic stroke in adults. Numerous risk factors for PAIS have been identified, but physiological factors unique to the perinatal period help account for the high risk of stroke in this population. Diagnosis requires a high index of suspicion and should be considered in neonates with seizures and older infants with early hand preference or other signs of hemiparesis. Neuroimaging is required to confirm a diagnosis of PAIS, and brain MRI is the most sensitive study for diagnosis of PAIS, especially in the acute period. Although initial treatment is supportive, rehabilitation therapies play a large role in facilitating functional improvement throughout childhood. The majority of children with PAIS have long-term motor, cognitive, or behavioral deficits or epilepsy, so there is a great opportunity to improve outcome with rehabilitative and educational interventions.

REFERENCES

1. Nelson KB. Perinatal ischemic stroke. *Stroke.* 2007;38(2 Suppl): 742-745.

2. Darmency-Stamboul V, Chantegret C, Ferdynus C, et al. Antenatal factors associated with perinatal arterial ischemic stroke. *Stroke.* 2012;43(9):2307-2312.

3. Grunt S, Mazenauer L, Buerki SE, et al. Incidence and outcomes of symptomatic neonatal arterial ischemic stroke. *Pediatrics.* 2015;135(5):e1220-e1228.

4. Lee J, Croen LA, Backstrand KH, et al. Maternal and infant characteristics associated with perinatal arterial stroke in the infant. *JAMA.* 2005;293(6):723-729.

5. Schulzke S, Weber P, Luetschg J, et al. Incidence and diagnosis of unilateral arterial cerebral infarction in newborn infants. *J Perinat Med.* 2005;33(2):170-175.

6. Schneider AT, Kissela B, Woo D, et al. Ischemic stroke subtypes: a population-based study of incidence rates among Blacks and Whites. *Stroke.* 2004;35(7):1552-1556.

7. Wu YW, Lindan CE, Henning LH, et al. Neuroimaging abnormalities in infants with congenital hemiparesis. *Pediatr Neurol.* 2006;35(3):191-196.

8. Kirton A, Armstrong-Wells J, Chang T, et al. Symptomatic neonatal arterial ischemic stroke: the International Pediatric Stroke Study. *Pediatrics.* 2011;128(6):e1402-e1410.

9. Estan J, Hope P. Unilateral neonatal cerebral infarction in full term infants. *Arch Dis Child Fetal Neonatal Ed.* 1997;76(2): F88-F93.

10. Lynch JK, Nelson KB. Epidemiology of perinatal stroke. *Curr Opin Pediatr.* 2001;13(6):499-505.

11. Golomb MR, Garg BP, Saha C, Azzouz F, Williams LS. Cerebral palsy after perinatal arterial ischemic stroke. *J Child Neuro.* 2008;23(3):279-286.

12. Benders MJ, Groenendaal F, Uiterwaal C, et al. Maternal and infant characteristics associated with perinatal arterial stroke in the preterm infant. *Stroke.* 2007;38(6):1759-1765.

13. Kirton A, Shroff M, Pontigon AM, et al. Risk factors and presentations of periventricular venous infarction vs arterial presumed perinatal ischemic stroke. *Arch Neurol.* 2010;67(7):842-848.

14. Golomb MR, MacGregor DL, Domi T, et al. Presumed pre- or perinatal arterial ischemic stroke: risk factors and outcomes. *Ann Neurol.* 2001;50(2):163-168.

15. Ozduman K, Pober BR, Barnes P, et al. Fetal stroke. *Pediatr Neurol.* 2004;30(3):151-162.

16. Wu YW, March WM, Croen LA, Grether JK, Escobar GJ, Newman TB. Perinatal stroke in children with motor impairment: a population-based study. *Pediatrics.* 2004;114(3):612-619.

17. Heier LA, Carpanzano CR, Mast J, Brill PW, Winchester P, Deck MD. Maternal cocaine abuse: the spectrum of radiologic abnormalities in the neonatal CNS. *AJNR Am J Neuroradiol.* 1991;12(5):951-956.

18. Harteman JC, Groenendaal F, Kwee A, Welsing PMJ, Benders MJ, de Vries L. Risk factors for perinatal arterial ischaemic stroke in full-term infants: a case-control study. *Arch Dis Child Fetal Neonatal Ed.* 2012;97(6):F411-F416.

19. Asakai H, Cardamone M, Hutchinson D, et al. Arterial ischemic stroke in children with cardiac disease. *Neurology.* 2015;85(23):2053-2059.

20. Chen J, Zimmerman RA, Jarvik GP, et al. Perioperative stroke in infants undergoing open heart operations for congenital heart disease. *Ann Thorac Surg.* 2009;88(3):823-829.

21. Werho DK, Pasquali SK, Yu S, et al. Epidemiology of stroke in pediatric cardiac surgical patients supported with extracorporeal membrane oxygenation. *Ann Thorac Surg.* 2015;100(5):1751-1757.

22. Raets MM, Dudink J, IJsselstijn H, et al. Brain injury associated with neonatal extracorporeal membrane oxygenation in the Netherlands: a nationwide evaluation spanning two decades. *Pediatr Crit Care Med.* 2013;14(9):884-892.

23. Salonen Ros H, Lichtenstein P, Bellocco R, Petersson G, Cnattingius S. Increased risks of circulatory diseases in late pregnancy and puerperium. *Epidemiology.* 2001;12(4):456-460.

24. Simchen MJ, Goldstein G, Lubetsky A, Strauss T, Schiff E, Kenet G. Factor V Leiden and antiphospholipid antibodies in either mothers or infants increase the risk for perinatal arterial ischemic stroke. *Stroke.* 2009;40(1):65-70.

25. Grabowski EF, Buonanno FS, Krishnamoorthy K. Prothrombotic risk factors in the evaluation and management of perinatal stroke. *Semin Perinatol.* 2007;31(4):243-249.

26. Kenet G, Lütkhoff LK, Albisetti M, et al. Impact of thrombophilia on risk of arterial ischemic stroke or cerebral sinovenous thrombosis in neonates and children: a systematic review and meta-analysis of observational studies. *Circulation.* 2010;121(16): 1838-1847.

27. Günther G, Junker R, Sträter R, et al; Childhood Stroke Study Group. Symptomatic ischemic stroke in full-term neonates: role of acquired and genetic prothrombotic risk factors. *Stroke.* 2000;31(10):2437-2441.

28. Curry CJ, Bhullar S, Holmes J, Delozier CD, Roeder ER, Hutchison HT. Risk factors for perinatal arterial stroke: a study of 60 mother-child pairs. *Pediatr Neurol.* 2007;37(2):99-107.

29. Kurnik K, Kosch A, Sträter R, Schobess R, Heller C, Nowak-Göttl U; Childhood Stroke Study Group. Recurrent thromboembolism in infants and children suffering from symptomatic neonatal arterial stroke: a prospective follow-up study. *Stroke.* 2003;34(12):2887-2892.

30. deVeber G, Monagle P, Chan A, et al. Prothrombotic disorders in infants and children with cerebral thromboembolism. *Arch Neurol.* 1998;55(12):1539-1543.

31. Amit M, Camfield PR. Neonatal polycythemia causing multiple cerebral infarcts. *Arch Neurol.* 1980;37(2):109-110.

32. Elbers J, Viero S, MacGregor D, deVeber G, Moore AM. Placental pathology in neonatal stroke. *Pediatrics.* 2011;127(3):e722-e729.

33. Cowan F, Mercuri E, Groenendaal F, et al. Does cranial ultrasound imaging identify arterial cerebral infarction in term neonates? *Arch Dis Child Fetal Neonatal Ed.* 2005;90(3):F252-F256.

34. Dudink J, Mercuri E, Al-Nakib L, et al. Evolution of unilateral perinatal arterial ischemic stroke on conventional and diffusion-weighted MR imaging. *AJNR Am J Neuroradiol.* 2009;30(5):998-1004.

35. van der Aa NE, Benders M, Vincken KL, Groenendaal F, de Vries LS. The course of apparent diffusion coefficient values following perinatal arterial ischemic stroke. *PLoS One.* 2013;8(2):e56784.

36. Küker W, Möhrle S, Mader I, Schöning M, Nägele T. MRI for the management of neonatal cerebral infarctions: importance of timing. *Childs Nerv Syst.* 2004;20(10):742-748.

37. Lequin MH, Peeters EAJ, Holscher HC, de Krijger R, Govaert P. Arterial infarction caused by carotid artery dissection in the neonate. *Eur J Paediatr Neurol.* 2004;8(3):155-160.

38. Murray DM, Boylan GB, Ali I, Ryan CA, Murphy BP, Connolly S. Defining the gap between electrographic seizure burden, clinical expression and staff recognition of neonatal seizures. *Arch Dis Child Fetal Neonatal Ed.* 2008;93(3):F187-F191.

39. Low E, Mathieson SR, Stevenson NJ, et al. Early postnatal EEG features of perinatal arterial ischaemic stroke with seizures. *PLoS One.* 2014;9(7):e100973.

40. Roach ES, Golomb MR, Adams R, et al. Management of stroke in infants and children: a scientific statement from a Special Writing Group of the American Heart Association Stroke Council and the Council on Cardiovascular Disease in the Young. *Stroke*. 2008;39(9):2644-2691.

41. Del Zoppo GJ, Saver JL, Jauch EC, Adams HP; American Heart Association Stroke Council. Expansion of the time window for treatment of acute ischemic stroke with intravenous tissue plasminogen activator: a science advisory from the American Heart Association/American Stroke Association. *Stroke*. 2009;40(8):2945-2948.

42. Harbert MJ, Tam EWY, Glass HC, et al. Hypothermia is correlated with seizure absence in perinatal stroke. *J Child Neurol*. 2011;26(9):1126-1130.

43. Chang YS, Mu D, Wendland M, et al. Erythropoietin improves functional and histological outcome in neonatal stroke. *Pediatr Res*. 2005;58(1):106-111.

44. Benders MJ, van der Aa NE, Roks M, et al. Feasibility and safety of erythropoietin for neuroprotection after perinatal arterial ischemic stroke. *J Pediatr*. 2014;164(3):481-486.

45. de Brito Brandao M, Gordon AM, Mancini MC. Functional impact of constraint therapy and bimanual training in children with cerebral palsy: a randomized controlled trial. *Am J Occup Ther*. 2012;66(6):672-681.

46. Kirton A, Anderson J, Herrero M, et al. Brain stimulation and constraint for perinatal stroke hemiparesis: The PLASTIC CHAMPS Trial. *Neurology*. 2016;86(18):1659-1667.

47. Lee J, Croen LA, Lindan C, et al. Predictors of outcome in perinatal arterial stroke: a population-based study. *Ann Neurol*. 2005;58(2):303-308.

48. Wu YW, Escobar GJ, Grether JK, et al. Chorioamnionitis and cerebral palsy in term and near-term infants. *JAMA*. 2003;290(20):2677-2684.

49. Golomb MR, deVeber GA, MacGregor DL, et al. Independent walking after neonatal arterial ischemic stroke and sinovenous thrombosis. *J Child Neurol*. 2003;18(8):530-536.

50. Kirton A, Deveber G. Life after perinatal stroke. *Stroke*. 2013;44(11):3265-3271.

51. Boardman JP, Ganesan V, Rutherford MA, Saunders DE, Mecuri E, Cowan F. Magnetic resonance image correlates of hemiparesis after neonatal and childhood middle cerebral artery stroke. *Pediatrics*. 2005;115(2):321-326.

52. Mercuri E, Barnett A, Rutherford M, et al. Neonatal cerebral infarction and neuromotor outcome at school age. *Pediatrics*. 2004;113(1):95-100.

53. de Vries LS, Van der Grond J, Van Haastert IC, Groenendaal F. Prediction of outcome in new-born infants with arterial ischaemic stroke using diffusion-weighted magnetic resonance imaging. *Neuropediatrics*. 2005;36(1):12-20.

54. Kirton A, Shroff M, Visvanathan T, deVeber G. Quantified corticospinal tract diffusion restriction predicts neonatal stroke outcome. *Stroke*. 2007;38(3):974-980.

55. van der Aa NE, Leemans A, Northington FJ, et al. Does diffusion tensor imaging-based tractography at 3 months of age contribute to the prediction of motor outcome after perinatal arterial ischemic stroke? *Stroke*. 2011;42(12):3410-3414.

56. McLinden A, Baird AD, Westmacott R, Anderson PE, deVeber G. Early cognitive outcome after neonatal stroke. *J Child Neurol*. 2007;22(9):1111-1116.

57. Ballantyne AO, Spilkin AM, Hesselink J, Trauner DA. Plasticity in the developing brain: intellectual, language and academic functions in children with ischaemic perinatal stroke. *Brain*. 2008;131(11):2975-2985.

58. Westmacott R, Askalan R, MacGregor D, Anderson P, deVeber G. Cognitive outcome following unilateral arterial ischaemic stroke in childhood: effects of age at stroke and lesion location. *Dev Med Child Neurol*. 2010;52(4):386-393.

59. Talib TL, Pongonis SJ, Williams LS, et al. Neuropsychologic outcomes in a case series of twins discordant for perinatal stroke. *Pediatr Neurol*. 2008;38(2):118-125.

60. Stiles J, Reilly J, Paul B, Moses P. Cognitive development following early brain injury: evidence for neural adaptation. *Trends Cogn Sci*. 2005;9(3):136-143.

61. Szaflarski JP, Allendorfer JB, Byars AW, et al. Age at stroke determines post-stroke language lateralization. *Restor Neurol Neurosci*. 2014;32(6):733-742.

62. Mercuri E, Anker S, Guzzetta A, et al. Neonatal cerebral infarction and visual function at school age. *Arch Dis Child Fetal Neonatal Ed*. 2003;89(2):F487-F491.

63. Smith SE, Chatterjee A. Visuospatial attention in children. *Arch Neurol*. 2008;65(10):1284-1288.

64. Trauner DA. Hemispatial neglect in young children with early unilateral brain damage. *Dev Med Child Neurol*. 2003;45(3):160-166.

65. Smith SE, Bloom JS, Minniti N. Cerebrovascular disease and disorders. In: Armstrong CLE, Morrow LAE, eds. *Handbook of Medical Neuropsychology*. New York, NY: Springer Verlag; 2010:101-121.

66. Paul B, Appelbaum M, Carapetian S, et al. Face and location processing in children with early unilateral brain injury. *Brain Cogn*. 2014;88:6-13.

67. Max JE, Fox PT, Lancaster JL, et al. Putamen lesions and the development of attention-deficit/hyperactivity symptomatology. *J Am Acad Child Adolesc Psychiatry*. 2002;41(5):563-571.

68. Benders MJ, Groenendaal F, De Vries LS. Preterm arterial ischemic stroke. *Semin Fetal Neonatal Med*. 2009;14(5):272-277.

69. van der Aa NE, Benders M, Nikkels PG, Groenendaal F, deVries LS. Cortical sparing in preterm ischemic arterial stroke. *Stroke*. 2016;47(3):869-871.

70. Wusthoff CJ, Kilaru Kessler S, Vossough A, et al. Risk of later seizure after perinatal arterial ischemic stroke: a prospective cohort study. *Pediatrics*. 2011;127(6):e1550-e1557.

71. Fox CK, Glass HC, Sidney S, Smith SE, Fullerton HJ. Neonatal seizures triple the risk of a remote seizure after perinatal ischemic stroke. *Neurology*. 2016;86(23):2179-2186.

72. Smith SE, Vargas G, Cucchiara AJ, Zelonis SJ, Beslow LA. Hemiparesis and epilepsy are associated with worse reported health status following unilateral stroke in children. *Pediatr Neurol*. 2015;52(4):428-434.

73. Bemister TB, Brooks BL, Dyck RH, Kirton A. Parent and family impact of raising a child with perinatal stroke. *BMC Pediatr*. 2014;14:182.

74. Gardner MA, Hills NK, Sidney S, Johnston SC, Fullerton HJ. The 5-year direct medical cost of neonatal and childhood stroke in a population-based cohort. *Neurology*. 2010;74(5):372-378.

SUGGESTED READINGS

Kenet G, Lütkhof LK, Albisetti M, et al. Impact of thrombophilia on risk of arterial ischemic stroke or cerebral sinovenous thrombosis in neonates and children: a systematic review and meta-analysis of observational studies. *Circulation*. 2010;121(16):1838-1847.

Kirton A, Deveber G. Life after perinatal stroke. *Stroke*. 2013;44(11):3265-3271.

Lee J, Croen LA, Backstrang KH, et al. Maternal and infant character-istics associated with perinatal arterial stroke in the infant. *JAMA.* 2005;293(6):723-729.

Lee J, Croen LA, Lindan C, et al. Predictors of outcome in peri-natal arterial stroke: a population-based study. *Ann Neurol.* 2005;58(2):303-308.

Roach ES, Golomb MR, Adams R, et al. Management of stroke in infants and children: a scientific statement from a Special Writing Group of the American Heart Association Stroke Council and the Council on Cardiovascular Disease in the Young. *Stroke.* 2008;39(9):2644-2691.

Wusthoff CJ, Kessler SK, Vossough A, et al. Risk of later seizure after perinatal arterial ischemic stroke: a prospective cohort study. *Pediatrics.* 2011;127(6):e1550-e1557.

Cerebral Sinovenous Thrombosis in Children

Mubeen F. Rafay, MB.BS, FCPS, MSc

Cerebral sinovenous thrombosis (CSVT) is both increasingly recognized and diagnosed, partly due to increased awareness and mainly due to advancements and improvements in neuroimaging techniques in children. As in adults, the childhood CSVT can occur with or without the presence of ischemic or hemorrhagic stroke. The objective demonstration of a clot in cortical vein(s) or dural venous sinus(es) is required for a confirmation of the diagnosis of CSVT. The thrombosis may involve the superficial venous system, the deep venous system, or both deep and superficial venous systems. In children, the small caliber of veins and venous sinuses can pose challenges in obtaining optimal vascular imaging.

Based on age, CSVT is defined as neonatal CSVT (occurring between 0 and 28 postnatal days of life) or childhood, or non-neonatal, CSVT (occurring over 28 days and up to 18 years of life). Across studies, neonatal CSVT represents 25% to 43% of all childhood CSVT cases.[1-3] Recent literature suggests that in some infants and young children, based on the patterns of ischemic infarction, it can be presumed that the incident event may have occurred remotely, either pre- or perinatally.[4] The clinical presentation varies based on the age of the child, location of venous thrombosis, degree of parenchymal involvement, and development of increased intracranial pressure. The mechanisms and etiologies responsible for the causation of CSVT in children are many. The absolute lack of randomized controlled trials and presence of controversial treatment approaches across pediatric patient populations and across countries has made management of these children quite challenging. The outcomes are significant, including death and disability in a significant proportion of children.[5] The following sections will discuss each of these topics in detail.

ANATOMY AND PATHOPHYSIOLOGY OF THE DURAL VENOUS SYSTEM

The dural venous system is the venous drainage system of the brain. It is composed of the superficial and deep cortical veins and the large venous channels or venous sinuses within the dural layers. The dural venous system drains by receiving blood from the cerebral cortical veins and by absorbing the cerebrospinal fluid (CSF) via the arachnoid granulations.

The cerebral dural venous system is categorized into two major subsystems: the superficial venous system (superficial cortical veins, the superior sagittal sinus, and the lateral or transverse sinus) and the deep venous system (the internal cerebral veins, the straight sinus, and the vein of Galen) within the subarachnoid space (Figure 3-1). The small protrusions of the arachnoid matter, called *arachnoid granulations* or *villi*, protrude into these venous channels allowing absorption and drainage of CSF into the bloodstream. These dural venous channels then lead the drainage of blood into the major cervical outflow tracts, namely internal jugular veins and the extrajugular venous collaterals. The presence of thrombus or flow interruption within any of the previously mentioned dural venous channels will lead to outflow obstruction or inadequate drainage, in turn leading to venous congestion in the affected

Atkinson HL, Nixon-Cave K, Smith SE, eds.
*Pediatric Stroke Rehabilitation: An Interprofessional and
Collaborative Approach* (pp 35-57).© 2018 Taylor & Francis Group.

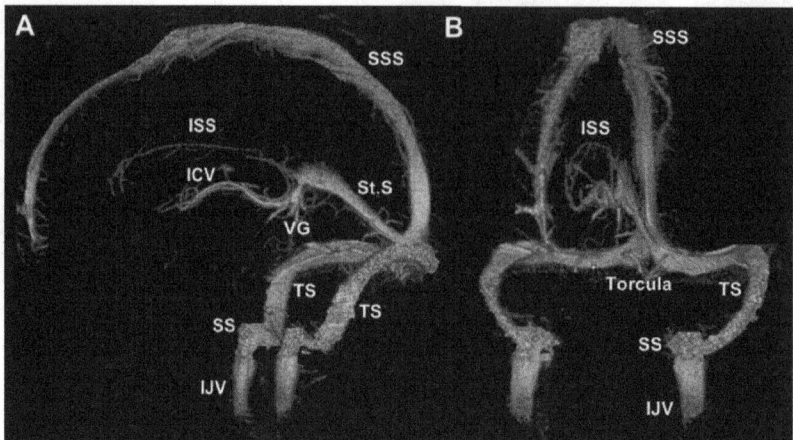

Figure 3-1. Cerebral dural venous sinus anatomy. (A) Lateral view. (B) Anteroposterior view. SSS: superior sagittal sinus; ISS: inferior sagittal sinus; St.S: straight sinus; SS: sigmoid sinus; TS: transverse sinus; ICV: internal cerebral vein; VG: vein of Galen; IJV: internal jugular vein

brain region and increase in CSF pressure. This then leads to extravasation of fluid into the affected regions, causing cerebral edema, venous congestion, intraventricular, intraparenchymal and extraparenchymal hemorrhage, or focal ischemic or hemorrhagic infarction. A vicious circle is then established because the already inadequate flow and increased pressure caused by the initial thrombosis in the venous system contributes to further propagation of the thrombosis, leading to further brain damage, unless the adequacy of the venous drainage is reestablished.

Incidence Estimates of Childhood Cerebral Sinovenous Thrombosis

In comparison to arterial ischemic stroke (AIS), CSVT is an uncommon form of stroke, representing 0.5% to 3% of all strokes. In adults, the incidence of CSVT is limited and is estimated to be 5 to 12.3 people/million annually.[6] As in adults, the incidence of CSVT is not well reported in children, and the data are limited to a few cohort studies and stroke registries. Based on these studies, the annual incidence of CSVT is estimated to be 0.25 to 0.67/100,000 children/year. For neonates with CSVT, data are also limited, and an annual incidence anywhere from 2.6 to 40.7/100,000 live births/year has been estimated (Table 3-1).[2,7-12] Interestingly, an 11-year study (1991-2001) of Chinese Hong Kong children with stroke reported an annual incidence for both ischemic and hemorrhagic stroke as 2.1/100,000 children/year, but noted no cases of CSVT in children. In this registry, neonates and children between the ages of 16 and 18 years were not included, and case ascertainment was based on the discharge diagnosis utilizing a centralized computerized database of only public

hospitals in Hong Kong. This approach may have missed children with CSVT, especially children without stroke and children seen at nonpublic or private hospitals.[13] The incidence of CSVT in children is likely underreported because many patients may be misdiagnosed or remain undiagnosed due to the nonspecific nature of its clinical presentation, challenges with availability and feasibility of appropriate vascular imaging techniques, inadequate visualization of sinovenous channels in young children, and known potential for spontaneous resolution of sinovenous thrombosis before detection in some patients.

Across studies, in children with CSVT neurological sequelae are reported in over 60% of survivors and death in 3% to 12%.[9-12,14] The extent of neurological impairment and mortality is largely dependent on the localization and severity of thrombosis and brain parenchymal involvement. The Canadian Pediatric Ischemic Stroke Registry (CPISR) studied 160 Canadian children, newborn to 18 years of age, with clinical symptoms and confirmed diagnosis of CSVT and noted that over 40% of CSVT cases occurred during the neonatal period, and over 55% presented without ischemic infarction and 28% with hemorrhage.[2] Recently, the largest multicenter cohort study among children with ischemic stroke, the International Pediatric Stroke Study (IPSS), enrolled 1187 ischemic stroke cases between 2003 and 2007 and reported isolated CSVT in 246 (14%) patients (162 with non-neonatal CSVT and 84 with neonatal CSVT). With childhood CSVT, they noted a male predominance of 60%, involvement of superficial venous system in 56%, both deep and superficial venous system in 24%, ischemic venous infarction in 37%, and intracranial hemorrhage in 31% of their cases. In neonates with CSVT, the IPSS reported involvement of the deep venous system in 21%, ischemic venous infarction in 6%, hemorrhagic infarction or other intracranial hemorrhage in 15%, and both infarction and hemorrhage in 31%.[15]

STUDIES	DURATION OF STUDY	ANNUAL INCIDENCE OF CHILDHOOD CEREBRAL SINOVENOUS THROMBOSIS*	ANNUAL INCIDENCE OF NEONATAL CEREBRAL SINOVENOUS THROMBOSIS†	TOTAL ISCHEMIC STROKE CASES WITH OR WITHOUT HEMORRHAGE	CEREBRAL SINOVENOUS THROMBOSIS CASES	ARTERIAL ISCHEMIC STROKE CASES
Canadian[2]	1992-1997	0.67	40.7	160	160	0.0
Hong Kong[13]	1991-2001	0.0	NI	50	0.0	36
Germany[7]	1995-2002	0.35	2.6	149	149	0.0
Australia[8]	1995-2001	0.34	0	NI	16	NI
Denmark[11]	1994-2006	0.25	10.7	251	40	211
Switzerland[9]	2000-2008	0.55	0.034	65	65	0.0

NI: Not included, *Cases/100,000 children population/year, † Cases/100,000 live births/year.

CLINICAL PRESENTATION

In children, the clinical presentation of CSVT is largely dependent on the age of the child, the severity and type of brain parenchymal involvement, and the increase in the intracranial pressure, which is in turn dependent on the location of the thrombus and the resultant impairment of venous drainage (either localized or diffuse). Often at the time of initial presentation, patients show clinical findings pertaining to both parenchymal involvement and the raised intracranial pressure. Clinical features characteristic of CSVT in both adults and children include headache, altered consciousness, seizures, and diffuse or focal neurologic deficits. Most of the clinical features are noted at presentation, but some may develop over the course of the illness, especially with progressive parenchymal involvement and propagation of sinovenous thrombosis. In addition, although some symptoms tend to occur at a young age and some in older children, none of the clinical features reported with CSVT are unique at any age.

As in adults, older children with CSVT present with diffuse symptoms and signs attributable to the increased intracranial pressure. These symptoms include headache, papilledema, visual impairment (often diplopia), cranial nerve palsies (commonly sixth nerve palsy), lethargy, and balance difficulties. Based on localized brain parenchymal involvement (due to infarction or hemorrhage), focal motor deficits and other cranial nerve palsies are also frequently reported. Seizures are noted, but not as commonly as in infants with CSVT. Compared with older children with CSVT, neonates and infants with CSVT more often present with seizures (50% to 70%) and diffuse and nonspecific signs (40% to 60%), including poor feeding, irritability/jitteriness, and alteration in consciousness. Focal neurological deficits are less frequently noted at this young age, mainly due to

inability to report symptoms and difficulty in recognizing these deficits in an irritable young child.[2,3,7,10,16-20]

Headache in CSVT is often abrupt onset and described as diffuse and progressive in severity. Older children report a variety of headache types, including migraine-type headache, dull constant pain, and the thunderclap headache (indicative of a subarachnoid hemorrhage) with poor response to analgesic medications. Headache occurs often in association with signs of increased intracranial pressure. However, isolated nonspecific headache without any focal neurological findings or papilledema is not uncommon. In children who present with the typical symptoms of increased intracranial hypertension (consisting of headache, papilledema, and/or diplopia caused by sixth nerve palsy), even without focal neurological signs, the diagnosis of CSVT should be considered and ruled out.

Seizures in CSVT can be seen at presentation or during the course of the illness, and are typically focal or generalized seizures. In childhood CSVT, focal seizures are commonly noted in neonates and with focal parenchymal brain injury.[2] The diffuse symptoms and signs (poor feeding, lethargy, and fever) noted in a significant proportion of children with CSVT are quite concerning for the treating physician. In the absence of focal neurological deficits, these diffuse symptoms are typically attributed to an infection or systemic illness, often resulting in a missed diagnosis of CSVT in children. It is important to note that infection or acute systemic illnesses are major players in increasing the risk of CSVT and therefore must always be considered with such childhood presentations.

The largest population-based study on childhood CSVT, published in 2001, the CPISR, enrolled 160 Canadian children, 91 non-neonates and 69 neonates, with a radiologically confirmed diagnosis of CSVT. The Canadian registry reported that among older children or non-neonates with

CSVT, 90% had diffuse neurological signs, including headaches in 59%, alteration in the level of consciousness in 49%, and papilledema on examination in 22%. Focal neurological signs were seen in 53%, including visual impairment in 18%, hemiparesis in 19%, other cranial nerve palsies in 11%, speech impairment in 7%, and ataxia in 7%. They reported that among 69 neonates with CSVT, the most frequently noted symptom was seizure (either localized or generalized) and occurred in 71%, followed by diffuse neurological symptoms and signs in 58% (including decreased level of consciousness in 36% and irritability/jitteriness in 20%) and focal neurological deficits in only 29%. In comparison to non-neonates with CSVT, the occurrence of seizures was significantly higher ($P=0.006$), and the frequency of diffuse neurological signs ($P=<0.001$) and focal neurological deficits ($P=0.004$) was lower in neonates with CSVT.[2] Infants with CSVT may later develop infantile spasms and reportedly had a poor outcome.[21]

More recently, a multicenter IPSS reported data on 170 children (non-neonates) with CSVT and 84 neonates with CSVT.[15,22] In children with CSVT, the IPSS reported headache in 70%, altered consciousness in 55%, seizures in 26%, and focal neurological deficits in 40%.[22] In neonates, the majority (61%) with CSVT presented during the first week of life in the IPSS cohort. The authors noted that in neonates with CSVT, the most commonly occurring presenting symptom was seizure (67%), followed by alteration in the level of consciousness (65%). Diffuse signs other than altered consciousness and including apnea, irritability, hypotonia, poor feeding, and vomiting were present in 13% and focal motor deficits in only 6% of their cohort of neonates with CSVT.[15] Several large cohort studies from different regions of the world have reported more or less similar clinical features in children and neonates with CSVT and are summarized in Tables 3-2 and 3-3.

Although most of the clinical features noted in CSVT are related to the severity and type of the parenchymal brain injury, the location and extent of sinovenous thrombosis largely dictates both the symptomatology and the parenchymal injury. The superficial venous system is the more commonly involved system, with predominant involvement of superior sagittal, transverse, and sigmoid sinuses.[2,7] Multiple sinuses may be involved in the same patient. Parenchymal brain injury occurs in at least half of the children with CSVT and includes diffuse or localized cerebral edema or congestion; venous infarction (both ischemic and hemorrhagic); and intraventricular, parenchymal, and extraparenchymal hemorrhage. The Canadian registry reported that the thrombosis involved the superficial venous system in 86% and deep venous system in 38%, with multiple sinuses involved in over half of the patients and no significant difference between the neonates and the non-neonates. In their cohort of children with CSVT, venous infarction was present in 66 (41%) children (29 neonates and 37 non-neonates), and of those with infarcts

there were hemorrhagic infarcts in 45 (68%) children. Extraparenchymal hemorrhage was noted in 9% of their total cohort.[2]

With regard to the relationship between the location of thrombosis and the clinical symptomatology in children, thrombosis involving the superior sagittal sinus typically causes bilateral hemispheric, usually parasagittal, venous infarction and/or hemorrhage and leads to signs and symptoms of increased intracranial pressure, such as headache, papilledema, and paraparesis. In addition, other focal motor deficits and seizures may occur as well as the presence of scalp edema and dilated scalp veins on examination. In children, transverse sinus thrombosis frequently occurs in association with middle ear and/or mastoid bone infection. Children with transverse sinus thrombosis therefore often appear sick and present with fever, unilateral or diffuse headache, ear pain or discharge, and swelling, redness, or pain in the mastoid region. The venous thrombosis and blockage of the deep cerebral venous system commonly results in intraventricular hemorrhage and thalamic or basal ganglia venous congestion and hemorrhagic infarction.[23] Children with deep venous system involvement often have rapid neurological deterioration, mainly decreased level of consciousness and coma.

Large cortical vein thrombosis is uncommon in children and, therefore, the clinical syndromes often seen in adults in association with cortical vein thrombosis are not frequently reported in children (such as temporal lobe hemorrhage associated with vein of Labbe thrombosis).

ETIOLOGIES AND RISK FACTORS

The etiologies and risk factors that are known to contribute to the occurrence of childhood CSVT are identified in over 80% of cases (Table 3-4). In many children with CSVT multiple risk factors may coexist.[7,16] Historically, etiologies for CSVT can be categorized as either infectious or non-infectious. The risk factors in neonates with sinovenous thrombosis are similar to risk factors seen in older children; however, maternal risk factors also contribute to the underlying etiology for perinatal CSVT cases.[1,15]

Infectious Risk Factors for Childhood Cerebral Sinovenous Thrombosis

In children, infection-related CSVT is very common as opposed to adults. At least 20% of childhood CSVT cases occur in association with an infectious cause or risk factor. The most common etiologies and risk factors that can lead to the thrombosis of venous sinuses include a systemic infection or septicemia and infections involving the head and neck (meningitis, encephalitis, otitis media, mastoiditis, or sinusitis). Across studies, a strong relationship has

TABLE 3-2. CHARACTERISTICS OF CHILDHOOD CEREBRAL SINOVENOUS THROMBOSIS †

CHARACTERISTICS	Barron 1992[24]	deVeber 2001[2]	Huisman 2001[26]	Carvalho 2001[3]	Heller 2003*[7]	Barnes 2004[8]	Kennet 2004[20]	Sebire 2005[10]	Sebire 2005*[10]	Kennet 2007*[25]	Wasay 2008*[28]	Mallick 2009[27]	Grunt 2010[9]	Vieira 2010*[29]	Ichord 2014*[22]
Demographics															
Study period	1980-1990	1992-1997	1994-1998	1986-1999	1995-2002	1995-2001	1996-2003	1994-2000	1992-2004	1996-2005	1992-2001	1997-2005	2000-2008	2001-2007	2003-2007
Country	USA	Canada	Switzerland	USA	Germany	Australia	Israel	UK	Argentina	Germany	USA	UK	Switzerland	Portugal	IPSS
Number of children	25	160	19	31	149	16	46	42	38	396	70	21	65	53	170
Age at presentation	2 d to 17 y	0 d to 1 y	14 d to 14 y	1 d to 13 y	0 d to 18 y	1.3 months to 16.4 y	1.1 to 10.1 y	3 weeks to 13 y	0.2 to 15.4 y	0 d to 18 y	6 d to 12 y	1.4 to 16.9 y	0.75 to 15.6 y	3 d to 17 y	1 month to 19 y
Male sex N (%)	7 (47)	86 (54)	9 (47)	21 (68)	84 (56)	8 (50)	29 (63)	27 (64)	27 (71)	236 (60)	28 (40)	10 (48)	44 (68)	30 (56)	102 (60)
Neonates N (%)	10	69 (43)	NR	19 (61)	40 (27)	0	8 (17)	NR	NR	75 (19)	25 (35)	0	21 (32)	6 (11)	NR
Clinical features of older children reported (%)															
Diffuse signs	47	90			33						29		61		
Drowsiness								43			51	19			
Poor feeding				17				12				14			
Fever			37	58		56		45			33				
Nausea/vomiting			21	50	33	50		28			29	29	59	28	
Headache	60	59	21	42	33	44		68	95		18	71	66	28	76
Altered consciousness	33	49	11	42	14	50		45	55		30	14	29.5	36	55
Seizures	20	48	42	33	56	25		40	47		59	10	20	23	26
Focal deficits	33	53			14	38		69	30		21	24	16		43
Visual abnormalities	27	18		58		13		11			34	76	20		

(continued)

TABLE 3-2 (CONTINUED). CHARACTERISTICS OF CHILDHOOD CEREBRAL SINOVENOUS THROMBOSIS †

CHARACTERISTICS	Barron 1992[24]	deVeber 2001[*2]	Huisman 2001[^26]	Carvalho 2001[3]	Heller 2003[*^7]	Barnes 2004[8]	Kennet 2004[*20]	Sebire 2005[*^10]	Sebire 2005[*^10]	Kennet 2007[*^25]	Wasay 2008[*^28]	Mallick 2009[27]	Grunt 2010[9]	Vieira 2010[*^29]	Ichord 2014[*22]
Radiological features (%)															
Location of thrombosis						NR	NR		NR						
Superficial venous system	93	90	100	100	65			76	100	67	85	100	66	94	56
Deep venous system	0	36	0	NR	1			14		4	6	29	34	40	19
Both	6	NR	16	NR	2	NR	NR	4	21	NR	9	NR	NR	NR	24
Parenchymal involvement	NR	40	42	33	NR			57	NR	16		14	16	NR	
Ischemic infarction		14	26	25				28.5		9	10	9.5	0		37
Hemorrhagic infarction		26	16	8				28.5		8	40	4.5	16		13
Extraparenchymal/other hemorrhage	NR	9	NR	NR	NR	NR	NR	NR	NR	0	NR	0	4.5	NR	15
Etiology and risk factors (%)															
Any risk factor	40	54	16	16	55	6	42	45	92	61	90				
Prothrombotic disorder		60		1	32			40	34		20	14	39	26	20
Underlying predisposing condition or comorbid disorder						NR	24		47		10	24	43	18	40
Recent cranial trauma			47			6		4	2				4.5		
Trauma not specified			2		9				5					2	11

(continued)

TABLE 3-2 (CONTINUED). CHARACTERISTICS OF CHILDHOOD CEREBRAL SINOVENOUS THROMBOSIS †

CHARACTERISTICS	Barron 1992[24]	deVeber 2001*[2]	Huisman 2001^[26]	Carvalho 2001[3]	Heller 2003*^[7]	Barnes 2004[8]	Kennet 2004*[20]	Sebire 2005*^[10]	Sebire 2005*^[10]	Kennet 2007*^[25]	Wasay 2008*^[28]	Mallick 2009[27]	Grunt 2010[9]	Vieira 2010^[29]	Ichord 2014*[22]
Any acute systemic illness		31		75									61		
Any infection	27	27	37	58	30	63	47	62	50		40		57	57	
Mastoiditis/ sinusitis/otitis media	20		32		9	44	42	47	50		25	62	52	43	
Meningitis/sepsis	6	4	26	1	9	44					15	10	11	7	8
Dehydration	6	21		1				21	5		4	14		4	17
Anemia								50			10	19			9
Any head/neck pathology	6	38	58	1		31	11							4	46
Outcome															
Any neurological morbidity	7	38	21	50	NR	42	21	74	32	NR	46	43	7	43	43
Death	0	^8	0.5	17	NR	0	5	12	0	3	13	5	2	0	4

† Case series reporting 10 or more children between 1990 and 2014 are included; *Multicenter studies; ^Neonates included; d=days; y=years; USA=United States of America; UK=United Kingdom

TABLE 3-3. CHARACTERISTICS OF NEONATAL CEREBRAL SINOVENOUS THROMBOSIS †

CHARACTERISTICS	Barron, 1992[24]	Deveber, 2001*[2]	Carvalho, 2001[3]	Wu, 2002[23]	Kennet, 2004*[20]	Fitzgerald, 2006[1]	Nwosu, 2008^[17]	Berfelo, 2010*[42]	Jordan, 2010*[15]	Grunt, 2010[9]	Moharir, 2011^^[18]	Kersbergen, 2011[19]
Demographics												
Study period	1980-1990	1992-1997	1986-1999	1989-2000	1996-2003	1986-2005	1986-2007	1999-2009	2003-2007	2000-2008	1992-2009	2002-2010
Country	USA	Canada	USA	USA	Israel	USA	USA	Netherlands	International	Switzerland	Canada	Netherlands
Number of neonates (preterm)	10	69	19	30 (1)	8	42 (6)	59 (12)	52 (5)	84	21 (4)	104	26 (6)
Age range (days)	2-30	NR	0-13			0-20	0-28	0-28	NR	0-27	0-27	0-28
Clinical features (%)												
Asymptomatic				13	12	5	3	13	0			NR
Diffuse signs	58	58		13		9	70		13			
Irritability/jittery	20	20					12	6				
Respiratory difficulties	20		42	7		19	73	17				
Poor feeding			21	30		12	59					
Fever			16									
Altered consciousness	10	36	16	10		7	42	2	65		53	
Seizures	80	71	68	65	88	57	69	56	67	57	69	
Focal deficits	20	29						3	6			
Radiological features (%)												
Location of thrombosis				NR	NR				NR			
Multiple sinuses	30	NR	37				71	50		76	82	81
Superior sagittal	62	62	47			67	75	23		81	57	65
Transverse/sigmoid	39	39	16			69	63	3		43	75	54

(continued)

TABLE 3-3 (CONTINUED). CHARACTERISTICS OF NEONATAL CEREBRAL SINOVENOUS THROMBOSIS[†]

CHARACTERISTICS	Barron, 1992[24]	Deveber, 2001*[2]	Carvalho, 2001[3]	Wu, 2002[23]	Kennet, 2004*[20]	Fitzgerald, 2006[1]	Nwosu, 2008^[17]	Berfelo, 2010*[42]	Jordan, 2010*[15]	Grunt, 2010[9]	Moharir, 2011^^[18]	Kersbergen, 2011[19]
Straight		30				33	31	15		62	34	85
Internal cerebral vein		12								38		
Vein of Galen		10				12	14			29		
Other	20	4				17	17	4		43	34	46
Parenchymal involvement	80	42	58			60	86			86		
Ischemic infarction	60	7	21	NR		7	12		6	10	40	19
Hemorrhagic infarction	NR	35	37	50		53	42	79	31	48	62	
Parenchymal bleeds	NR			36	12			48	14	33	71	58
Ventricular hemorrhage	NR			33	12	19	19	56		38	28	77
Risk factors (%)												
Any risk factor		99	74	87		62			51		48	NR
Any Infection	20	26	21	10		17	24	15			88	
Meningitis/sepsis	20	16	16	3			17	2		38	10	
Dehydration/diarrhea	30	30	26		12	26			13		13	
Perinatal complications		51		57		82[¥]	71[¥]	67	70	57	46	
Prothrombotic state	0	20	‡	17	63	17	59	33	10	29	20	
Cardiac disorder		0	21	23		26	37	2	21	10	10	

(continued)

TABLE 3-3 (CONTINUED). CHARACTERISTICS OF NEONATAL CEREBRAL SINOVENOUS THROMBOSIS†

CHARACTERISTICS	Barron, 1992[24]	Deveber, 2001*[2]	Carvalho, 2001[3]	Wu, 2002[23]	Kennet, 2004*[20]	Fitzgerald, 2006[1]	Nwosu, 2008^[17]	Berfelo, 2010*[42]	Jordan, 2010*[15]	Grunt, 2010[9]	Moharir, 2011^^[18]	Kersbergen, 2011[19]
Major medical disorder				67	12		32			19		
Outcome (%)		‡		NR								
Normal	50		26		63	22		45	64		39	78
Neurologic impairment	50		58		25	48		48	33	54	61	12
Cognitive impairment	NR		5		NR	38		NR	NR	73	27	11
Epilepsy	NR		NR		NR	17		21	NR	38	18	11
Death (preterm)	0		10	NR	12	2		19	3	5	5	23 (4)

† Case series reporting 10 or more neonates between 1990 and 2014 are included; * Multicenter studies; ^42 neonates reported previously from the same center by Fitzgerald et al in 2006; ^^83 neonates reported previously from the same center in 2010,; ‡ Not reported separately for neonates; ¥Maternal risk factors included

TABLE 3-4. ETIOLOGIES AND RISK FACTORS FOR CEREBRAL SINOVENOUS THROMBOSIS IN CHILDREN	
INFECTIOUS RISK FACTORS	**NONINFECTIOUS LOCAL RISK FACTORS**
Fever	Local compression of venous sinuses
Septicemia	Tumor invasion of venous sinuses
Head and neck infections (eg, otitis media, mastoiditis, sinusitis, abscess, upper respiratory tract infections)	**PROTHROMBOTIC DISORDERS AND STATES**
Meningitis/encephalitis	*Inherited Causes*
NONINFECTIOUS SYSTEMIC RISK FACTORS	Protein C deficiency
Dehydration	Protein S deficiency
Malignancy	Activated protein C resistance
Head and neck injury	Antithrombin III deficiency
Cranial surgery	Lupus anticoagulant presence
Iron-deficiency anemia	Antiphospholipid antibodies presence
Paroxysmal nocturnal hemoglobinuria	Hyperhomocysteinemia
Polycythemia	Factor V Leiden mutation
Thrombocythemia	Prothrombin 20210A mutation
Thrombotic thrombocytopenic purpura	Methylene tetrahydrofolate reductase gene mutation
Heparin-induced thrombocytopenia	*Acquired Causes*
Systemic lupus erythematosus	Cancer
Sarcoidosis	Procoagulant drugs (eg, L-asparaginase, steroids)
Inflammatory bowel disease	Nephrotic syndrome
Behcet's disease	Cyanotic congenital or acquired heart disease
Thyroid disorders	Exogenous hormones
Pregnancy	

been reported between head and neck infections and CSVT, with most of the pediatric literature reporting otitis media, mastoiditis, and meningitis in 20% to 65% of all childhood CSVT cases.[2,3,7-11,20,24-31]

Noninfectious Risk Factors for Childhood Cerebral Sinovenous Thrombosis

Many chronic and comorbid disorders have been reported to increase the risk of both cerebral and systemic thrombosis in children. However, the mechanisms by which the noninfectious risk factors initiate thrombosis are poorly understood. In general, the underlying noninfectious risk factors for CSVT are either acquired or genetic (see Table 3-4).

The acquired noninfectious risk factors include surgery, head trauma, dehydration secondary to increased fluid loss or decreased intake, congenital heart disease, iron-deficiency anemia, exogenous hormones, procoagulant drugs (eg, L-asparaginase, oral contraceptives) or states (eg, cancer, pregnancy),[2,10,20,25,32,33] and chronic systemic diseases such as inflammatory bowel disease, nephrotic syndrome, Behcet's disease, systemic lupus erythematosus, thyrotoxicosis, etc.[34-37] The correlation of cancer, commonly hematologic malignancies, to childhood CSVT has been speculated for some time. The CPISR has reported that 8% of cases of childhood CSVT have some type of cancer.[2] The likely mechanisms associated with cancer in children with CSVT include direct tumor compression, tumor invasion of cerebral sinuses, and the hypercoagulable states associated with cancer and chemotherapeutic and hormonal agents used for cancer treatment. Other uncommon causes that have been related to CSVT include paroxysmal nocturnal hemoglobinuria, thrombocythemia, heparin-induced thrombocytopenia, and thrombotic thrombocytopenic purpura.[6]

The genetic risk factors include inherited thrombophilias such as deficiency of antithrombin III, protein C, and protein S; hyperhomocysteinemia; and mutations in factor V Leiden, prothrombin gene, and rarely, homozygous mutation of the thermolabile variant of the methylene tetrahydrofolate reductase (MTHFR) gene,[2,6,30,38-41] In comparison to adults, inherited thrombophilias have been reported to occur in 20% to 80% of childhood CSVT cases.[2,6,38-40] The wide variation in the reported occurrence of hypercoagulable abnormalities across studies is due to the nature and extent of investigations undertaken, types of ischemic stroke investigated, and geographic and ethnic disparities between studies. Presence of a similar hypercoagulable disorder or a tendency for one or more of the family members to form clots may be present and helpful in guiding further investigations. Several studies in children with CSVT have shown that the presence of more than two genetic inherited thrombophilia traits confer a greater risk of thrombosis in children.[16] Most helpful is the recent meta-analysis by Kenet and colleagues that investigated both inherited and acquired thrombophilic disorders in children (0 to 18 years of age) who had suffered an initial ischemic stroke event of any type (ie, both ischemic stroke subtypes: AIS and CSVT.[16] Twenty-two studies met inclusion criteria and included a total of 1764 patients (1526 AIS, 238 CSVT) and 2799 control subjects. They found that for each thrombophilia trait investigated, a statistically significant association with first stroke existed. In addition, they found no difference between AIS and CSVT patients. The summary odds ratios for each trait investigated included antithrombin III deficiency, 7.06 (95% CI, 2.44 to 22.42); protein C deficiency, 8.76 (95% CI, 4.53 to 16.96); protein S deficiency, 3.20 (95% CI, 1.22 to 8.40), factor V G1691A, 3.26 (95% CI, 2.59 to 4.10); factor II G20210A, 2.43 (95% CI, 1.67 to 3.51); MTHFR C677T, 1.58 (95% CI, 1.20 to 2.08); antiphospholipid antibodies, 6.95 (95% CI, 3.67 to 13.14), elevated lipoprotein (a), 6.27 (95% CI, 4.52 to 8.69), and combined thrombophilias, 11.86 (95% CI, 5.93 to 23.73).[42]

Maternal and Perinatal Risk Factors for Neonatal Cerebral Sinovenous Thrombosis

In neonates with CSVT, several maternal and neonatal risk factors can confer increased risk for CSVT. During the perinatal period, commonly reported maternal risk factors include the presence of a prothrombotic condition (mainly positive antiphospholipid antibody status, history of deep vein thrombosis), prolonged second stage of labor, pre- or postdate deliveries, pre-eclampsia/eclampsia, gestational

diabetes, tobacco use, breech presentation, emergent caesarian section, instrument-assisted delivery, prolonged rupture of membranes, maternal fever, and group B streptococcal infection.[1,15] Neonatal risk factors include birth trauma, resuscitation at birth, meningitis, sepsis, acute systemic illness, dehydration, congenital heart diseases, and prothrombotic states.[1,15,23,43-45]

The American Heart Association (AHA) recommendations for the investigation of children with CSVT diagnosis[6] include the following:

1. Class I Recommendations (evidence for and/or general agreement that the procedure or treatment is useful and effective), Level of Evidence C (consensus opinion of experts, case studies, or standard of care):

a. Complete blood count is appropriate, mainly to rule out infection and anemia (Class I, Level of Evidence C).

2. Class II Recommendations (conflicting evidence and/ or a divergence of opinion about the usefulness/efficacy of a procedure or treatment), Level of Evidence B (data derived from a single randomized trial or nonrandomized studies):

a. Investigation for underlying infections with blood cultures and head and neck radiographs (Class IIb, Level of Evidence B).

b. Hypercoagulable screen to identify underlying prothrombotic risk factors because some disorders can affect the risk of recurrent thrombosis and therapeutic choices (Class IIb, Level of Evidence B).

DIAGNOSIS: CLINICAL AND IMAGING ASPECTS

When the clinical findings are suggestive of CSVT, specific imaging methods are necessary for diagnosing the condition accurately and promptly. Early and specific neuroimaging is important because in some individuals recanalization of venous sinuses may occur early, even before the detection of thrombosis, and hence creating challenges in correctly identifying the underlying cause of the child's symptoms.[10,25] In older children, the progression is often slow, leading to later appearance of symptoms and hence causing delays in CSVT diagnosis and treatment. The frequent presence of various nonspecific symptoms and risk factors for CSVT further contribute to these challenges. Several important clinical features that contribute in distinguishing CSVT from other cerebrovascular abnormalities include focal or generalized seizures, changes in the level of consciousness without focal neurological findings, objective signs of raised intracranial pressure, and bilateral brain involvement.

The diagnosis of CSVT requires neuroimaging evidence of thrombus or lack of flow in the cerebral veins or venous sinuses either by head computed tomography venogram (CTV) or magnetic resonance venogram (MRV) with contrast, with or without evidence of parenchymal involvement (either by infarction or hemorrhage) (Figures 3-2 through 3-4). In recent years, the widespread availability of neuro-imaging tests, in particular magnetic resonance imaging (MRI), has allowed improved detection and diagnosis of ischemic stroke in children. Head computed tomography (CT) alone may miss the presence of infarct and/or venous sinus involvement. A noncontrast CT or MRV can often lead to the erroneous diagnosis of CSVT. A false-positive result on noncontrast imaging may be due to the increased hematocrit in neonates and most commonly slow blood flow in the cerebral venous system. In the CPISR, initial noncontrast head CT scan missed the diagnosis of CSVT in over 15% of patients.[2] In other studies, the initial CT scan missed the diagnosis in at least 40%.[24,46,47]

The characteristic findings that suggest CSVT on a noncontrast CT include *dense triangle* or the *cord sign*, which indicates hyperdense thrombus in the sinovenous channels. On the contrast-enhanced MRV or CTV, an empty triangle, or the *delta sign*, represents a clot in the venous sinuses (see Figure 3-2). The ability to detect early parenchymal lesions by diffusion-weighted MRI sequences and lack of flow and presence of thrombus with increased specificity and sensitivity by brain MRI and gadolinium-enhanced MRV (without radiation effects) have made these the diagnostic imaging modalities of choice for CSVT at many pediatric hospitals.[16,48,49]

The AHA recommendations for the diagnosis and monitoring of children with suspected CSVT[6] include the following:

1. Class I Recommendations (evidence for and/or general agreement that the procedure or treatment is useful and effective), Level of Evidence C (consensus opinion of experts, case studies, or standard of care):

   a. A plain CT or MRI is useful in the initial evaluation of patients with suspected CSVT, and a CTV or MRV, preferably contrast enhanced, is required to confirm or rule out a diagnosis of CSVT (Class I, Level of Evidence C).

   b. An early follow-up CTV or MRV is recommended in CSVT patients with persistent or progressive symptoms indicative of propagation of thrombus (Class I, Level of Evidence C).

2. Class II Recommendations (conflicting evidence and/or a divergence of opinion about the usefulness/efficacy of a procedure or treatment), Level of Evidence B (data derived from a single randomized trial or nonrandomized studies) or C:

   a. Repeat the neuroimaging studies in children with CSVT to confirm vessel recanalization or recurrence of the thrombus (Class II, Level of Evidence C).

   b. MRI gradient echo T2 susceptibility-weighted images can be useful to improve the accuracy of CSVT diagnosis (Class II, Level of Evidence B).

   c. Catheter cerebral angiography can be useful in patients with strong clinical suspicion for CSVT if the CTV or MRV fails to confirm the diagnosis (Class II, Level of Evidence C).

TREATMENT

There is an absolute lack of randomized multicenter clinical trials for the treatment of childhood CSVT. In children, the treatment of this disabling disorder is mainly based on the adult ischemic stroke literature or on management approaches published in the pediatric studies. Limited data regarding treatment of CSVT in children led to the emergence of the recently published expert consensus-based guidelines for the management of childhood ischemic stroke (including CSVT and AIS).[6] It should be noted that the evidence for most of the recommendations in these guidelines are Class I (evidence or agreement that the procedure or treatment is useful and effective) or Class II (conflicting evidence of a divergence of opinion about the usefulness/efficacy of the procedure or treatment) with Level of Evidence C (expert opinion or case studies).

As with AIS, the treatment of CSVT is multifaceted and includes multidisciplinary care involving many pediatric subspecialties. The treatment of CSVT mainly consists of general supportive measures and anticoagulant therapy. In addition, treatment of the underlying etiology is extremely important, such as prompt treatment of infections, dehydration, and anemia. The following section discusses in detail the therapeutic approaches for the treatment of childhood CSVT.

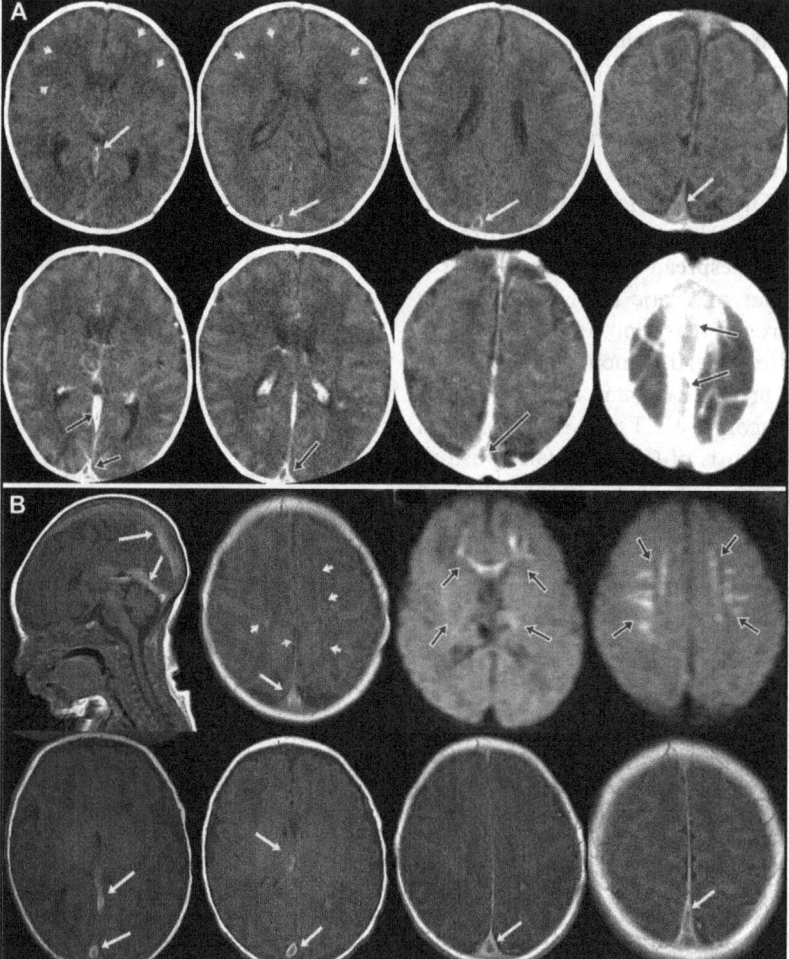

Figure 3-2. Eleven-day-old neonate, born at 35-weeks' gestation with uneventful birth history, presented with recurrent apneic spells and seizures consisting of eye blinking and jerking of limbs. (A) CT head noncontrast images demonstrating diffuse cerebral edema (white arrowheads), hyperintensity along the cerebral falx indicating hemorrhage, and hypodensity in the superior sagittal sinus (white arrows) suggestive of thrombus in the superior sagittal sinus (empty delta sign). CT head contrast-enhanced images demonstrating filling defects confirming thrombus in the straight and superior sagittal sinuses (black arrows). (B) MRI brain sagittal and axial T1 sequences demonstrating both hyperintense signal abnormalities indicative of thrombus in the superior sagittal, inferior sagittal and straight sinuses, internal cerebral vein and torcula (white arrows), and hyperintense signal abnormality along the falx and bilateral periventricular white matter indicative of hemorrhage (white arrowheads). MRI brain diffusion-weighted sequences demonstrating restricted diffusion in the bilateral periventricular white matter and corpus callosum, internal and external capsule, basal ganglia, and thalami (black arrows). MRI brain axial T1 contrast-enhanced images demonstrating filling defect indicative of extensive thrombosis involving the superior sagittal, straight and transverse sinuses, internal cerebral vein, and torcula (white arrows).

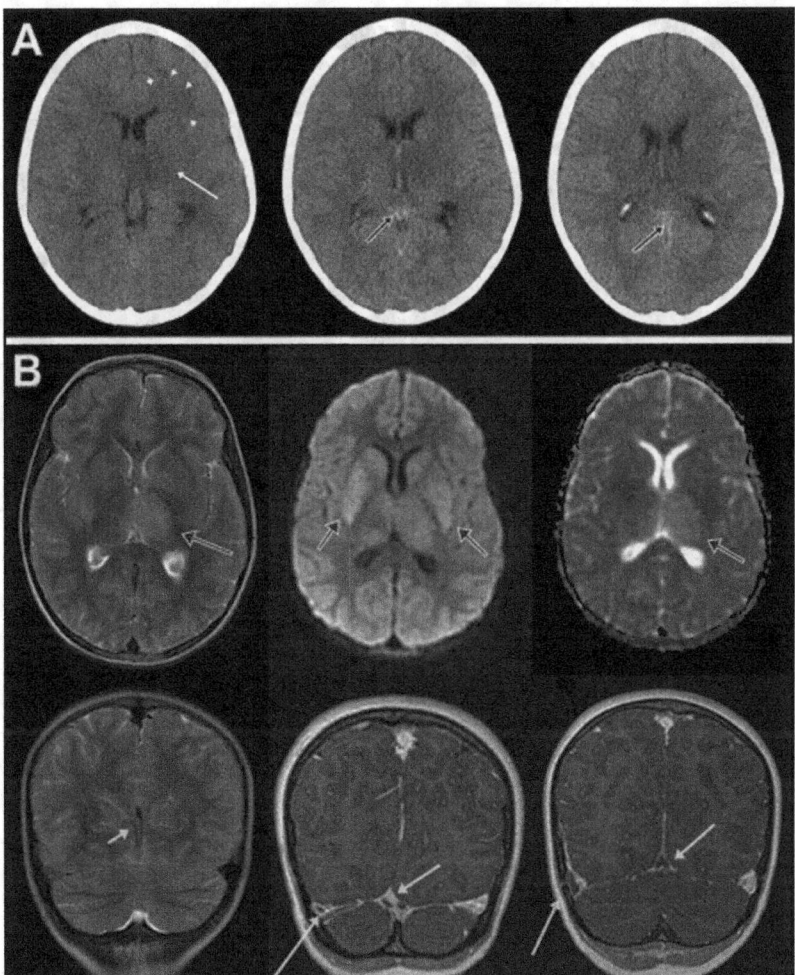

Figure 3-3. Nine-year-old girl with abdominal pain, vomiting, blood in stools, loss of appetite, and marked anemia and was subsequently diagnosed with inflammatory bowel disease. In hospital, she deteriorated with decreasing level of alertness, headaches, right arm and leg weakness, and abnormal movements suspected of possible seizure-like activity. (A) Initial noncontrast head CT scan revealed ischemic infarction in the left thalamus and basal ganglia (white arrow) with surrounding significant edema (white arrowheads) and evidence of blood involving the cerebral falx and possible thrombus in the straight sinus (black arrows). (B) MRI brain confirmed the presence of bilateral, left more than right, thalamic infarction; axial T2, diffusion-weighted, and apparent diffusion coefficient sequences (black arrows). There was evidence of several filling defects on the gadolinium-enhanced sequences indicating thrombus in the straight sinus, right sigmoid sinus, transverse sinus, and bilateral internal cerebral veins (white arrows). (C) Follow-up MRI brain after 3 months on anticoagulant therapy show old ischemic infarction in the left thalamus and the basal ganglia (white arrows) and almost complete resolution of thrombus in the dural venous sinuses, except minimal nonocclusive thrombus in the right transverses sinus (black arrows).

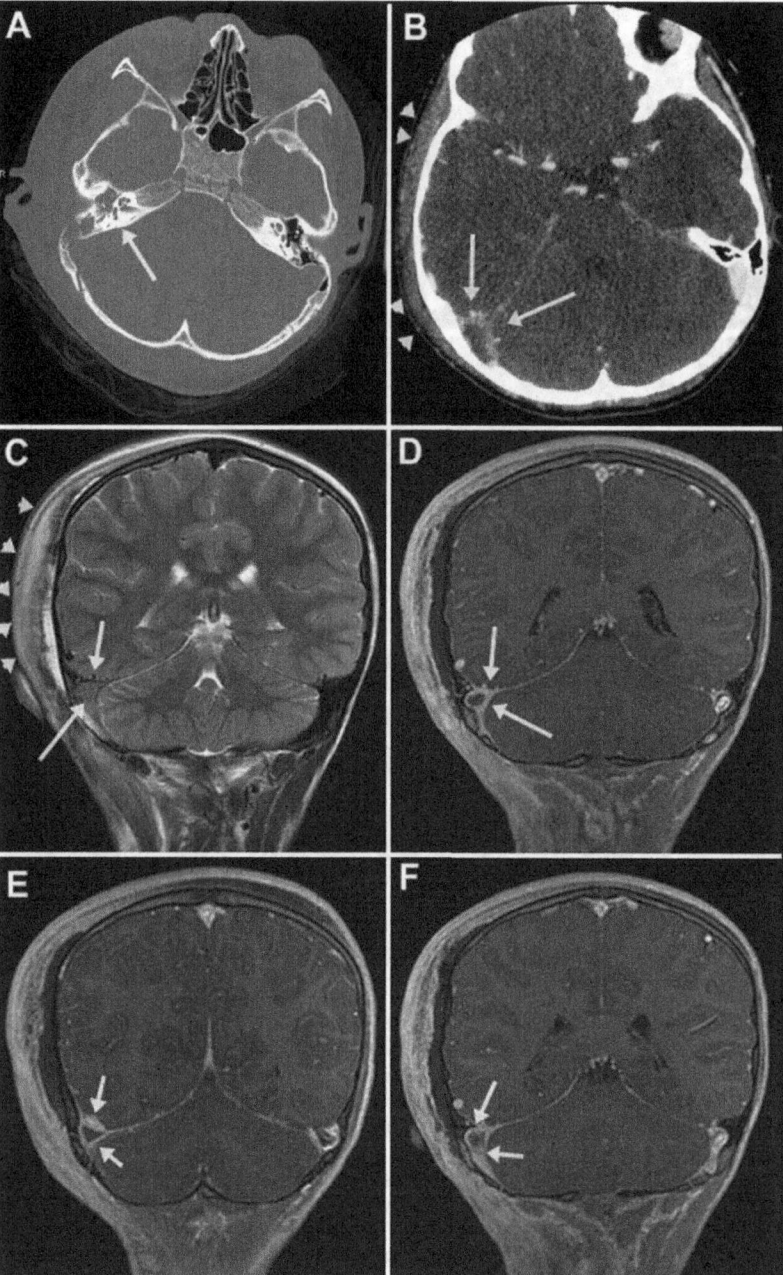

Figure 3-4. Eight-year-old girl with right ear pain and swelling of right side of face with trouble chewing and swallowing. (A) CT head bone window demonstrates extensive destruction of the mastoid septae and opacification of the mastoid air cells on the right side, indicative of right mastoid abscess (arrow). (B) Noncontrast CT head demonstrates marked scalp swelling overlying the right temporal and parietal bones, suggesting a large scalp abscess overlying the right temporal and parietal bones (arrowheads). (C) Postoperative MRI brain on coronal T2 nonenhanced image reveals hyperintense signal abnormality involving the cutaneous and subcutaneous soft tissues overlying the right parietal and temporal bone, indicative of soft tissue swelling and residual exudate or fluid collection following the abscess drainage (arrows). (D, E, and F) Postoperative MRI brain coronal contrast-enhanced images demonstrate a filling defect within the lateral aspect of the right transverse sinus extending into the right sigmoid sinus (arrows), indicating occlusive thrombus within these sinuses.

Supportive Therapy

The general supportive measures are the mainstay in the management of children with CSVT and are targeted at decreasing the increased intracranial pressure, treating seizures, and promptly treating underlying etiologies and associated conditions. The most comprehensive recommendations for supportive care are provided by the published AHA guidelines on the management of children with CSVT[6] and are based on opinions of pediatric stroke experts and available published case studies of childhood CSVT. The AHA recommendations on the management of children with CSVT diagnosis[6] include the following:

1. Class I Recommendations (evidence for and/or general agreement that the procedure or treatment is useful and effective), Level of Evidence C (consensus opinion of experts, case studies, or standard of care):

   a. Appropriate hydration of the child, including treatment of dehydration with intravenous fluids (Class I, Level of Evidence C).

   b. In case of seizure occurrence, prompt control of epileptic seizures with age-appropriate anticonvulsant therapy for usually a brief defined duration is advised to prevent further seizures (Class I, Level of Evidence C). Due to the increased risk of anoxic brain damage, anticonvulsant treatment even after a single seizure is reasonable. In the absence of seizures, the prophylactic use of antiepileptic medications is not advised because the risk of side effects may outweigh the benefits of treatment.

   c. Treatment of fever and suspected and confirmed bacterial infection with appropriate use of antibiotics (Class I, Level of Evidence C).

   d. Close monitoring for signs and symptoms related to increased intracranial pressure, including persistent and progressive headache, nausea, vomiting, alterations in level of alertness, visual impairment (including papilledema and third or sixth nerve palsies), and progressively increasing head circumference in infants (Class I, Level of Evidence C). Because long-standing intracranial hypertension can potentially lead to visual loss and may be difficult to identify early in young children, periodic examinations for visual fields and acuity are advised (Class I, Level of Evidence C).

2. Class II Recommendations (conflicting evidence and/or a divergence of opinion about the usefulness/efficacy of a procedure or treatment), Level of Evidence B (data derived from a single randomized trial or nonrandomized studies):

   a. Because frequent seizures are reported in children with acute CSVT, continuous electroencephalographic monitoring may be considered in children with decreased level of consciousness or who are paralyzed and mechanically ventilated (Class IIb, Level of Evidence C).

   b. If increased intracranial pressure is noted, appropriate and prompt measures should be undertaken to control elevated intracranial pressure and its complications such as hydrocephalus and visual impairment.

There are no randomized trials to guide the optimal treatment of increased intracranial pressure in children with CSVT. Rational management of increased intracranial pressure includes the following:

- Lumbar puncture with removal of CSF with aim to achieve a normal CSF closing pressure. However, the use of anticoagulants and the presence of markedly increased pressure with potential for brain herniation can be limiting factors. Refractory chronic intracranial hypertension may require lumboperitoneal shunting.

- Acetazolamide, a carbonic anhydrase inhibitor, is a diuretic and decreases CSF production. It is often used for the treatment of significant intracranial hypertension with CSVT in children.

- Although used occasionally, corticosteroids are not effective and carry risk of infections and high blood glucose levels, which are injurious to ischemic brain.

- Prompt treatment of venous outflow obstruction with anticoagulation and possibly thrombolytic treatment may result in resolution of intracranial hypertension.

- Optic nerve fenestration decompression or shunts is a treatment option to decrease optic nerve pressure and halt progressive visual loss.

- In patients with neurological deterioration due to severe mass effect or intracranial hemorrhage causing intractable intracranial hypertension, decompressive craniotomy may be considered, although limited evidence is available on the role of decompressive craniotomy in CSVT.

Antithrombotic Therapy

Although recent advances in the field of childhood ischemic stroke have resulted in promising avenues, one needs to be mindful of evidence-based treatment approaches. In children with CSVT, there are currently no multicenter randomized double-blind studies on which to base treatment with antithrombotic therapy, either antiplatelet or anticoagulant therapy. The rationale for treatment with antithrombotic therapy is based on its potential to prevent further propagation of clot with resultant improvement in venous outflow tract obstruction and further neurological deterioration and recurrence, but its use is challenged with the fact that it can cause and exacerbate hemorrhages.

Adult studies on the use of anticoagulation with heparin in CSVT cases have revealed conflicting data. The first randomized placebo-controlled study in adults with CSVT showed no clinical benefit with intravenous unfractionated heparin (UFH), and in fact, in their cohort of patients increased mortality was noted, resulting in early termination of the trial. The second randomized placebo-controlled study, which examined low-molecular-weight heparin (LMWH) in adults with CSVT, found a trend toward clinical efficacy with improved outcome. Following that several case studies and a recent Cochrane review of adult CSVT cases reported that use of anticoagulants is safe and can be effective in the treatment of CSVT.[6,50] Most recently, the AHA statement on the management of adults with CSVT endorsed the use of anticoagulants and recommended initial anticoagulation with UFH or LMWH in therapeutic anticoagulant doses, with or without the presence of intracranial hemorrhages (Class II; Level of Evidence B).

In children, published data on safety and efficacy of antithrombotic therapy consist of mainly case reports and series that have also demonstrated similar safety and efficacy of antithrombotic treatment in childhood CSVT as in adults.[6,10,46,47] A Canadian study, published in 1998, was the first to examine the effects of anticoagulant therapy in a prospective cohort of 30 children with CSVT. In their cohort, 22 children were treated with anticoagulant therapy (10 UFH and 12 LMWH) and 8 children were ineligible for anticoagulant therapy (mainly due to either associated intracranial hemorrhage or increased bleeding risk). They reported 3 deaths in the untreated group compared to 0 symptomatic intracranial hemorrhages and deaths in the treated group.[47] A European multicenter cohort study, published more recently in 2007, followed 396 consecutively enrolled patients with CSVT with a median follow-up of 36 months. They treated 250 children (65%) with anticoagulation during the acute period and continued anticoagulation prophylaxis in 165 (43%) children. Of the 396 children enrolled, 12 died within 2 weeks of presentation (one of whom was treated with anticoagulation) and 22 (6%) had recurrent venous thrombosis (6/22 children with recurrence were receiving anticoagulation). Their data suggested that recurrence rate among untreated children is higher than the children treated with anticoagulants. In their study, because death was relatively uncommon later in the disease process, the effect of treatment on mortality could not be assessed.

There are no concrete data on the use of antiplatelet therapy, thrombolysis, or thrombectomy in adults or children with CSVT except a single nonrandomized study in adults that compared urokinase thrombolysis to heparin and reported a better functional outcome in patients who underwent thrombolysis, but risk of intracranial hemorrhage was high.[51]

The absolute lack of randomized controlled studies regarding the use of anticoagulant treatment in children with CSVT led to treatment variations across centers and countries. This led to the emergence of 2 simultaneously published guidelines in 2004 for the management of ischemic stroke in children: the United Kingdom Royal College of Physicians Pediatric Stroke Working group (UK) and the American College of Chest Physicians (ACCP) practice guidelines (this guideline was subsequently updated in 2008). Both guidelines were consensus or working group recommendations among physicians with expertise in pediatric stroke (including neurologists, hematologists, neurosurgeons and physiatrists, and rehabilitation therapists).[33,52] Subsequent to these 2 guidelines, the AHA guideline was published for the management of stroke and CSVT in infants and children.[6,46] In accordance with the published guidelines on the management of childhood CSVT, for children with CSVT (outside the neonatal age group) and without evidence of significant intracranial hemorrhage, both ACCP and AHA guidelines recommend treatment with anticoagulation for a duration of 3 to 6 months, with reassessment of recanalization at 3 months. With significant intracranial hemorrhage, only close monitoring with serial neuroimaging is advised, and in case of clot propagation in these patients, treatment with anticoagulation is advised to be considered. However, in neonates, there is no consensus. The ACCP guidelines recommend treatment with anticoagulation in neonates without large ischemic infarction or intracerebral hemorrhage, and radiographic monitoring for children with intracerebral hemorrhage with the recommendation to initiate anticoagulation if the extension of thrombosis occurs.[52] The AHA recommendations are to provide supportive therapy, such as treatment of dehydration, infection, raised intracranial pressure, and seizures. The AHA recommends that anticoagulation may be considered in selected neonates who show clinical or radiological propagation CSVT in spite of supportive therapy.[46]

The choice of anticoagulant agent during the acute phase (either intravenous UFH or subcutaneous LMWH) is usually based on a health center's and physician's preference and level of comfort with its use. Some centers prefer to use intravenous UFH for the initial 5 to 7 days with subsequent switch to subcutaneous LMWH because of the ability of intravenous UFH to achieve rapid clinical effect (as monitored by activated partial thromboplastin time) as well as quick reversal of its effect in case of deleterious hemorrhage. However, in the recent past, subcutaneous LMWH has gained favor in children because of ease of its administration and ability to monitor and achieve steady anti-Xa levels without much fluctuation compared to heparin. In older children after an initial treatment with LMWH, switch to an oral vitamin K agonist, such as warfarin, is favored by some physicians for the remainder of the treatment period. The exact duration of therapy is variable and is based on venous channels' recanalization rates (maximal time to recanalization in neonates is 3 months and within 3 to 6 months in older children). The recommended duration of therapy is therefore 3 to 6 months and can be stopped as early as 3 months if complete recanalization has occurred or after a maximum period of 3 months in neonates and 6 months in non-neonates.[6,46] In one multicenter European study of children with CSVT, with median follow-up of 6 months, the rates of complete recanalization were 46% and of partial recanalization were 42%.[25] The guidelines on the management of children with CSVT advise follow-up serial MRV or CTV to assess recanalization or persistence of sinovenous occlusion for at least a year after the initial CSVT event, usually at 3-, 6-, and 12-month intervals.[6]

There are no systematic studies on the role of chronic prophylactic anticoagulant therapy in both adults and children with CSVT.[6] Long-term treatment with an anticoagulant agent in prophylactic doses is only advised in selected individuals with CSVT in whom a specific prothrombotic tendency or deficiency and an associated increased risk of recurrent thrombosis is present (such as protein C and S deficiencies).

Following is the summary of the published guidelines on the management of childhood CSVT:

UK guidelines[33]:

- Providing there is no hemorrhage on brain imaging, anticoagulation should be considered in children with CSVT.

- Neonates were not addressed separately in the UK guidelines.

Chest guidelines[52]:

- For children with CSVT, initial treatment with either UFH or LMWH for 5 to 7 days, followed by LMWH or vitamin K agonists such as warfarin (target international normalized ratio [INR], 2.5; INR range, 2.0 to 3.0) for 3 to 6 months even in the presence of a localized hemorrhagic infarct (Grade 2C).

- For neonates with CSVT and without large ischemic infarctions or intracranial hemorrhage, initial treatment with either UFH or LMWH, followed by LMWH therapy for 3 months is advised (Grade 2C).

- For neonates with CSVT and with large ischemic infarcts or intracranial hemorrhage, serial radiographic monitoring is advised. Commencement of anticoagulation therapy is advised if further propagation of CSVT is noted (Grade 2C).

AHA guidelines[6,46]:

- In children with CSVT, it is reasonable to initiate either intravenous UFH or subcutaneous LMWH, irrespective of secondary hemorrhage, followed by warfarin for 3 to 6 months (Class IIb, Level of Evidence C). In addition, the AHA recommended that in selected children with CSVT who clinically deteriorate quickly and fail to respond to anticoagulation, the administration of a thrombolytic agent may be considered (Class IIb, Level of Evidence C).

- In neonates with CSVT, anticoagulation is not routinely advised because the AHA felt that until additional information on the safety and efficacy of anticoagulation is available in this specific age group, a recommendation on the use of anticoagulation cannot be made except in selected neonates with clinical or radiographic evidence of propagating CSVT, in whom the AHA recommends consideration for anticoagulation with either UFH or LMWH (Class II, Level of Evidence C).

REHABILITATIVE APPROACHES

Cognitive and neurological sequelae are frequent with childhood CSVT and may require rehabilitation therapy. As in adults, traditional rehabilitative therapies are generally considered to be beneficial in children with neurological sequelae secondary to CSVT in enhancing recovery and improving function, perhaps more effective in children due to the amazing brain plasticity at this young age. In spite of the paucity of systematic studies for these rehabilitative approaches, there is general consensus that during the acute stroke phase, these assessments should be obtained to determine need for both acute and long-term rehabilitative services, including physiotherapy, occupational therapy, and speech and language therapy (if required).[46] In children who have suffered parenchymal infarction, psychological and cognitive assessments and processes to support their adequate placement or settlement in the school (development of an individualized education program, educational assistance, etc.) as well as in the community are important factors to consider in this regard. As in AIS, other well-recognized therapies such as tendon-lengthening procedures and local botulinum toxin A injections for spasticity may improve functional outcome in children with motor impairment due to CSVT.

OUTCOME

In children with CSVT, permanent motor or cognitive disabilities have been reported in over 60% of survivors and death in 3% to 12%.[5,9-12,14] Most frequently reported neurological sequelae include visual impairment, such as impaired visual acuity and sixth cranial nerve palsy; sensorimotor impairments; speech, cognitive, and behavioral deficits; developmental delays; and learning disabilities.[9-12,14] Other long-term sequelae in children with CSVT include chronic headache, long-term epilepsy, and movement disorders.[2,5] One of the largest follow-up studies of children with CSVT was published by the CPISR, which followed 160 children with CSVT for a mean follow-up interval of 20 months and noted neurological deficits in 38% and death in 8% of the children.[2] Decreased quality of life reportedly occurs in over 50% of survivors of childhood ischemic stroke, which affects not just the individual but the entire family and the community at large.[53] Children with neonatal CSVT are at greater risk of developmental delays, learning disabilities, motor impairments ranging from mild hemiplegia to severe quadriplegia, and cerebral palsy (long-term motor deficits are noted in 6% to 28% and developmental delays in at least 58%).[2,3,5,14] Survivors of neonatal CSVT reportedly have epilepsy beyond the neonatal age in up to 20% of cases.[46]

The poor prognostic indicators of childhood CSVT include young age at the time of stroke (in particular neonates), presence of parenchymal hemorrhage or infarction (in particular neonates), lack of treatment with anticoagulation, deep cerebral venous system thrombosis involvement, and presence of markedly increased intracranial pressure.[9-12,14]

Recurrent symptomatic or cerebral venous thrombotic events are reported in 10% to 20% of children with CSVT.[9-12,14] The long-term follow-up data on thrombosis recurrence are scant. One European multicenter study of 396 consecutive children with CSVT with a mean follow-up interval of 36 months found that 22 children (6%) had recurrent thrombotic episodes (13 children with recurrent CSVT and 9 with systemic venous thrombosis). The predictors of recurrent thrombosis in their study included persistent occlusion on follow-up venography, heterozygosity for the G20210A prothrombin gene mutation, and the lack of anticoagulant treatment. In their cohort of children, children with initial CSVT occurrence under the age of 2 years did not have any recurrent thrombosis, indicating an extremely low risk of recurrence in young infants and neonates.[25]

FAMILY FOCUS BOX

1. The chapter provides epidemiological information regarding CSVT. Of the ischemic stroke population, children with CSVT constitute at least 20% of all cases, and this condition is more common in young children.

2. The clinical signs of CSVT can be nonspecific and subtle, especially in infants and young children. Seizures, irritability, and feeding problems are common symptoms in young children, whereas headache, lethargy, and altered consciousness are common in older children.

3. A significant proportion of both neonates and non-neonates have motor and cognitive difficulties after CSVT. Poor outcomes are noted in young children and in patients with diffuse and multifocal parenchymal brain injuries, markedly increased intracranial pressure, and deep venous sinus thrombosis.

4. The use of anticoagulant medication in children with no obvious contraindications and with evidence of propagation may lead to early recanalization of occluded venous channels, thereby improving clinical outcomes.

CASE STUDY

A 9-year-old girl presented with abdominal pain, vomiting, blood in stools, loss of appetite, and marked anemia for one week. She was subsequently diagnosed with inflammatory bowel disease. In hospital, she deteriorated with decreasing level of alertness, headaches, right arm and leg weakness, and abnormal movements suspected of possible seizure-like activity. Initial noncontrast head CT scan revealed evidence of blood involving the cerebral falx, possible thrombus in the straight sinus, and ischemic infarction in the left thalamus and basal ganglia with surrounding significant edema. This was followed by a brain MRI with gadolinium enhancement, which confirmed the presence of bilateral, left more than right, thalamic infarction on axial T2, diffusion-weighted, and apparent diffusion coefficient sequences. There was evidence of several filling defects on the gadolinium-enhanced sequences indicating thrombus in the straight sinus, right sigmoid sinus, transverse sinus, and bilateral internal cerebral veins. She was treated with subcutaneous LMWH therapy. Follow-up brain MRI after 3 months on anticoagulant therapy showed old ischemic infarction in the left thalamus and the basal ganglia and almost complete resolution of thrombus in the dural venous sinuses, except minimal nonocclusive thrombus in the right transverse sinus (Figure 3-3). Clinical follow-up 3 and 12 months after the initial presentation demonstrated full clinical recovery with normal neurological examination.

SUMMARY

Clinicians face many practical challenges in the recognition of CSVT in children. The clinical signs of childhood CSVT can be nonspecific and easily missed or mistaken for other diagnoses. A significant proportion of children with CSVT have resultant long-term motor and cognitive difficulties. Diagnostic and therapeutic interventions vary among centers and countries due to lack of randomized studies in childhood CSVT. Most management strategies are extrapolated from the adult data. Systematic approaches for the application of a variety of diagnostic and therapeutic interventions are at very early stages of research in children with CSVT. The recently published guidelines on the management of children with CSVT clearly indicate the urgent need for systematic randomized studies in this field. Under the umbrella of the IPSS, a collaborative group of physicians and investigators around the globe are working together to address some of the important management questions and controversies in the area of pediatric ischemic stroke (https://app3.ccb.sickkids.ca/cstrokestudy/). In particular, researchers are targeting studies to improve the clinical care and outcome of children with CSVT, as well as improve our understanding of this significantly disabling disorder in children. One of these remarkable efforts includes determining the safety and efficacy of anticoagulant therapy in neonates with CSVT. It is hoped that the resultant global multicenter collaboration will facilitate further systematic management approaches and research in children with ischemic stroke due to CSVT.

ACKNOWLEDGMENTS

Dr. Jens Wrogemann, Section of Pediatric Radiology, Department of Radiology, Children's Hospital, Winnipeg, University of Manitoba, for assistance with figures.

REFERENCES

1. Fitzgerald KC, Williams LS, Garg BP, Carvalho KS, Golomb MR. Cerebral sinovenous thrombosis in the neonate. *Arch Neurol.* 2006;63(3):405-409.
2. deVeber G, Andrew M, Adams C, et al. Cerebral sinovenous thrombosis in children. *N Engl J Med.* 2001;345(6):417-423.
3. Carvalho KS, Bodensteiner JB, Connolly PJ, Garg BP. Cerebral venous thrombosis in children. *J Child Neurol.* 2001;16(8):574-580.
4. Kirton A, deVeber G, Pontigon AM, MacGregor D, Shroff M. Presumed perinatal ischemic stroke: vascular classification predicts outcomes. *Ann Neurol.* 2008;63(4):436-443.
5. deVeber GA, MacGregor D, Curtis R, Mayank S. Neurologic outcome in survivors of childhood arterial ischemic stroke and sinovenous thrombosis. *J Child Neurol.* 2000;15(5):316-324.
6. Saposnik G, Barinagarrementeria F, Brown RD Jr, et al. Diagnosis and management of cerebral venous thrombosis: a statement for healthcare professionals from the American Heart Association/American Stroke Association. *Stroke.* 2011;42(4):1158-1192.
7. Heller C, Heinecke A, Junker R, et al. Cerebral venous thrombosis in children: a multifactorial origin. *Circulation.* 2003;108(11):1362-1367.
8. Barnes C, Newall F, Furmedge J, Mackay M, Monagle P. Cerebral sinus venous thrombosis in children. *J Paediatr Child Health.* 2004;40(1-2):53-55.
9. Grunt S, Wingeier K, Wehrli E, et al. Cerebral sinus venous thrombosis in Swiss children. *Dev Med Child Neurol.* 2010;52(12):1145-1150.
10. Sebire G, Tabarki B, Saunders DE, et al. Cerebral venous sinus thrombosis in children: risk factors, presentation, diagnosis and outcome. *Brain.* 2005;128(Pt 3):477-489.
11. Tuckuviene R, Christensen AL, Helgestad J, Johnsen SP, Kristensen SR. Paediatric arterial ischaemic stroke and cerebral sinovenous thrombosis in Denmark 1994-2006: a nationwide population-based study. *Acta Paediatr.* 2011;100(4):543-549.
12. Christerson S, Stromberg B. Childhood stroke in Sweden I: incidence, symptoms, risk factors and short-term outcome. *Acta Paediatr.* 2010;99(11):1641-1649.
13. Chung B, Wong V. Pediatric stroke among Hong Kong Chinese subjects. *Pediatrics.* 2004;114(2):e206-e212.
14. Moharir MD, Shroff M, Stephens D, et al. Anticoagulants in pediatric cerebral sinovenous thrombosis: a safety and outcome study. *Ann Neurol.* 2010;67(5):590-599.
15. Jordan LC, Rafay MF, Smith SE, et al. Antithrombotic treatment in neonatal cerebral sinovenous thrombosis: results of the International Pediatric Stroke Study. *J Pediatr.* May;156(5):704-710.
16. Kenet G, Lutkhoff LK, Albisetti M, et al. Impact of thrombophilia on risk of arterial ischemic stroke or cerebral sinovenous thrombosis in neonates and children: a systematic review and meta-analysis of observational studies. *Circulation.* 2010;121(16):1838-1847.
17. Nwosu ME, Williams LS, Edwards-Brown M, Eckert GJ, Golomb MR. Neonatal sinovenous thrombosis: presentation and association with imaging. *Pediatr Neurol.* 2008;39(3):155-161.
18. Moharir MD, Shroff M, Pontigon AM, et al. A prospective outcome study of neonatal cerebral sinovenous thrombosis. *J Child Neurol.* 2011;26(9):1137-1144.
19. Kersbergen KJ, Groenendaal F, Benders MJ, de Vries LS. Neonatal cerebral sinovenous thrombosis: neuroimaging and long-term follow-up. *J Child Neurol.* 2011;26(9):1111-1120.
20. Kenet G, Waldman D, Lubetsky A, et al. Paediatric cerebral sinus vein thrombosis. A multi-center, case-controlled study. *Thromb Haemost.* 2004;92(4):713-718.
21. Soman TB, Moharir M, deVeber G, Weiss S. Infantile spasms as an adverse outcome of neonatal cortical sinovenous thrombosis. *J Child Neurol.* 2006;21(2):126-131.
22. Ichord RN, Benedict SL, Chan AK, Kirkham FJ, Nowak-Goettl U. Paediatric cerebral sinovenous thrombosis: findings of the International Paediatric Stroke Study. *Arch Dis Child.* 2014;100(2):174-179.
23. Wu YW, Hamrick SE, Miller SP, et al. Intraventricular hemorrhage in term neonates caused by sinovenous thrombosis. *Ann Neurol.* 2003;54(1):123-126.
24. Barron TF, Gusnard DA, Zimmerman RA, Clancy RR. Cerebral venous thrombosis in neonates and children. *Pediatr Neurol.* 1992;8(2):112-116.
25. Kenet G, Kirkham F, Niederstadt T, et al. Risk factors for recurrent venous thromboembolism in the European collaborative paediatric database on cerebral venous thrombosis: a multicentre cohort study. *Lancet Neurol.* 2007;6(7):595-603.
26. Huisman TA, Holzmann D, Martin E, Willi UV. Cerebral venous thrombosis in childhood. *Eur Radiol.* 2001;11(9):1760-1765.
27. Mallick AA, Sharples PM, Calvert SE, et al. Cerebral venous sinus thrombosis: a case series including thrombolysis. *Arch Dis Child.* 2009;94(10):790-794.
28. Wasay M, Dai AI, Ansari M, Shaikh Z, Roach ES. Cerebral venous sinus thrombosis in children: a multicenter cohort from the United States. *J Child Neurol.* 2008;23(1):26-31.
29. Vieira JP, Luis C, Monteiro JP, et al. Cerebral sinovenous thrombosis in children: clinical presentation and extension, localization and recanalization of thrombosis. *Eur J Paediatr Neurol.* 2010;14(1):80-85.
30. Bonduel M, Sciuccati G, Hepner M, Torres AF, Pieroni G, Frontroth JP. Prethrombotic disorders in children with arterial ischemic stroke and sinovenous thrombosis. *Arch Neurol.* 1999;56(8):967-971.
31. Ozyurek E, Balta G, Degerliyurt A, Parlak H, Aysun S, Gurgey A. Significance of factor V, prothrombin, MTHFR, and PAI-1 genotypes in childhood cerebral thrombosis. *Clin Appl Thromb Hemost.* 2007;13(2):154-160.
32. James AH, Bushnell CD, Jamison MG, Myers ER. Incidence and risk factors for stroke in pregnancy and the puerperium. *Obstet Gynecol.* 2005;106(3):509-516.
33. Paediatric Stroke Working Group. *Stroke in Childhood: Clinical Guidelines for Diagnosis, Management And Rehabilitation.* London, United Kingdom: Royal College of Physicians of London; 2004. http://icnapedia.org/guidelines/open/f98c6540-a541-4bed-837d-ef293ac458bf.pdf. Accessed March 28, 2017.
34. Uziel Y, Laxer RM, Blaser S, Andrew M, Schneider R, Silverman ED. Cerebral vein thrombosis in childhood systemic lupus erythematosus. *J Pediatr.* 1995;126(5 Pt 1):722-727.
35. Standridge S, de los Reyes E. Inflammatory bowel disease and cerebrovascular arterial and venous thromboembolic events in 4 pediatric patients: a case series and review of the literature. *J Child Neurol.* 2008;23(1):59-66.
36. Fluss J, Geary D, deVeber G. Cerebral sinovenous thrombosis and idiopathic nephrotic syndrome in childhood: report of four new cases and review of the literature. *Eur J Pediatr.* 2006;165(10):709-716.
37. Borhani-Haghighi A, Samangooie S, Ashjazadeh N, et al. Neurological manifestations of Behcet's disease. *Neurosciences (Riyadh).* 2006;11(4):260-264.
38. Ganesan V, McShane MA, Liesner R, Cookson J, Hann I, Kirkham FJ. Inherited prothrombotic states and ischaemic stroke in childhood. *J Neurol Neurosurg Psychiatry.* 1998;65(4):508-511.
39. Heller C, Heinecke A, Junker R, et al. Cerebral venous thrombosis in children: a multifactorial origin. *Circulation.* 2003;108(11):1362-1367.

40. Riikonen RS, Vahtera EM, Kekomaki RM. Physiological anticoagulants and activated protein C resistance in childhood stroke. *Acta Paediatr.* 1996;85(2):242-244.

41. Bonduel M, Sciuccati G, Hepner M, et al. Arterial ischemic stroke and cerebral venous thrombosis in children: a 12-year Argentinean registry. *Acta Haematol.* 2006;115(3-4):180-185.

42. Kenet G, Lutkhoff LK, Albisetti M, et al. Impact of thrombophilia on risk of arterial ischemic stroke or cerebral sinovenous thrombosis in neonates and children: a systematic review and meta-analysis of observational studies. *Circulation.* 2010;121(16):1838-1847.

43. Fitzgerald KC, Golomb MR. Neonatal arterial ischemic stroke and sinovenous thrombosis associated with meningitis. *J Child Neurol.* 2007;22(7):818-822.

44. Berfelo FJ, Kersbergen KJ, van Ommen CH, et al. Neonatal cerebral sinovenous thrombosis from symptom to outcome. *Stroke.* 2010;41(7):1382-1388.

45. Hunt RW, Inder TE. Perinatal and neonatal ischaemic stroke: a review. *Thromb Res.* 2006;118(1):39-48.

46. Roach ES, Golomb MR, Adams R, et al. Management of stroke in infants and children: a scientific statement from a Special Writing Group of the American Heart Association Stroke Council and the Council on Cardiovascular Disease in the Young. *Stroke.* 2008;39(9):2644-2691.

47. deVeber G, Chan A, Monagle P, et al. Anticoagulation therapy in pediatric patients with sinovenous thrombosis: a cohort study. *Arch Neurol.* 1998;55(12):1533-1537.

48. Teksam M, Moharir M, deVeber G, Shroff M. Frequency and topographic distribution of brain lesions in pediatric cerebral venous thrombosis. *AJNR Am J Neuroradiol.* 2008;29(10):1961-1965.

49. Medlock MD, Olivero WC, Hanigan WC, Wright RM, Winek SJ. Children with cerebral venous thrombosis diagnosed with magnetic resonance imaging and magnetic resonance angiography. *Neurosurgery.* 1992;31(5):870-876.

50. Stam J, de Bruijn SF, deVeber G. Anticoagulation for cerebral sinus thrombosis. *Cochrane Database Syst Rev* 4[CD002005]. 2002.

51. Wasay M, Bakshi R, Kojan S, Bobustuc G, Dubey N, Unwin DH. Nonrandomized comparison of local urokinase thrombolysis versus systemic heparin anticoagulation for superior sagittal sinus thrombosis. *Stroke.* 2001;32(10):2310-2317.

52. Monagle P, Chalmers E, Chan A, et al. Antithrombotic therapy in neonates and children: American College of Chest Physicians Evidence-Based Clinical Practice Guidelines (8th ed). *Chest.* 2008;133(6 Suppl):887S-968S.

53. Friefeld S, Yeboah O, Jones JE, deVeber G. Health-related quality of life and its relationship to neurological outcome in child survivors of stroke. *CNS Spectr.* 2004;9(6):465-475.

4

Intracerebral Hemorrhage in Neonates and Children

Shih-Shan Lang, MD and Gregory G. Heuer, MD, PhD

Similar to adults, the two major types of childhood stroke are ischemic (arterial or venous infarction) and hemorrhagic. For the purposes of this chapter, we will focus on nontraumatic intracerebral hemorrhage (ICH), which includes both intraparenchymal (Figure 4-1) and intraventricular hemorrhage, as well as nontraumatic subarachnoid hemorrhage (SAH). Hemorrhagic transformation of ischemic stroke, traumatic ICH, and extradural hematomas will not be discussed in this chapter, as these entities are not usually considered true hemorrhagic strokes. Unlike adults, childhood ICH usually occurs in otherwise healthy children with occult vascular malformations, with a smaller percentage attributed to underlying hematological disorders or tumors. SAH commonly occurs in healthy children with aneurysms or vascular malformations. Starting at the time of presentation of an ICH, a multidisciplinary team approach is usually the best strategy for achieving the best outcome.

EPIDEMIOLOGY

Despite being an uncommonly described entity, childhood stroke is not rare. The incidence is reported to be 2 to 3/100,000 children.[1-5] The incidence of hemorrhagic stroke is 1.1/100,000 person-years, vs 1.2/100,000 person-years for ischemic stroke.[1,4-7] The most common underlying causes for childhood ICH are vascular lesions, including ruptured arteriovenous malformations (AVMs) (Figure 4-2), cavernomas (Figure 4-3), and aneurysms, with AVMs accounting for the majority of cases.[8,9] In a large cohort study spanning more than a decade, the incidence of these malformations and/or other risk factors were as follows: 31% cerebral AVMs, 13% cerebral aneurysms, 15% cavernous malformations, 14% medical etiologies, 2.5% brain tumors, and 25% undetermined.[10] The less common etiologies of ICH in children are hematological abnormalities, including coagulopathies, brain tumors, hypertension, and cerebral infections.[11,12] There is a subset of the population for whom, even after extensive evaluation, the etiology of the ICH is considered idiopathic.[10,12,13]

CLINICAL PRESENTATION

The initial clinical presentation of ICH and SAH in children can vary widely. Depending on location and size, presentations can occur either rapidly over minutes to hours or slowly over days, which can make diagnosis difficult. Younger patients may have more generalized and less specific symptoms, which also makes timely diagnosis complicated.[12] Over half of children present with headache and a decreased level of consciousness.[8,13] Other common presenting symptoms are also not specific to this disease

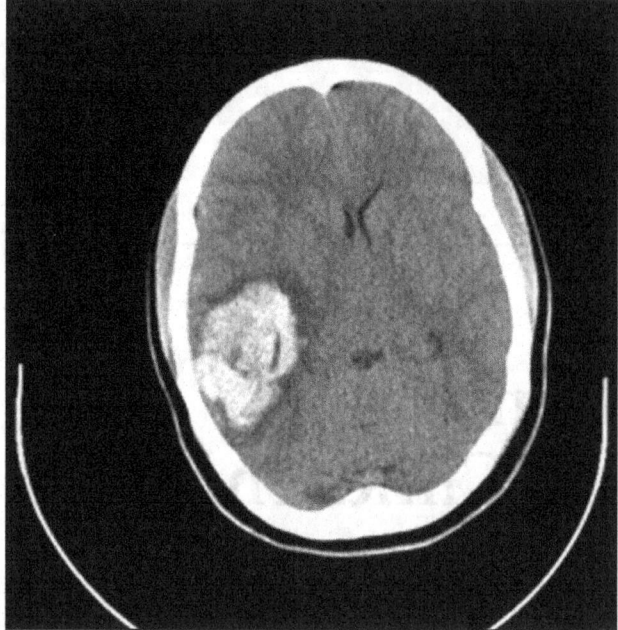

Figure 4-1. Axial noncontrast head computed tomography (HCT) showing a right frontal-parietal acute intraparenchymal hemorrhage.

process; these include nausea, vomiting, seizures, and focal neurological deficits such as hemiparesis.[8,13]

RISK FACTORS AND
SPECIAL POPULATIONS

As mentioned earlier, retrospective case series suggest that ICH and SAH in childhood is most often due to vascular malformations, hematologic abnormality, or brain tumors. Vascular malformations will be discussed under the diagnostic studies section.

Hematological abnormalities such as thrombocytopenia and hemophilia are thought to be a major contributor in nearly a quarter of all ICH.[2,6,14,15]

Idiopathic Thrombocytopenia Purpura

Idiopathic thrombocytopenia purpura (ITP) is an autoimmune condition with antibodies against platelets. Platelets normally help form clots when bleeding; therefore, patients with this disorder tend to bleed due to low platelets. A small percentage of children (< 1%) with ITP present with ICH.[16,17] In a review of the literature for ITP with ICH, 75 cases were reported.[16] Most of these children had an ICH within 6 months of diagnosis of ITP; however, it was extremely rare for ICH to be the presenting symptom. Not surprisingly, almost three-quarters of these patients had a platelet count of less than

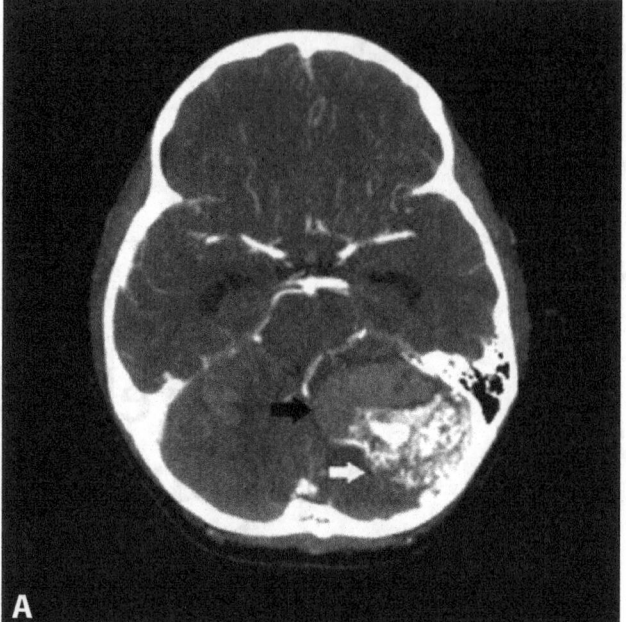

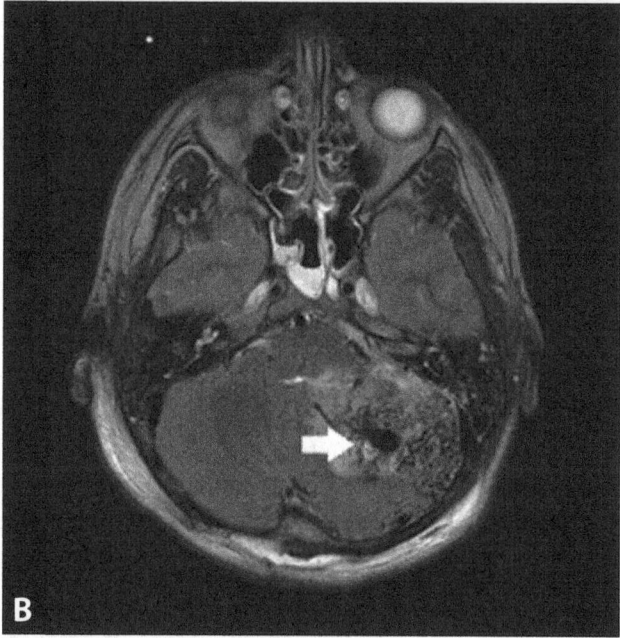

Figure 4-2. (A) Axial head computed tomography angiogram depicting a large left cerebellar ruptured arteriovenous malformation (AVM; white arrow) with associated hemorrhage (black arrow). (B) Magnetic resonance angiogram (MRA) showing the same ruptured AVM with flow voids (white arrow).

10,000, and only one patient had a platelet count greater than 20,000. Unfortunately, the mortality for children with ITP and ICH was approximately 50%.[18]

Hemophilia and Other Congenital Bleeding Disorders

In general, hemophilia and other bleeding diatheses are due to a qualitative or quantitative deficiency of components of the coagulation cascade. Therefore, these disorders carry an increased risk of ICH as well as extradural hematomas, usually in the setting of trauma. The prevalence of any intracranial hemorrhage in hemophiliac children has been reported to be between 2.9% and 12%.[19-21] Medical management should be aimed toward replacement therapy of specific coagulation factors that are decreased or absent as part of the underlying disorder.[22]

Common factor deficiencies associated with bleeding are factor VIII and IX, which are named hemophilia A and B, respectively. Another common bleeding disorder, von Willebrand disease, is not a direct factor in the coagulation cascade; however, von Willebrand factor is attached to factor VIII in order for it to activate correctly in the cascade.

Sickle Cell Disease

Children with sickle cell disease (SCD) have a nearly 67-fold increased risk of hemorrhagic stroke, with this risk increasing as age increases.[23] Hemorrhagic stroke in this population of children has been associated with a history of hypertension or recent blood transfusions or treatment with corticosteroids. There are guidelines for exchange transfusions in children suffering from acute arterial ischemic stroke; however, there are no studies or consensus on the use of transfusion in patients with ICH.[24,25] Patients with SAH and IPH with arterial ischemia on imaging do often undergo transfusion therapy.[26] SCD is associated with vascular malformations, especially in the posterior circulation, so additional vascular imaging should be obtained for any child with ICH or SAH.[27] A better understanding of modifiable risk factors in this population may help prevent major neurological compromise.

Malignancy

There are few reports describing ICH in children with malignancy. Recent reports indicate that hemorrhagic stroke and ischemic stroke occur with approximately equal frequency of 1% in children with cancer. In addition, children with leukemia and brain tumors are at greatest risk.[28] Other intracranial hemorrhages, such as epidural and subdural hemorrhages, can occur in this population in addition to SAH and ICH. The mortality related to ICH is high (50%) for children who hemorrhage directly into a primary or metastatic brain tumor.[29]

Neonatal and Newborn Intracerebral Hemorrhage

The neonatal population is grouped separately because ICH in premature infants is typically caused by germinal matrix hemorrhages rather than an underlying vascular disorder or lesion. Germinal matrix hemorrhage is bleeding into the subependymal germinal matrix surrounding

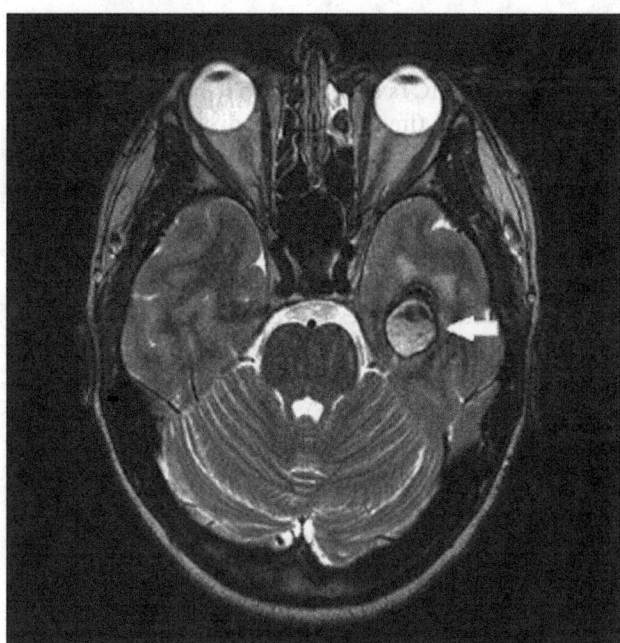

Figure 4-3. Axial T2-weighted MRI depicting a left temporal cavernoma (white arrow) with associated hemorrhage.

the lateral ventricles. The germinal matrix is the site where neuronal and glial precursors are located in the neonate and is highly vascular and fragile.[30] The population of near-term infants with ICH is more often due to hemorrhagic transformation of ischemic infarcts than germinal matrix hemorrhage.[31] In concordance with this, the largest identifiable risk factors in term infants are congenital heart disease and fetal distress.[31,32]

ICH in the newborn is associated with prolonged delivery, use of adjunct tools in the delivery such as forceps or suction,[33] and potentially vitamin K deficiency.[34] Vitamin K deficiency is an acquired coagulopathy in infants because of the inability to activate the coagulation cascade that requires vitamin K because of the low amount of that is found in a newborn. It is the current standard that all hospital-born infants are given an intramuscular injection of vitamin K at birth. Studies show that a deficiency in vitamin K can lead to increased risk of ICH in the newborn that may lead to devastating neurological outcomes.[34-36]

INITIAL EVALUATION AND MANAGEMENT

The initial evaluation of the child in which an ICH is suspected should be geared toward diagnosis of the hemorrhage, assessment for the presence of increased intracranial pressure (ICP), and correction of any underlying coagulopathy. No randomized controlled trials exist for childhood ICH or SAH management. Therefore, guidelines are taken from retrospective studies and adult randomized controlled trials.[37-41] Usually, the initial imaging study of choice by the emergency department or the intensive care unit is an HCT. HCTs are widely available in any hospital, with a rapid scan time that clearly distinguishes between hemorrhagic and ischemic stroke. It can also usually be performed in children without sedation.[9] However, in the case of SAH, HCT can miss a certain percentage of cases due to the age of the bleed or the fact that there is a small amount of blood below the detection limit.[14,42,43] Even with more recent advances in technology in HCT and CT angiography, a lumbar puncture is still suggested if SAH is suspected despite a negative HCT.[14,42,43] As in adults, the cerebrospinal fluid (CSF) from the lumbar puncture should be spun down to evaluate for xanthochromia, a bilirubin breakdown product found in SAH. Detection of xanthochromia is consistent with SAH and allows for differentiation from a traumatic lumbar puncture. In addition, red blood cell counts (RBCs) from the first and fourth tubes should be assessed; there should be a large discrepancy in RBCs between these tubes in a traumatic lumbar puncture vs no appreciable decrease in a true SAH.

Other than the initial imaging and diagnostic studies, laboratory studies should be drawn that include electrolytes, a complete blood count with platelets, prothrombin time (PT), international normalized ratio, activated partial thromboplastin time (aPTT), and fibrinogen. Any apparent coagulopathies or thrombocytopenia should be corrected as quickly as possible.[24,40] A hematologist should be consulted for any patient with hematologic abnormalities. In addition, a hematologist should be consulted to guide evaluation for a bleeding diathesis if no structural cause of hemorrhage is found (ie, vascular malformation, tumor). Common laboratory tests that are typically sent in initial workup include thrombin time, aPTT, PT, and platelet count. If any of these are abnormal, a hematologist can provide expertise in the next step of laboratory studies to obtain in order to diagnose the bleeding diathesis.

Children taking medication for anticoagulation should have their anticoagulation reversed after careful discussion of the risks and benefits with the anticoagulation provider.

Those children who present with seizures should receive an anticonvulsant medication to help reduce the possibility of recurrent seizures in order to help control any increased ICP. A neurosurgeon should be consulted immediately once an ICH is diagnosed.

REPRESENTATIVE NEUROIMAGING

As mentioned previously, if an ICH or SAH is suspected, HCT is considered the initial imaging study of choice because it is widely available in hospitals and is a quick study that almost always identifies the acute hemorrhage. The other most common imaging, MRI, is not universally available in all hospitals and may require some experience

with interpreting the images. In addition, the scanning time is much longer than an HCT and so sedation may be required in children.[44]

In almost all circumstances, except in impending herniation, given a diagnosis of ICH or SAH, dedicated cerebrovascular imaging is of utmost importance. The specific studies are often patient specific, as there is no perfect imaging study for all lesions. One study found that a combination of MRI, MRA, and magnetic resonance venogram images identified an underlying lesion and the cause for ICH in only 66% of the children.[45] However, in this study there were two false-negative MRIs: one child with a mycotic aneurysm and another with an AVM. Interestingly, in this study, the gold standard of cerebrovascular imaging, a conventional cerebral angiogram (CCA), only identified a cause for the ICH in 61% of the patients.[45] CCA is a form of imaging used to visualize the blood vessels of the brain. This involves inserting a catheter into the femoral (inner thigh) artery that is threaded into the neck. Contrast is injected while using real-time x-ray to create a picture of the blood vessels in the brain. Another series had a higher diagnostic yield for ICH in patients who underwent CCAs. In this series, the cause of nontraumatic ICH was found in 97% of children who underwent CCA compared to 80% who did not undergo a CCA.[8] Even if noninvasive imaging suggests the presence of an underlying lesion or vascular malformation, most neurosurgeons and interventional radiologists will recommend a CCA to further characterize the lesion in order to determine the optimal management option. Many times this diagnostic CCA leads to an intervention that requires angiography to coil or embolize an AVM or aneurysm (Figure 4-4). Embolization and coil are minimally invasive alternatives to open craniotomy and surgery that can be done in certain situations. Embolization or coil basically prevents blood flow to an area of the body. After embolizing or coiling an AVM or aneurysm, blood flow is diverted back to the normal blood vessels instead of into the AVM or aneurysm, which greatly reduces the chances of rupture. If surgery is required, preoperative embolization of an AVM greatly decreases the risk of intraoperative bleeding because blood flow has been diverted away from the AVM. In a recent report of children who underwent surgical resection of an AVM, intraoperative angiography was useful in identifying any residual AVM that may need to be resected before finishing the operation.[46] This usually requires comparison of a preoperative CCA in order to determine if and where the residual AVM is. In the adult population, intraoperative angiography for aneurysm clipping and AVM resections is considered the standard of care.[47]

There are certainly risks to any procedure; however, the published rate of major complications of pediatric CCAs is relatively low at 0.5%.[48] The risk of CCA often is less than missing a potentially life-threatening lesion. Occasionally, vascular malformations are not evident for weeks or even

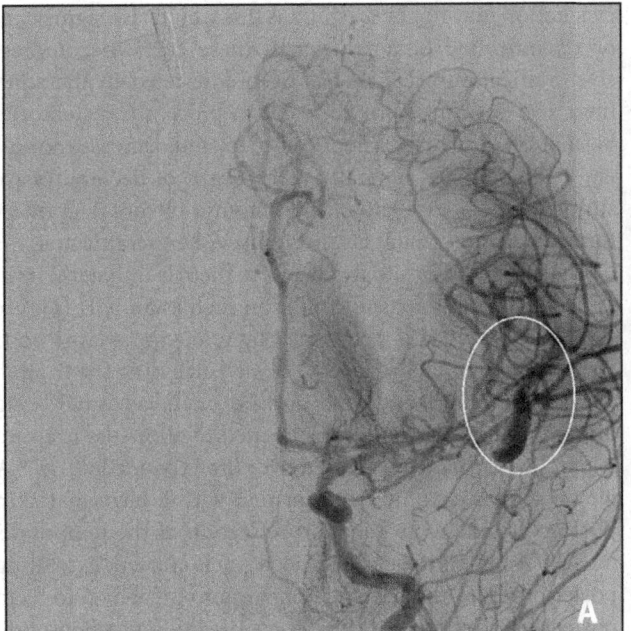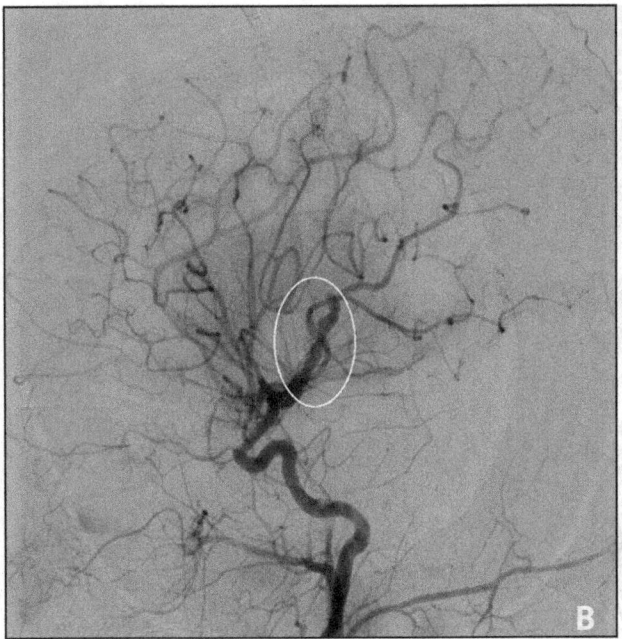

Figure 4-4. Digital subtraction angiogram (A) AP view and (B) lateral view demonstrating a left middle cerebral artery fusiform aneurysm (white circle). The patient underwent coiling of the fusiform aneurysm.

months after the acute hemorrhage. A large hemorrhage may compress the vessels associated with the lesion, which becomes evident after the ICH resolves. Most centers will repeat the vascular imaging once the hemorrhage has been absorbed, usually within 4 to 6 weeks of the original hemorrhage. The optimal timing and choice of modality have not been sufficiently studied.[49-51]

TREATMENT

Medical Management of Elevated Intracerebral Hemorrhage

Signs and symptoms of elevated ICP include declining mental status, headache, vomiting, cranial nerve palsies, irritability, and papilledema. The classic Cushing triad of hypertension, bradycardia, and irregular respirations is a late finding and usually means the child is in imminent danger of herniation. Typically, the first-line treatment for ICP monitoring is an external ventricular device (EVD). An EVD is a plastic tube placed into the ventricle of the brain and is usually done emergently at the bedside or in the operating room. It is usually placed on the right side of the brain into the frontal horn of the lateral ventricle. This allows for ICP measurement and for CSF drainage to help decrease ICP. If an EVD cannot be placed, an intracranial monitor can be placed for ICP monitoring. An intracranial monitor is a fiber-optic catheter that can be placed into any subdural space or anywhere in the parenchyma of the brain. It does not have to be in the position of an EVD because it

does not need to be in the ventricle. The catheter has capabilities to measure continuous ICP without CSF drainage.

Initially, to promote cerebral venous outflow, the head of the bed should be at 30 degrees. If the patient is intubated, hyperventilating the patient to a PCO_2 of 25 to 30 will help reduce ICP. In addition, diuresis through pharmacological agents such as mannitol or hypertonic saline should be considered. Electrolytes and osmolarity must be closely monitored when administering these medications. Lastly, sedation and/or paralytics may be needed for refractory ICP management. Sedatives decrease ICP by eliminating the transient elevations in ICP that are related to agitation, response to pain, and anxiety.

Surgical Management of Elevated Intracranial Pressure and Hemorrhage

Many patients continue to have persistently elevated ICP or cerebral edema that isrefractory to first-line medical therapies. When elevated ICP is clinically diagnosed and imaging studies indicate the presence of an ICH with no underlying vascular malformation, some adult studies report improved outcomes following aggressive surgical evacuation of the hematoma.[52,53] However, recent studies such as The Surgical Trial in Intracerebral Hemorrhage (STICH) and STICH 2 demonstrated that in adult patients with spontaneous supratentorial ICH, emergent surgical evacuation of hematoma within 72 hours of bleeding onset did not improve outcome when compared with best medical management.[37,38] Of course, these studies may not be directly translatable to the pediatric population. Children may require more urgent intervention to reduce elevated

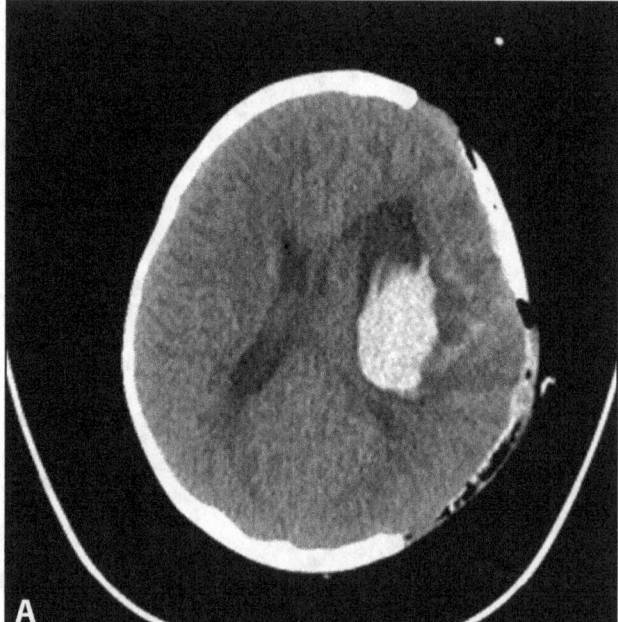

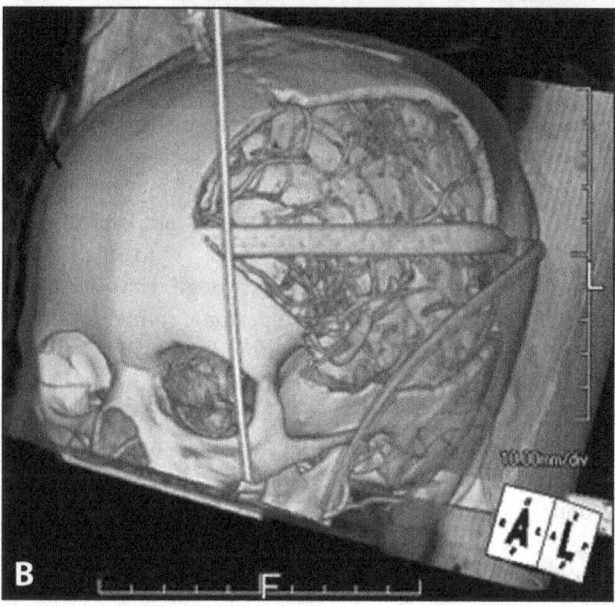

Figure 4-5. (A) Axial noncontrast HCT showing a left DCH performed for elevated ICP secondary to the ICH. (B) HCT reconstruction post-DCH.

ICP in order to prevent brain herniation because they do not have the cerebral atrophy found in older adults. A few pediatric studies have shown that children with cerebellar hemorrhage may need evacuation to prevent herniation.[54,55] In addition, the pediatric brain may respond differently to the insult of the ICH, potentially having greater ability to recover, and thus making the STICH trial data not applicable to this population.

Occasionally, a hemorrhage is in an area of eloquent cortex and cannot be evacuated without risking significant neurological deficits. Also, if an underlying AVM is present that the surgeon is not prepared to treat, emergent

evacuation may not be feasible, as this would risk significant or uncontrolled hemorrhage. In these cases, decompressive craniectomy (DCH) has been advocated in the adult literature as a lifesaving measure to prevent transtentorial herniation, decrease ischemic burden, and decrease mortality.[56,57] There are generally three forms of decompressive surgical operations: hemicraniectomy, bifrontal craniectomy, and suboccipital craniectomy. A hemicraniectomy is often performed in situations where there is unilateral injury or a focal pathological condition such as an ICH (Figure 4-5). Briefly, DCH is performed by removing a large bone flap with a diameter of at least 12 cm (including the frontal, parietal, temporal, and parts of the occipital squama).[58] No brain is removed, the dura is opened to allow the brain to expand, and the skin is closed over the expanded dura.[59] A bifrontal craniectomy is performed with a bicoronal skin incision (from ear to ear) and reflection of the temporalis muscle. A large bifrontal craniectomy is created, extending posteriorly into the parietal bones approximately 3 to 5 cm posterior to the coronal sutures and including the temporal bone and the frontal bone down to the orbit rims. This type of craniectomy is preferred for patients with frontal or bifrontal lesions. A suboccipital craniectomy is performed in patients with hematomas in the posterior fossa (Figure 4-6). This is done through a midline incision with the patient prone. Although DCH has been shown to be effective in reducing increased ICP, studies disagree on whether DCH improves overall outcome in adults.[58,60]

There are no Class I evidence reports of DCH in children with ICH. However, most neurosurgeons will consider this surgery in patients with a large ICH and declining neurological exam. A few small studies showed a positive outcome in a few children who underwent DCH for intractable elevated ICP.[13,59,61]

OUTCOME

Although there are several reports of neurological outcome after arterial ischemic stroke in children,[62,63] outcome measures besides simple mortality after ICH have not been well reported. Average mortality in older literature ranges widely from 7% to 54%,[4,15] whereas newer studies show a lower rate of mortality of around 5%.[64] Improvements in pediatric critical care and neurosurgical techniques may account for some of this reduction in mortality.[65] Infratentorial location, Glasgow Coma Scale <7, age <3 years, an underlying hematological disorder, larger ICH volume, and altered mental status within 6 hours of hospital presentation have all been reported to predict poor outcome.[11-13,66]

Little attention has been paid to cognitive outcomes, with the exception of one retrospective cohort study.[6] This study spanned 20 years and had a long-term follow-up of approximately 10 years with an overall mortality of 64%.

In the patients who completed neuropsychological testing and intelligence quotient (IQ) testing, the mean IQ was not below average or left-shifted. However, the standard deviation was large, indicating quite a range of IQs. Forty-eight percent of patients had signs of cognitive deficits in comparison to their academic abilities before the ICH and 23% had moderate to severe deficits. In another study, over two-thirds of the patients had a sensorimotor deficit, but all were ambulatory and able to communicate.[67]

The risk of long-term epilepsy after ICH is a topic with very little data in the literature. A large prospective study showed that the risk for developing epilepsy is 13% in patients at 2-year follow-up. The largest risk factors for epilepsy and remote seizures were elevated ICP requiring acute neurosurgical intervention.[67] One study showed that the quality of life perception by patients and their parents following unilateral stroke or ICH was lower for patients who had neurological impairments such as hemiparesis and epilepsy.[68]

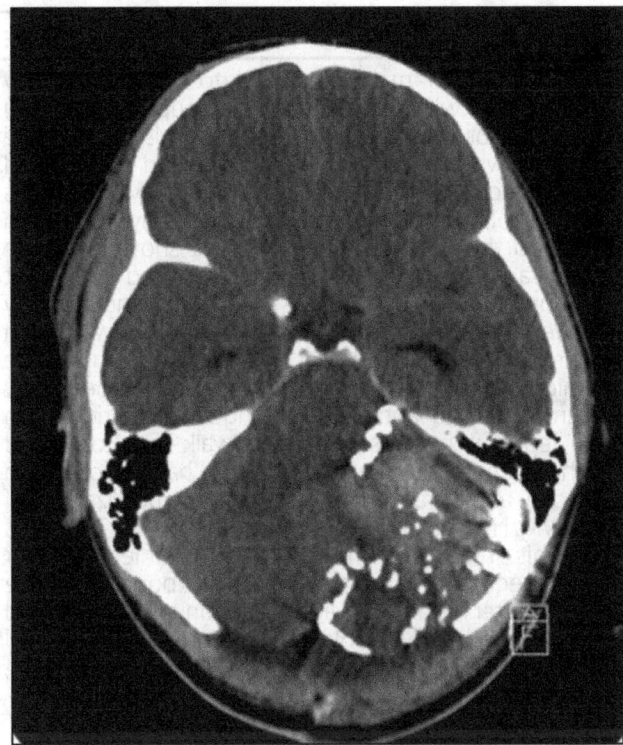

Figure 4-6. Axial noncontrast HCT demonstrating a suboccipital craniectomy for a cerebellar hemorrhage secondary to an AVM (white arrow) with associated hemorrhage.

FAMILY FOCUS BOX
1. Nontraumatic ICH (bleeding in the brain), also known as hemorrhagic stroke, may affect any infant, child, or teenager, even those who are otherwise healthy. Hemorrhagic strokes affect more than 1/100,000 children/year.
2. Abnormal blood vessels in the brain are responsible for the majority of cases of hemorrhagic stroke in children. These include AVMs, cavernous malformations (cavernomas), and aneurysms. Children with an inherited or acquired bleeding tendency are also at higher risk of intracerebral hemorrhage.
3. Common symptoms of ICH include severe headache, sleepiness or loss of consciousness, vomiting, weakness of part of the body, difficulty speaking or understanding language, and seizures. ICH is a medical emergency requiring urgent diagnosis and treatment. Diagnosis is made by imaging the brain and blood vessels in and around the brain. Common tests include HCT, brain MRI, and cerebral angiogram. Blood tests are done to check for a bleeding tendency.
4. Treatment often requires surgery to remove the blood and/or the abnormal blood vessels responsible for the hemorrhagic stroke. Some children develop hydrocephalus (increased fluid in the brain), which must be drained. Many children have persistent weakness or learning difficulties, and some have seizures. The potentially devastating outcomes affect all family members and require a tertiary hospital and specialized team of health care workers in order to provide the best care for the affected child.

CASE STUDY

An 11-year-old male presented to the trauma bay unresponsive with a unilateral dilated pupil (*blown pupil*) suggestive of brain herniation. He was in his normal state of health while playing a soccer game and complained of a headache. He progressively became drowsy and was unarousable upon arrival to the trauma bay. HCT upon arrival to the emergency department showed a large left intraparenchymal hemorrhage centered in the left temporal-parietal lobe (Figure 4-7) and CT angiography showed the cause for the ICH was an AVM. He was taken emergently to the operating room for a decompressive hemicraniectomy and clot evacuation. Postoperatively he improved to antigravity strength of his right arm and leg, but he was unable to walk and continued to have moderate hemiparesis. He had a follow-up cerebral angiogram and subsequent embolization of the AVM. He was taken to the operating room 2 months after his initial decompressive hemicraniectomy for AVM resection and replacement of his bone flap. Nine months after his hemorrhage, he continued to have mild hemiparesis but was able to walk independently and complete 75% of his daily activities, such as showering, independently.

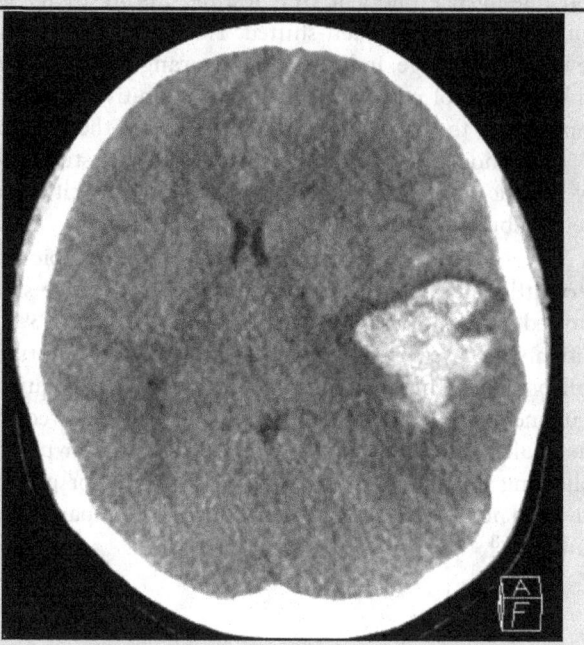

Figure 4-7. Axial noncontrast HCT demonstrating a large temporal-parietal ICH.

SUMMARY

Hemorrhagic stroke and SAH are uncommon, but very important, causes of pediatric neurological morbidity and mortality. Vascular malformations are the most common causes of ICH in children and require a multidisciplinary team and specialized tertiary care center to optimize care. Additional research studies are needed to evaluate the optimal management of pediatric ICH and SAH in order to minimize long-term neurological deficits.

REFERENCES

1. Fullerton HJ, Wu YW, Zhao S, Johnston SC. Risk of stroke in children: ethnic and gender disparities. *Neurology.* 2003;61(2):189-194.
2. Giroud M, Lemesle M, Madinier G, Manceau E, Osseby GV, Dumas R. Stroke in children under 16 years of age. Clinical and etiological difference with adults. *Acta Neurol Scand.* 1997;96(6):401-406.
3. Lynch JK, Hirtz DG, deVeber G, Nelson KB. Report of the National Institute of Neurological Disorders and Stroke workshop on perinatal and childhood stroke. *Pediatrics.* 2002;109(1):116-123.
4. Beslow LA, Jordan LC. Pediatric stroke: the importance of cerebral arteriopathy and vascular malformations. *Childs Nerv Syst.* 2010;26(10):1263-1273.
5. Jordan LC, Hillis AE. Hemorrhagic stroke in children. *Pediatr Neurol.* 2007;36(2):73-80.
6. Blom I, De Schryver EL, Kappelle LJ, Rinkel GJ, Jennekens-Schinkel A, Peters AC. Prognosis of haemorrhagic stroke in childhood: a long-term follow-up study. *Dev Med Child Neurol.* 2003;45(4):233-239.
7. Lynch JK, Han CJ. Pediatric stroke: what do we know and what do we need to know? *Semin Neurol.* 2005;25(4):410-423.
8. Al-Jarallah A, Al-Rifai MT, Riela AR, Roach ES. Nontraumatic brain hemorrhage in children: etiology and presentation. *J Child Neurol.* 2000;15(5):284-289.
9. Broderick J, Talbot GT, Prenger E, Leach A, Brott T. Stroke in children within a major metropolitan area: the surprising importance of intracerebral hemorrhage. *J Child Neurol.* 1993;8(3):250-255.
10. Jordan LC, Johnston SC, Wu YW, Sidney S, Fullerton HJ. The importance of cerebral aneurysms in childhood hemorrhagic stroke: a population-based study. *Stroke.* 2009;40(2):400-405.
11. Jordan LC, Kleinman JT, Hillis AE. Intracerebral hemorrhage volume predicts poor neurologic outcome in children. *Stroke.* 2009;40(5):1666-1671.
12. Meyer-Heim AD, Boltshauser E. Spontaneous intracranial haemorrhage in children: aetiology, presentation and outcome. *Brain Dev.* 2003;25(6):416-421.
13. Beslow LA, Licht DJ, Smith SE, et al. Predictors of outcome in childhood intracerebral hemorrhage: a prospective consecutive cohort study. *Stroke.* 2010;41(2):313-318.
14. Adams HP Jr, Kassell NF, Torner JC, Sahs AL. CT and clinical correlations in recent aneurysmal subarachnoid hemorrhage: a preliminary report of the Cooperative Aneurysm Study. *Neurology.* 1983;33(8):981-988.
15. Livingston JH, Brown JK. Intracerebral haemorrhage after the neonatal period. *Arch Dis Child.* 1986;61(6):538-544.
16. Butros LJ, Bussel JB. Intracranial hemorrhage in immune thrombocytopenic purpura: a retrospective analysis. *J Pediatr Hematol Oncol.* 2003;25(8):660-664.

17. Lilleyman JS. Intracranial haemorrhage in idiopathic thrombocytopenic purpura. Paediatric Haematology Forum of the British Society for Haematology. *Arch Dis Child.* 1994;71(3):251-253.

18. Woerner SJ, Abildgaard CF, French BN. Intracranial hemorrhage in children with idiopathic thrombocytopenic purpura. *Pediatrics.* 1981;67(4):453-460.

19. Nagel K, Pai MK, Paes BA, Chan AK. Diagnosis and treatment of intracranial hemorrhage in children with hemophilia. *Blood Coagul Fibrinolysis.* 2013;24(1):23-27.

20. Klinge J, Auberger K, Auerswald G, Brackmann HH, Mauz-Korholz C, Kreuz W. Prevalence and outcome of intracranial haemorrhage in haemophiliacs—a survey of the paediatric group of the German Society of Thrombosis and Haemostasis (GTH). *Eur J Pediatr.* 1999;158 Suppl 3:S162-165.

21. Yoffe G, Buchanan GR. Intracranial hemorrhage in newborn and young infants with hemophilia. *J Pediatr.* 1988;113(2):333-336.

22. Amin C, Sharathkumar A, Griest A. Bleeding diathesis and hemophilias. *Handb Clin Neurol.* 2014;120:1045-1059.

23. Earley CJ, Kittner SJ, Feeser BR, et al. Stroke in children and sickle-cell disease: Baltimore-Washington Cooperative Young Stroke Study. *Neurology.* 1998;51(1):169-176.

24. Roach ES, Golomb MR, Adams R, et al. Management of stroke in infants and children: a scientific statement from a Special Writing Group of the American Heart Association Stroke Council and the Council on Cardiovascular Disease in the Young. *Stroke.* 2008;39(9):2644-2691.

25. Strouse J, Hulbert M, DeBaun M, Jordan L, Casella J. Primary hemorrhagic stroke in children with sickle cell disease is associated with recent transfusion and use of corticosteroids. *Pediatrics.* 2006;118(5):1916-1924.

26. Atweh GF, DeSimone J, Saunthararajah Y, et al. Hemoglobinopathies. *Hematology Am Soc Hematol Educ Program.* 2003:14-39.

27. Preul MC, Cendes F, Just N, Mohr G. Intracranial aneurysms and sickle cell anemia: multiplicity and propensity for the vertebrobasilar territory. *Neurosurgery.* 1998;42(5):971-977; discussion 977-978.

28. Noje C, Cohen K, Jordan LC. Hemorrhagic and ischemic stroke in children with cancer. *Pediatr Neurol.* 2013;49(4):237-242.

29. Kyrnetskiy EE, Kun LE, Boop FA, Sanford RA, Khan RB. Types, causes, and outcome of intracranial hemorrhage in children with cancer. *J Neurosurg.* 2005;102(1 Suppl):31-35.

30. Ballabh P. Pathogenesis and prevention of intraventricular hemorrhage. *Clin Perinatol.* 2014;41(1):47-67.

31. Bruno CJ, Beslow LA, Witmer CM, et al. Haemorrhagic stroke in term and late preterm neonates. *Arch Dis Child Fetal Neonatal Ed.* 2014;99(1):F48-F53.

32. Goodman S, Pavlakis S. Pediatric and newborn stroke. *Curr Treat Options Neurol.* 2008;10(6):431-439.

33. Brouwer AJ, Groenendaal F, Koopman C, Nievelstein RJ, Han SK, de Vries LS. Intracranial hemorrhage in full-term newborns: a hospital-based cohort study. *Neuroradiology.* 2010;52(6):567-576.

34. Schulte R, Jordan LC, Morad A, Naftel RP, Wellons JC III, Sidonio R. Rise in late onset vitamin K deficiency bleeding in young infants because of omission or refusal of prophylaxis at birth. *Pediatr Neurol.* 2014;50(6):564-568.

35. Ijland MM, Pereira RR, Cornelissen EA. Incidence of late vitamin K deficiency bleeding in newborns in the Netherlands in 2005: evaluation of the current guideline. *Eur J Pediatr.* 2008;167(2):165-169.

36. Demiroren K, Yavuz H, Cam L. Intracranial hemorrhage due to vitamin K deficiency after the newborn period. *Pediatr Hematol Oncol.* 2004;21(7):585-592.

37. Mendelow AD, Gregson BA, Rowan EN, Murray GD, Gholkar A, Mitchell PM. Early surgery versus initial conservative treatment in patients with spontaneous supratentorial lobar intracerebral haematomas (STICH II): a randomised trial. *Lancet.* 2013;382(9890):397-408.

38. Mendelow AD, Gregson BA, Fernandes HM, et al. Early surgery versus initial conservative treatment in patients with spontaneous supratentorial intracerebral haematomas in the International Surgical Trial in Intracerebral Haemorrhage (STICH): a randomised trial. *Lancet.* 2005;365(9457):387-397.

39. Morgenstern LB, Hemphill JC III, Anderson C, et al. Guidelines for the management of spontaneous intracerebral hemorrhage: a guideline for healthcare professionals from the American Heart Association/American Stroke Association. *Stroke.* 2010;41(9):2108-2129.

40. Broderick J, Connolly S, Feldmann E, et al. Guidelines for the management of spontaneous intracerebral hemorrhage in adults: 2007 update: a guideline from the American Heart Association/American Stroke Association Stroke Council, High Blood Pressure Research Council, and the Quality of Care and Outcomes in Research Interdisciplinary Working Group. *Stroke.* 2007;38(6):2001-2023.

41. Wang YF, Wu JS, Mao Y, Chen XC, Zhou LF, Zhang Y. The optimal time-window for surgical treatment of spontaneous intracerebral hemorrhage: result of prospective randomized controlled trial of 500 cases. *Acta Neurochir Suppl.* 2008;105:141-145.

42. Bakker NA, Groen RJ, Foumani M, et al. Appreciation of CT-negative, lumbar puncture-positive subarachnoid haemorrhage: risk factors for presence of aneurysms and diagnostic yield of imaging. *J Neurol Neurosurg Psychiatry.* 2013;85(8):885-888.

43. Horstman P, Linn FH, Voorbij HA, Rinkel GJ. Chance of aneurysm in patients suspected of SAH who have a 'negative' CT scan but a 'positive' lumbar puncture. *J Neurol.* 2012;259(4):649-652.

44. Kidwell CS, Chalela JA, Saver JL, et al. Comparison of MRI and CT for detection of acute intracerebral hemorrhage. *JAMA.* 2004;292(15):1823-1830.

45. Liu AC, Segaren N, Cox TS, et al. Is there a role for magnetic resonance imaging in the evaluation of non-traumatic intraparenchymal haemorrhage in children? *Pediatr Radiol.* 2006;36(9):940-946.

46. Lang SS, Beslow LA, Bailey RL, et al. Follow-up imaging to detect recurrence of surgically treated pediatric arteriovenous malformations. *J Neurosurg Pediatr.* 2012;9(5):497-504.

47. Goren O, Monteith SJ, Hadani M, Bakon M, Harnof S. Modern intraoperative imaging modalities for the vascular neurosurgeon treating intracerebral hemorrhage. *Neurosurg Focus.* 2013;34(5):E2.

48. Burger IM, Murphy KJ, Jordan LC, Tamargo RJ, Gailloud P. Safety of cerebral digital subtraction angiography in children: complication rate analysis in 241 consecutive diagnostic angiograms. *Stroke.* 2006;37(10):2535-2539.

49. Woodfield J, Rane N, Cudlip S, Byrne JV. Value of delayed MRI in angiogram-negative subarachnoid haemorrhage. *Clin Radiol.* 2014;69(4):350-356.

50. Delgado Almandoz JE, Kadkhodayan Y, Crandall BM, et al. Diagnostic yield of delayed neurovascular imaging in patients with subarachnoid hemorrhage, negative initial CT and catheter angiograms, and a negative 7 day repeat catheter angiogram. *J Neurointerv Surg.* 2013;34(4):833-839.

51. Dalyai R, Chalouhi N, Theofanis T, et al. Subarachnoid hemorrhage with negative initial catheter angiography: a review of 254 cases evaluating patient clinical outcome and efficacy of short- and long-term repeat angiography. *Neurosurgery.* 2013;72(4):646-652.

52. Zuccarello M, Brott T, Derex L, et al. Early surgical treatment for supratentorial intracerebral hemorrhage: a randomized feasibility study. *Stroke.* 1999;30(9):1833-1839.

53. Lau D, El-Sayed AM, Ziewacz JE, et al. Postoperative outcomes following closed head injury and craniotomy for evacuation of hematoma in patients older than 80 years. *J Neurosurg.* 2012;116(1):234-245.

54. Kumar R, Shukla D, Mahapatra AK. Spontaneous intracranial hemorrhage in children. *Pediatr Neurosurg.* 2009;45(1):37-45.

55. Chadduck WM, Duong DH, Kast JM, Donahue DJ. Pediatric cerebellar hemorrhages. *Childs Nerv Syst.* 1995;11(10):579-583.

56. Delashaw JB, Broaddus WC, Kassell NF, et al. Treatment of right hemispheric cerebral infarction by hemicraniectomy. *Stroke.* 1990;21(6):874-881.

57. Weiner GM, Lacey MR, Mackenzie L, et al. Decompressive craniectomy for elevated intracranial pressure and its effect on the cumulative ischemic burden and therapeutic intensity levels after severe traumatic brain injury. *Neurosurgery.* 2010;66(6):1111-1118; discussion 1118-1119.

58. Vahedi K, Hofmeijer J, Juettler E, et al. Early decompressive surgery in malignant infarction of the middle cerebral artery: a pooled analysis of three randomised controlled trials. *Lancet Neurol.* 2007;6(3):215-222.

59. Montgomery AK, Maixner WJ, Wallace D, Wray A, Mackay MT. Decompressive craniectomy in childhood posterior circulation stroke: a case series and review of the literature. *Pediatr Neurol.* 2012;47(3):193-197.

60. Cooper DJ, Rosenfeld JV, Murray L, et al. Decompressive craniectomy in diffuse traumatic brain injury. *N Engl J Med.* 2011;364(16):1493-1502.

61. Smith SE, Kirkham FJ, Deveber G, et al. Outcome following decompressive craniectomy for malignant middle cerebral artery infarction in children. *Dev Med Child Neurol.* 2011;53(1):29-33.

62. Hetherington R, Tuff L, Anderson P, Miles B, deVeber G. Short-term intellectual outcome after arterial ischemic stroke and sinovenous thrombosis in childhood and infancy. *J Child Neurol.* 2005;20(7):553-559.

63. Ganesan V, Hogan A, Shack N, Gordon A, Isaacs E, Kirkham FJ. Outcome after ischaemic stroke in childhood. *Dev Med Child Neurol.* 2000;42(7):455-461.

64. Fullerton HJ, Wu YW, Sidney S, Johnston SC. Recurrent hemorrhagic stroke in children: a population-based cohort study. *Stroke.* 2007;38(10):2658-2662.

65. Fullerton HJ, Chetkovich DM, Wu YW, Smith WS, Johnston SC. Deaths from stroke in US children, 1979 to 1998. *Neurology.* 2002;59(1):34-39.

66. Adil MM, Qureshi AI, Beslow LA, Malik AA, Jordan LC. Factors associated with increased in-hospital mortality among children with intracerebral hemorrhage. *J Child Neurol.* 2015;30(8):1024-1028.

67. Beslow LA, Abend NS, Gindville MC, et al. Pediatric intracerebral hemorrhage: acute symptomatic seizures and epilepsy. *JAMA Neurol.* 2013;70(4):448-454.

68. Smith SE, Vargas G, Cucchiara AJ, Zelonis SJ, Beslow LA. Hemiparesis and epilepsy are associated with worse reported health status following unilateral stroke in children. *Pediatr Neurol.* 2015;52(4):428-434.

Suggested Readings

Jordan LC, Hillis AE. Hemorrhagic stroke in children. *Pediatr Neurol.* 2007;36(2):73-80.

Jordan LC, Kleinman JT, Hillis AE. Intracerebral hemorrhage volume predicts poor neurologic outcome in children. *Stroke.* 2009;40(5):1666-1671.

Zuccarello M, Brott T, Derex L, et al. Early surgical treatment for supratentorial intracerebral hemorrhage: a randomized feasibility study. *Stroke.* 1999;30(9):1833-1839.

5

The Provision of Rehabilitation Medicine Across the Continuum of Care in Pediatric Stroke

Phillip R. Bryant, DO

The continuum of care for stroke management spans the clinical course of a patient from their acute episode to their long-term management. This continuum of stroke care involves primary prevention and health promotion, as well as public awareness and education. It involves the acute management of stroke episodes, most notably exemplified by the availability of stroke alerts within hours of an episode at multiple medical centers and stroke centers where highly trained and experienced stroke specialists provide acute medical management in intensive care units. After acute medical stabilization, the continuum of care incorporates stroke rehabilitation assessment and therapeutic intervention as tolerated by the patient.

Stroke rehabilitation initially begins in the acute care setting after the diagnosis of stroke is established and life-threatening complications are under acceptable control. It subsequently transitions to a postacute environment, which includes home, inpatient rehabilitation, day hospital rehabilitation, outpatient rehabilitation, long-term skilled facility care, or palliative care. The continuum also includes secondary prevention measures, particularly in those patients in whom a recurrent stroke event is highly likely and measures are available to decrease the risk. For some patients, the anticipated goal is eventual community reintegration. This includes return to home, school, or pre-morbid work environment (applicable to older adolescents already engaged in the work force), or an alternative work site if residual deficits preclude return to their work.

The goals of stroke rehabilitation in the acute care setting include the following: timely participation in the acute care management of patients who have incurred an acute stroke in collaboration with the attending physician; the identification of precautions and the early implementation of preventive measures applicable to the patient; the prevention of medical and psychological complications; the assessment, documentation, and prescription of interventions to address residual impairments; and the prescription of selective rehabilitation therapies, orthotics, and assistive devices as deemed appropriate. Secondary prevention is fundamental to minimizing the potential for recurrent strokes. Standardized evaluations and valid assessment tools are essential and add credibility to the development of a comprehensive rehabilitation treatment plan. Evidence-based interventions are optimally based on both medical and functional goals.

Ideally, pediatric patients requiring stroke rehabilitation have access to an interprofessional, well-experienced, and well-coordinated team of rehabilitation specialists. This coordinated care is not always addressed by a multiprofessional approach where multiple individuals work in parallel but fail to collaboratively work toward a common goal. Such fragmented care can actually hinder rather than promote functional recovery by fostering sometimes conflicting goals, by creating vulnerability to miscommunication, and by disrupting the proper sequence of care, thus creating confusion in the care plan. An interprofessional team, on the other hand, works collaboratively, synergistically, and collectively to facilitate a patient's transition from the acute to postacute phases of their stroke recovery and optimize a patient's clinical and functional outcomes. The latter approach is much more likely to promote a timely and more appropriate sequence of rehabilitation interventions.

Atkinson HL, Nixon-Cave K, Smith SE, eds.
Pediatric Stroke Rehabilitation: An Interprofessional and Collaborative Approach (pp 69-88). © 2018 Taylor & Francis Group.

Such an interprofessional team typically includes an admission coordinator, pediatric rehabilitation physician specialist (pediatric physiatrist), rehabilitation nurses, dietitian, social worker, case manager, rehabilitation psychologist, physical and occupational therapists, and speech and language pathologist. In some inpatient rehabilitation units, a nurse practitioner or pediatric hospitalist may also be an integral part of this team. In those centers where the resources are available, a school teacher, child life specialist, and music and art therapist add incremental value to the quality of care provided.

It is imperative to involve the patient, when cognitively and behaviorally capable, and the family and/or caregiver in the poststroke assessment and management process. Family education, including periodic family meetings, leads to improved and informed decision making; minimizes miscommunication; avoids misunderstandings regarding expectations; and aligns the patient, family, and rehabilitation team toward shared goals, which hopefully results in an improved functional outcome and an appropriate disposition.

Well-functioning and coordinated interprofessional rehabilitation teams also effectively utilize community resources, including school services, to help a patient reintegrate back into the community. Patients poststroke may have significant residual medical problems or complications that require ongoing medical surveillance or intervention, as well as formal accommodations to permit their return to the school or work environment. Timely and prompt management of these medical challenges and associated risk factors is essential to preventing complications, including recurrent strokes.

REHABILITATION IN THE ACUTE CARE SETTING

Rehabilitation medicine is typically perceived as an intervention that occurs in the postacute care phase of a patient's stroke management. In actuality, the process of rehabilitation medicine should be implemented shortly after a patient's onset of a stroke in the acute care setting. Ideally, stroke rehabilitation occurs as soon as the patient's life-threatening acute care issues are stabilized and effectively controlled. The initial rehabilitation intervention may be limited to a brief assessment only if the patient is significantly medically compromised and marginally stable. However, as the patient recovers, the intensity and frequency of intervention of rehabilitation services should correspondingly increase to facilitate functional recovery.

The highest priorities during the early phase of a patient's recovery include the prevention of life-threatening medical problems and the prevention of recurrent stroke and its associated complications. Examples of potential clinical priorities include prompt medical interventions to prevent recurrent ischemic or hemorrhagic stroke, the identification and management of hydrocephalus, the prompt treatment of respiratory compromise, the avoidance of hemodynamic complications (including hyper- or hypotension), the management of electrolyte imbalances, the improvement of suboptimal nutritional intake, the prevention of deep vein thrombosis and pulmonary emboli, precautions to prevent aspiration pneumonia, and the avoidance of falls.

Although not typically life threatening and therefore not the highest initial priority, the prevention of pressure sore development and joint contractures has high importance as the patient recovers and proceeds through his or her rehabilitation course because of the morbidity, pain, and high costs associated with their occurrence. The proper management of poststroke depression, emotional lability, and behavioral disturbances also merits focused attention, and this attention should begin early in a patient's course. Optimally, the management of these problems begins in the acute care setting and extends into the postacute care phase. The patient's emotional and cognitive status can have a significant influence on a patient's willingness to participate in rehabilitation therapies, their capacity to learn, and their ability to retain what they have been taught, including carryover into their daily functional activities. In addition, deterioration of executive-level skills, such as impaired immediate, short-term, and/or long-term memory and expressive and receptive language skills deficits, as well as deficiencies in judgment, problem solving, and motor planning, merit formal attention early in a patient's course but typically require a more prolonged course of therapeutic intervention, which often extends beyond the acute and subacute phases of stroke rehabilitation.

Rehabilitation services in the acute care setting are provided by acute care therapists (physical and occupational therapists, and speech and language pathologists). The frequency of the rehabilitation therapies are limited in the acute care setting by the medical stability of the patient and the number of therapists available to provide the service. Nevertheless, the early introduction of rehabilitation therapies in a patient's course can significantly facilitate their functional recovery and prevent the multiple complications associated with immobilization, including deconditioning, joint contractures, pressure sore development, weakness, and deep vein thrombosis. In addition, the emotional health of the patient may be enhanced by the early intervention of these therapists.

INPATIENT REHABILITATION

When the patient transitions to the inpatient rehabilitation unit, more comprehensive and more frequent rehabilitation services are provided. Such services include rehabilitation nursing provided 24 hours/day, physician rounds daily,

TABLE 5-1. PRINCIPLES OF REHABILITATION
■ Prevent poststroke complications
■ Minimize functional impairments
■ Maximize function and encourage resumption of premorbid, age-appropriate self-care activities
■ Promote independence in the performance of activities of daily life
■ Provide early assessment and intervention by a team of rehabilitation specialists
■ Promote and apply evidence-based interventions based on functional outcomes
■ Acknowledge and incorporate the patient, the family, and other caregivers in the recovery and rehabilitation process
■ Provide ongoing patient, family, and other caregiver education regarding the medical and rehabilitation interventions
■ Collaboratively and synergistically work as a rehabilitation team to optimize a patient's functional outcome and well-being
■ Utilize hospital and community resources to promote functional recovery and community integration
■ Provide ongoing medical surveillance and intervention as clinically warranted while simultaneously progressing functionally
■ Address risk factors and manage co-morbidities, including implementation of prevention measures, to prevent or minimize a recurrent stroke
These principles are applicable to both the adult and pediatric populations.

dietary evaluation and recommendations by a dietitian as clinically appropriate, physical and occupational therapy—each typically provided twice/day for 5 to 7 days/week—and speech and language therapy at a frequency dependent on a patient's specific needs. Likewise, social work, case management, and psychology services are typically provided at a frequency warranted by the patient's condition. In addition, school services are provided on the inpatient unit at a frequency based on a patient's functional progress and their availability relative to the other services being provided.

Although the multiple professionals and the frequency of their services provided to the patient in the inpatient rehabilitation setting is of particular significance, of comparable value is the communication and coordination of these services among these disciplines. The Agency for Healthcare Policy and Research Guideline for Post-Stroke Rehabilitation concluded[1]:

> A considerable body of evidence, mainly from countries in Western Europe, indicates that better clinical outcomes are achieved when patients with acute stroke are treated in a setting that provides coordinated, multidisciplinary stroke-related evaluation and services. Skilled staff, better organization of services, and earlier implementation of rehabilitation interventions appear to be important components.

The value of interprofessional teams in addressing patients incurring a stroke is well-established. Early rehabilitation following a stroke has been acknowledged to be an effective intervention in enhancing functional recovery and minimizing disability.[2] Specific principles of rehabilitation are particularly applicable to the pediatric population (Table 5-1).

In addition, the type of inpatient rehabilitation (interprofessional vs multiprofessional) is a predictor of outcome following a stroke. An interdisciplinary setting is one in which clinical services are provided by diverse professionals who communicate regularly and collaboratively use their respective areas of expertise and experience to work toward a common goal. This is in contrast to multidisciplinary settings in which the participating clinical professionals may have less consistent communication and less deliberate alignment of goals. Interdisciplinary, in contrast to multidisciplinary, inpatient rehabilitation is strongly associated with improved functional outcome, shorter length of stay, and decreased costs and mortality.[3] Other predictors for improved outcome at hospital discharge and follow-up are increased functional skills on admission to rehabilitation and early initiation of rehabilitation services.

The well-organized and well-coordinated team approach among the various health care providers in the inpatient rehabilitation unit should be continued for patients discharged to a home-based, day hospital rehabilitation, or outpatient rehabilitation clinic setting. Deliberate and coordinated utilization of community resources for stroke rehabilitation can augment the care initiated in the acute care and rehabilitation unit settings and provide valuable support to further improve or sustain functional gains achieved in the acute and subacute phases of a patient's rehabilitation course.

The highly variable clinical presentations, particularly in the pediatric population, and the equally variable functional outcomes make it impractical to offer a single clinical pathway for children and adolescents who incur a stroke. However, general principles of stroke rehabilitation management are applicable and appropriate for the majority of these patients.

ROLE OF THE PEDIATRIC REHABILITATION PHYSICIAN SPECIALIST (PEDIATRIC PHYSIATRIST)

Early inpatient consultation by a pediatric rehabilitation physician specialist (*pediatric physiatrist*) on a patient in the acute care setting allows him or her to assess the severity of the patient's initial clinical presentation and participate in the diagnostic workup. It also offers the pediatric physiatrist an opportunity to suggest and implement early rehabilitation measures to assist in a patient's acute care, including recommendations to prevent potential complications. It additionally permits the pediatric physiatrist to participate in facilitating patient flow from the acute to the postacute care setting. Subsequent follow-up in the acute care setting as a patient progresses allows the pediatric physiatrist, in coordination with the inpatient attending physician, to identify the most appropriate time for discharge from the acute care setting. It also allows the consultant an opportunity to participate in the decision regarding disposition to the most appropriate level of care for the patient. The participation of the pediatric physiatrist in the acute care setting also helps identify pertinent precautionary measures that may require carryover into the post-acute care setting, such as weight-bearing precautions, exercise and range-of-motion restrictions, deep vein thrombosis and systemic embolic prophylaxis, aspiration precautions, hemodynamic parameters, seizure prophylaxis, and special wound care measures, if applicable.

ROLE OF REHABILITATION NURSES

Rehabilitation nurses play a critical role in the care of the pediatric stroke patient. Their close daily surveillance of the child's medical stability and administration of their specific nursing care needs are particularly important in the early identification and prevention of potential medical complications. They also serve a pivotal role in educating patients and families regarding their medical care and, in coordination with the rehabilitation therapists, help prepare patients and families for transition to home or an alternative patient care facility. They may also cotreat patients in coordination with the rehabilitation therapists to facilitate a patient's recovery of their activities of daily living skills.

ROLE OF THE DIETITIAN

Many pediatric stroke patients experience significant dysphagia and require special attention to ensuring they receive adequate nutritional intake. Because their dietary needs and mode of delivery of nutrition may change over time, periodic re-evaluation of their nutritional needs is required during their inpatient course and may also be necessary postdischarge on an outpatient basis.

ROLE OF ACUTE CARE REHABILITATION THERAPISTS

Early referral for evaluation and therapeutic intervention by rehabilitation therapists, including physical and occupational therapists, as well as speech and language therapists, in the acute care setting permits them an opportunity to initiate appropriate rehabilitation services early in the clinical course as soon as the patient is medically stable enough to accommodate such intervention. Physical therapists perform baseline and follow-up assessments of a patient's motor abilities, focus on providing exercises and activities to facilitate functional mobility, normalize gait patterns to the extent possible, increase core and extremity strength, improve balance and gross motor coordination, and provide progressive endurance training. Occupational therapists perform baseline and follow-up assessments of a patient's upper extremity fine motor function, strength, and coordination and provide exercises and activities to optimize functional independence in the performance of their age-appropriate activities of daily living. Speech and language therapists perform baseline evaluations and follow-up assessments of a patient's swallowing function and speech and language skills, including higher-level executive functions, and provide recommendations and precautions to progressively enhance a child's swallowing function.

Rehabilitation therapy services can be critical in mobilizing patients sooner in their recovery, thus preventing the multiple complications associated with immobilization, including deconditioning, muscle atrophy, contractures, deep vein thromboses, constipation, pressure sores, and aspiration. Close communication between the pediatric physiatrist and the rehabilitation therapists on patients on whom they are mutually consulted is important to ensure that the patient receives well-coordinated, timely, and appropriate rehabilitation services. Close communication also helps minimize the potential for conflicting recommendations to the attending medical team. The acute rehabilitation therapists and pediatric rehabilitation physician consultant ideally also communicate on an ongoing basis regarding the optimal level of care necessary for a patient when they transition out of the acute care setting. Close collaboration between the rehabilitation therapists and pediatric rehabilitation consultant helps avoid potential conflicting recommendations regarding rehabilitation management and discharge disposition.

ROLE OF THE CASE MANAGER (OR SOCIAL WORKER)

The case manager or social worker in the acute care setting should typically begin preparation for a patient's discharge shortly after his or her arrival in the acute care setting. Multiple factors are involved in the disposition of patients, including medical stability, willingness to participate in rehabilitation therapies, the motivation of the family and patient to transition to a postacute setting, the patient's ability to participate and progress in rehabilitation, and insurance status. If it is deemed by the pediatric physiatrist consultant that a patient's clinical presentation warrants inpatient rehabilitation, the case manager in the acute care setting works closely with the admission coordinator and case manager on the inpatient rehabilitation unit to facilitate the transition of the patient from the acute to the postacute care setting. When a patient has completed the inpatient rehabilitation program, the case manager in the rehabilitation unit actively assists in the patient's preparation for discharge, which may be to a day hospital setting, if it is available and deemed necessary, or to home. On occasion, the case manager in the rehabilitation setting may assist in the patient's preparations for discharge to a long-term facility. Alternatively, a patient who has residual deficits requiring ongoing rehabilitation therapies may be best served by outpatient rehabilitation therapies in the community, optimally in close proximity to his or her home.

ROLE OF THE ADMISSIONS COORDINATOR/LIAISON

Some inpatient rehabilitation programs employ a liaison who serves as an admission coordinator (AC). He or she often has a nursing background but may include individuals with prior social work, case management, or rehabilitation therapy training and experience. He or she communicates with case managers and referring providers in the acute care setting regarding patients potentially appropriate for inpatient rehabilitation. He or she also communicates on a frequent basis with the pediatric rehabilitation physician assigned to perform inpatient consultations in the acute care setting and with the attending physician on the inpatient rehabilitation unit.

The AC is responsible for care coordination and the transition of appropriate patients from the acute care hospital to the acute inpatient rehabilitation unit. The AC may be solely focused on facilitating admission to the inpatient rehabilitation unit from the acute care hospital in which the rehabilitation unit is integrated. In other health systems, the AC also has a regional role and helps to facilitate patient admissions from other hospitals in the region.

The AC maintains a close relationship with patient referral sources and the case management team to facilitate timely communication and eliminate delays in admission. He or she also often serves as the central point of contact for inpatient and day hospital rehabilitation referrals and triage referrals to the appropriate interdisciplinary team member. They gather intake information such as patient demographics, insurance information, updated medical status, diagnosis, social contact, and current functional status. They review all patient referrals based upon established rehabilitation admission criteria and consultations by the rehabilitation clinical team. They periodically provide the rehabilitation interprofessional team with a status update on the discharge readiness of the patients and potential patient referrals from the acute care setting. They discuss challenges and potential barriers anticipated with some referrals, such as need for social clearances, psychosocial issues, insurance considerations, and medical readiness for a rehabilitation admission. They collaborate with the interprofessional rehabilitation team, including both the acute care therapists and the attending physician and the therapists on the inpatient rehabilitation unit, in the decision-making process to admit or deny a given patient, or offer alternative recommendations for disposition to the referring source. They schedule the admission of patients to the inpatient rehabilitation unit when medical readiness and insurance clearances are obtained and a bed is available. They also coordinate with the bed management staff to assure appropriate bed assignment.

INPATIENT REHABILITATION ADMISSION CRITERIA

It is important that an inpatient rehabilitation unit establish admission criteria appropriate for their particular unit. Basic principles of admission apply to most inpatient rehabilitation units, including the following: 1) the ability to participate in the rehabilitation therapies; 2) the ability to tolerate the rehabilitation therapies; 3) the patient's willingness to participate in the rehabilitation therapies;

TABLE 5-2. INPATIENT REHABILITATION ADMISSION CRITERIA: MEDICAL GUIDELINES
■ Patient is medically stable at the time of admission.
□ Stable, clear airway
◘ May have a tracheostomy tube, but does not require pressure support via a ventilator
□ Stable oxygen requirements for the past 24 hours
□ Oxygen requirement of 40% oxygen supplementation or less
□ No fever within last 24 hours (unless due to central fevers)
□ No worsening neutropenia
□ Stable blood pressure and heart rate without need for pressors for the past 48 hours (no acute interventions)
□ No unexplained worsening of the neurological status within the past 24 hours
□ Not actively experiencing ketoacidosis
□ Baseline labs within an acceptable range for at least 48 hours
□ Platelets > 30,000
■ Patient requires close medical surveillance and potential periodic intervention to maintain clinical stability and enhance recovery.
An example of potential criteria for admission to an inpatient rehabilitation unit.

4) the patient's medical stability; 5) the patient's potential for functional recovery; and 6) anticipated disposition to home. The specific details regarding medical stability may, however, vary between one pediatric rehabilitation unit and another. The variation will depend on the scope of care of the nursing and medical staff; the expertise and experience of the nursing, medical staff, and rehabilitation therapists; the nature of the physical environment; the resources available to the unit patients; specific hospital rules, regulations, and policies; the availability of medical coverage; the availability of pediatric specialists; and the availability of radiology, ultrasound, laboratory services, and other diagnostic studies. Table 5-2 illustrates one example of medical guidelines for admission criteria. Table 5-3 is an example of potential exclusion criteria.

As noted earlier, the specific admission criteria may vary among rehabilitation units, but formally establishing and periodically revising the criteria as necessary will help ensure consistency in the admission process and minimize confusion for referring services regarding a patient's appropriateness for admission to the inpatient rehabilitation unit. For example, patients who are persistently febrile may harbor an underlying infectious process that may require additional workup and medical management in the acute care setting. Patients with excessively low platelets may be prone to bleeding in their joints with aggressive range-of-motion and resistive exercises. Immunosuppressed patients with significant neutropenia may be at high risk of an infectious process and may require special precautions that limit their ability to fully engage in their inpatient rehabilitation program. Also, patients who have unstable airways, high oxygen requirements, or become cyanotic with minimal exercise often have markedly limited endurance and an inability to actively engage in progressive, intensive inpatient rehabilitation therapies. They may be more appropriately managed in a setting with lower-intensity rehabilitation therapies.

Functional appropriateness for admission to an inpatient rehabilitation unit requires consideration of a number of variables. Table 5-4 outlines several of these key variables when making this decision. Table 5-5 is a checklist of questions that may be helpful when assessing a patient for appropriateness for admission. Some pediatric rehabilitation services have special programs, resources, and expertise that permit them to accommodate selected patient populations (Table 5-6).

Approval for admission to an inpatient rehabilitation unit requires medical necessity for ongoing medical management or surveillance and rehabilitation justification for comprehensive rehabilitation therapies. Figure 5-1 describes a typical process involved in admitting a patient from the acute care setting to an inpatient rehabilitation unit. A formal interprofessional rehabilitation care plan is necessary to justify continuation of the rehabilitation services in an inpatient rehabilitation unit. The care plan is typically

TABLE 5-3. INPATIENT REHABILITATION EXCLUSION CRITERIA: MEDICAL GUIDELINES

- Predominantly psychiatric or severe, functionally limiting psychiatric condition
- Medical condition(s) that disrupts the ability of therapists to consistently provide rehabilitation therapies
- Medical condition(s) that limits the patient's ability to receive consistent rehabilitation therapies

Potential criteria for exclusion from admission to an inpatient rehabilitation unit.

TABLE 5-4. INPATIENT ADMISSION: FUNCTIONAL APPROPRIATENESS

- Patient demonstrates a favorable potential for progressive functional improvement through rehabilitative therapies at the time of admission.
- Patient has needs and goals that can be met by the rehabilitation services/programs offered.
- Patient will be capable of tolerating the rehabilitation therapy frequency, duration, and intensity provided in the inpatient rehabilitation program.
- Patient has functional impairment(s) that will improve with physical, occupational, and/or speech therapy, with an interdisciplinary team approach.

Key variables affecting a patient's appropriateness for admission to an inpatient rehabilitation unit.

TABLE 5-5. CHECKLIST OF QUESTIONS FOR POTENTIAL INPATIENT REHABILITATION PATIENTS

- Does the patient have a favorable prognosis for functional improvement?
- Would he or she benefit from the intensity and comprehensive services provided in an inpatient rehabilitation setting?
- Does he or she have additional diagnostic work-up pending?
- What additional diagnostic workup is required and how long will it take to accomplish?
- Are the results of the workup likely to affect whether or not the patient is a candidate for inpatient rehabilitation?
- Does he or she have additional therapeutic intervention(s) required prior to admission to inpatient rehabilitation?
- Will he or she require additional diagnostic, surgical, or other invasive intervention(s) within a short period of time after admission to the rehabilitation unit?
- Is the family interested and willing to come to inpatient rehabilitation?
- Is the patient interested and willing to come to inpatient rehabilitation?
- Does the family live in or outside of the region?
- Are all pertinent rehabilitation therapies ordered?
- Are rehabilitation therapies being done at sufficient frequency to warrant inpatient rehabilitation (need for daily therapies are required by some insurances)?
- What is the recommendation of the rehabilitation therapists regarding inpatient rehabilitation vs day hospital rehabilitation vs outpatient therapies vs return to home?
- Is he or she a better candidate for day hospital admission?
- Is he or she a better candidate for outpatient rehabilitation?

(continued)

TABLE 5-5 (CONTINUED). CHECKLIST OF QUESTIONS FOR POTENTIAL INPATIENT REHABILITATION PATIENTS
■ What rehabilitation therapies will he or she need when he or she arrives on the inpatient rehabilitation unit, including any need for a psychology consultation?
■ What medical management/surveillance will he or she need when he or she arrives on the inpatient rehabilitation unit?
■ What specialist(s) should be consulted upon arrival to the inpatient rehabilitation unit?
■ When will he or she be ready for admission to inpatient rehabilitation?
■ How long do you anticipate he or she will need inpatient rehabilitation?
■ Are there any major patient and/or family psychosocial issues that are likely to impact on admission and duration of stay?
■ Are there any major financial/insurance barriers to admitting the patient on the inpatient rehabilitation service?
■ Will the patient require a formal appeal for admission to inpatient rehabilitation following a denial?
Checklist of questions that may be helpful when assessing a patient for appropriateness for admission to an inpatient rehabilitation unit.

TABLE 5-6. SPECIAL PROGRAMS
■ Stable but ventilator-dependent respiratory insufficiency
■ Stable but complex medical and post-operative conditions
□ Heart transplant
□ Lung transplant
□ Liver transplant
□ Tumor resection
□ Complex orthopedic procedures, including spine surgery
■ Severe but stable spinal cord injuries and disorders
■ Minimally responsive post-brain injury or disease (but with anticipation of functional improvement)
■ Neuromuscular disorders (such as Duchenne muscular dystrophy, congenital myopathies, and spinal muscular atrophy)
■ Neurodegenerative disorders (for evaluation of functional status and equipment needs in preparation for transition back to home)
■ Day hospital (for patients requiring comprehensive rehabilitation therapies on a daily basis but who are stable enough to return to their home at night)
Some pediatric rehabilitation services have special programs, resources, and expertise that permit them to accommodate selected patient populations based on their underlying diagnoses.

discussed in an interprofessional team meeting held within a reasonable time after a patient's admission. Planning for discharge begins at the time of the patient's admission.

Whenever feasible, diagnostic workup should typically be done in the acute care setting prior to discharge and admission to an inpatient rehabilitation unit. The patient's willingness to consistently participate in his or her inpatient rehabilitation therapies and the parents' support in the rehabilitation process are critical to ensuring successful functional gains and outcomes.

HANDOFF OF COMMUNICATION

One of the most important transitions in a patient's continuum of care is the discharge from the acute care setting to the inpatient rehabilitation unit. When the inpatient rehabilitation unit is an integral part of the acute care hospital from which the patient is referred, there is sometimes confusion as to whether or not the patient is transferred or discharged and admitted to the inpatient rehabilitation. As

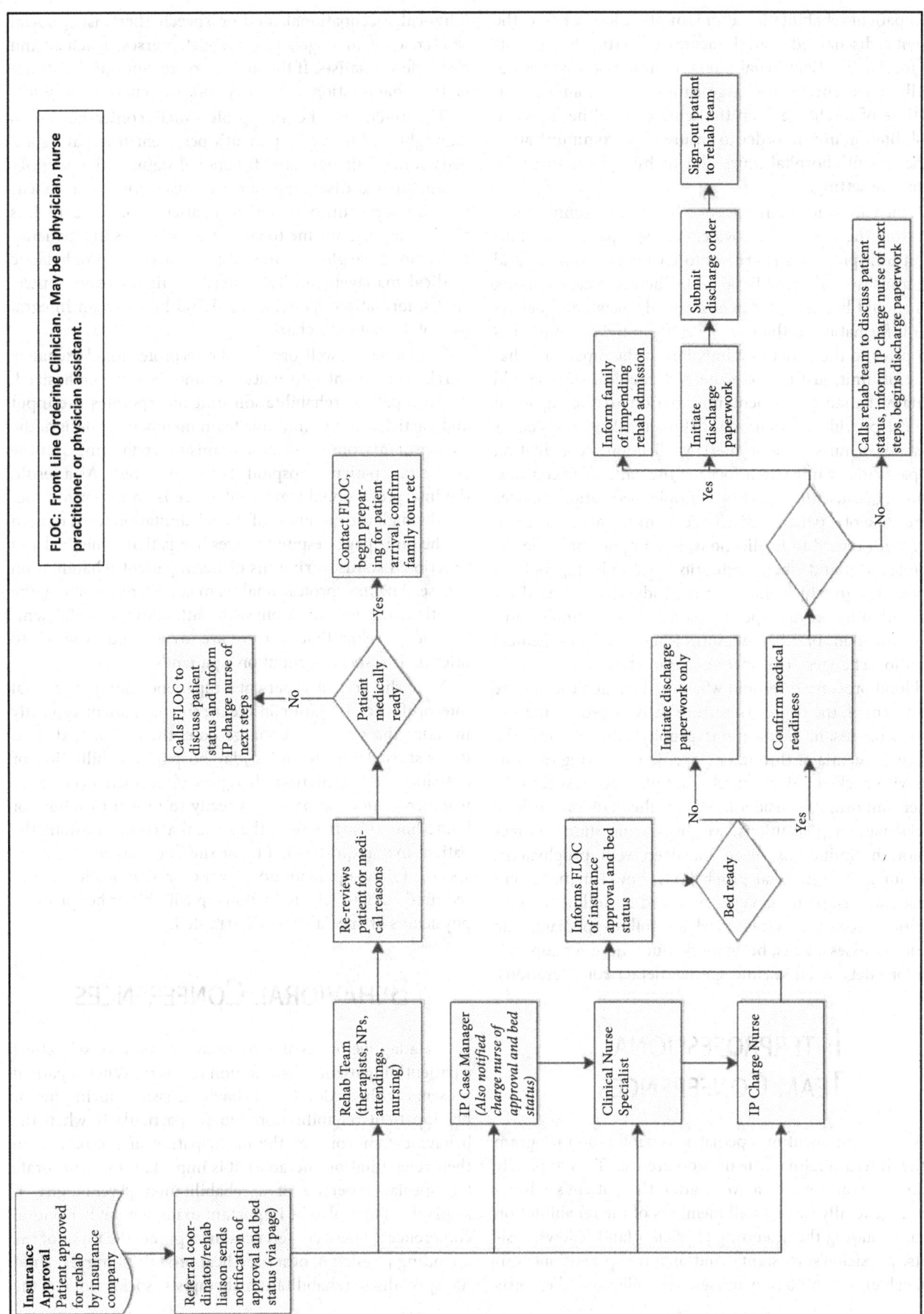

Figure 5-1. An example of a typical process involved in admitting a patient from the acute care setting to an inpatient rehabilitation unit. (NP = nurse practitioner; IP = inpatient)

the inpatient rehabilitation unit is another level of care, the patient is discharged from the acute care setting and admitted to the inpatient rehabilitation unit, not transferred. Ideally, an accurate discharge summary is completed at the time of discharge from the acute care to the inpatient rehabilitation unit in order to ensure clear communication of the patient's hospital course during his or her care in the acute care setting.

A formal rather than informal handoff of communication from the acute care providers to the inpatient rehabilitation unit providers is critical to ensuring a smooth and safe transition of care (Table 5-7). The acute care nursing staff should handoff pertinent medical, social, and behavioral information to the nursing staff on the rehabilitation unit prior to the patient's admission to the inpatient rehabilitation unit, just as the acute care medical staff should formally handoff pertinent information to the inpatient medical providers (attending, fellow, resident, physician's assistant, or nurse practitioner). Medication reconciliation is a particularly important focus of the handoff of communication because there may be multiple medication changes at the time of a patient's discharge from the acute care setting. With regard to medications, it is important to clearly understand if and when medications are to be tapered off, the manner in which the taper is conducted, the need for medication levels, and specific parameters for implementing medications or other measures when a patient's medical condition changes. The specific parameters could include the blood pressure threshold when cardiac medications are implemented, the degree of seizure activity prompting use of anticonvulsant medications prophylactically, and the degree of anemia or thrombocytopenia prompting transfusion with packed red blood cells and platelets, respectively. Other important considerations in the handoff include special patient precautions, weight-bearing status, range-of-motion limitations, need for deep vein prophylaxis, need for gastrointestinal prophylaxis, bowel management considerations, pain management, need for follow-up with specific specialty services, need for follow-up diagnostic studies or assessments, behavioral issues, need for supervision for safety, allergies, and special dietary considerations.

INTERPROFESSIONAL TEAM CONFERENCES

A key component of a pediatric rehabilitation program is the interdisciplinary team conference. This typically occurs several days to a week after the patient's admission. It generally involves all members of the rehabilitation team, including the attending physician (and fellows, residents, physician's assistants, and/or nurse practitioners, if applicable), rehabilitation nurses, rehabilitation therapists

(physical, occupational, and/or speech therapists), social worker, case manager, psychologist, nurses, teacher, and child life specialists. If therapeutic recreation specialists are on the rehabilitation team, they, too, are generally included.

The intent of the interprofessional conference is to highlight and update a patient's pertinent medical issues, behavioral challenges, and functional status and to identify an anticipated discharge date and disposition. It is essentially an opportunity to update a patient's plan of care. It is also an important time to clarify any changes in a patient's restrictions, weight-bearing status, or need for prophylactic medical management. The interdisciplinary team conference information is documented and becomes an integral part of the patient's chart.

The value of a well-organized interprofessional exchange of relevant patient information cannot be overemphasized. As an inpatient rehabilitation unit incorporates the input and participation of multiple team members by design, the chance of miscommunication or misunderstanding over the course of a patient's hospital stay is quite high. As a result, the interprofessional team conference is an important tool by which all the members of the rehabilitation team remain on the same page despite changes in a patient's medical and functional status during his or her inpatient rehabilitation course. The interprofessional team conference is led by the inpatient rehabilitation physician attending, but all members of the rehabilitation team are invited and expected to offer their respective input on a patient's status.

Near the end of a patient's inpatient course, the final interprofessional team conference for the patient typically includes the specific discharge date, the anticipated need for postdischarge therapies (day hospital rehabilitation or outpatient rehabilitation therapies if deemed necessary), whether or not the patient is ready to return to school or home-bound instruction, the special accommodations the patient may require when he or she does return to school, special follow-up laboratory work or diagnostic studies required, and anticipated follow-up with his or her primary physicians or specialists, as warranted.

BEHAVIORAL CONFERENCES

Maladaptive or disruptive behavior can adversely affect a patient's inpatient rehabilitation recovery. When a patient presents with or develops behavioral issues during his or her inpatient rehabilitation course, particularly when the behavior compromises the participation of the patient in their rehabilitation therapies, it is important to incorporate the special expertise of a rehabilitation psychologist, if available. It may also be important to implement behavioral conferences. These conferences incorporate the input of the attending physician, other medical providers, nurses, child life specialists, rehabilitation therapists, social worker, the psychologist directly involved in the child's care, and the input and approval of the patient's family to generate a behavioral plan while the patient is undergoing his or her rehabilitation therapies.

The purpose of the behavioral conferences is to identify and define the behavior in question, to establish specific behavioral management goals and objectives to address it, to design a specific behavioral plan, and to implement the behavioral plan in a consistent manner. The impact of the behavioral plan is then closely observed and documented. Follow-up behavioral conferences may be required depending on the patient's response to the initial behavioral plan. The behavioral plan may need periodic modification depending on the child's response. This interdisciplinary team approach to behavioral management can be an effective means of managing even difficult behaviors and may minimize or even eliminate the need for medicinal approaches to behavioral management.

FAMILY CONFERENCES

One of the most important interactions on the inpatient rehabilitation unit is the relationship and communication of the rehabilitation team members with the patient's family and the patient. Although daily rounds service to maintain communication with the patient and family on an ongoing basis, the interaction is typically brief and limited.

The family conference offers an opportunity for a more in-depth update of a patient's medical and functional status and a chance for families to express their concerns regarding the care received to date, including clarification of the goals of care when necessary. It may also include discussion regarding functional prognosis, medical and rehabilitation equipment needs, anticipated need for therapies after discharge, need for supervision when discharged to home, and clarification of the date of disposition.

COMMUNICATION WITH THE PRIMARY PHYSICIAN

A patient often presents abruptly with an acute stroke. His or her care is frequently emergent and may be complicated. As the focus is on the acute care management of the patient, the patient's primary pediatrician may not be promptly notified and updated regarding the patient's status. However, it is strongly advisable to do so because of his or her understandable concern for his or her patient and the family, but also because the primary pediatrician may offer additional insight and history pertinent to the care of the patient. Likewise, the primary care pediatrician should be notified by the rehabilitation medical team when the

TABLE 5-7. HANDOFF OF COMMUNICATION AT THE TIME OF ADMISSION TO THE INPATIENT REHABILITATION UNIT: KEY CONSIDERATIONS

- Medication reconciliation
- Fall precautions
- Aspiration precautions
- Seizure precautions
- Contact precautions
- Wound care concerns and precautions
- Range-of-motion restrictions
- Weight-bearing limitations and duration
- Deep venous thrombosis prophylaxis
- Systemic emboli prophylaxis
- Allergies
- Nutritional restrictions
- Special parameters for changes in medical condition
- Behavioral status
- Need for supervision for patient safety
- Social considerations
- Anticipated disposition
- Anticipated need for future diagnostic work-up
- Anticipated need for follow-up post discharge

Key considerations when performing handoff of communication from acute care providers to inpatient rehabilitation unit providers.

patient transitions from the acute care team to the inpatient rehabilitation unit. Incorporating the primary pediatrician early in the inpatient rehabilitation hospital course permits him or her to be an integral part of the medical team while the patient is still undergoing his or her inpatient rehabilitation care and helps ensure the patient's safe discharge to his or her home environment.

POSTDISCHARGE CONSIDERATIONS

At the time of discharge from the inpatient rehabilitation unit, a formal discharge summary is completed. It includes a summary of the patient's medical condition and his or her acute hospital course, as well as a summary of his or her inpatient rehabilitation course. In addition, it outlines the medical and rehabilitation equipment that the patient has received or is anticipated to receive after discharge. It also includes an updated medication list and follow-up appointments with the primary pediatrician and other specialists involved in the patient's care or expected to be involved after discharge.

DAY HOSPITAL REHABILITATION

In some hospital settings, a day hospital rehabilitation program may be available for patients who have experienced a functionally debilitating stroke. The day hospital program has similar admission criteria as the inpatient admission except that the patient no longer requires daily medical surveillance in an inpatient setting to ensure his or her medical stability and safety. Day hospital rehabilitation programs typically offer comprehensive rehabilitation services, including physical, occupational, and speech and language therapy, nursing, and psychological services, but do so during the weekdays, typically Monday through Friday. The patients return to their homes at night and do not receive formal therapies on the weekend; although, they may have instructions to perform a home program of stretching and active exercises during the weekend. The day hospital program is typically ideal for the patient who has already undergone comprehensive inpatient rehabilitation therapy and no longer requires ongoing medical management in an inpatient setting, but will continue to benefit from comprehensive inpatient rehabilitation services.

OUTPATIENT REHABILITATION THERAPIES, HOME PROGRAM, AND SCHOOL-BASED REHABILITATION SERVICES

Based on their functional outcomes, some children can transition from the inpatient rehabilitation unit to outpatient rehabilitation therapies or directly to home with a home program of rehabilitation exercises, as instructed by the rehabilitation therapists. In neonates with perinatal stroke, motor deficits are rarely present at stroke onset, and inpatient rehabilitation is not developmentally appropriate, so rehabilitation begins in the community setting after hospital discharge. In many communities, early intervention programs provide home-based physical, occupational, and speech and language therapy programs for children from 0 to 3 years of age. When children reach 3 years of age, comparable intermediate care services are provided through the local school district if needed. When children reach school age, school-based rehabilitation services, including physical, occupational, speech and language, and vision therapy, and special education services, can be provided based on a child's specific needs. Please see Chapter 12 for more information. Ongoing follow-up with a pediatric neurologist, and in many cases a pediatric physiatrist, will continue throughout childhood, and those specialists will make updated recommendations regarding the need for therapy and other treatments as a child develops.

PRINCIPLES OF STROKE REHABILITATION

There are a wide range of etiologies and a broad spectrum of risk factors in children who experience strokes. In addition, the clinical presentations can be highly variable even among children with a stroke due to the same etiology. See Chapters 1 to 4 for details about stroke subtypes in children. The majority of children experiencing a stroke will have some degree of residual neurological deficits and functional impairment. This may manifest as spasticity, weakness, movement disorders, seizures, speech and language impairments, swallowing dysfunction, visual deficits, musculoskeletal abnormalities, cognitive challenges, and/or behavioral abnormalities. These impairments can adversely affect a child's normal developmental progress. Therefore, the rehabilitation of children who incur a stroke requires an understanding of normative growth parameters, as well as normal cognitive, motor, and speech and language development and associated milestones. Please see Section II for further discussion regarding rehabilitation of neuromotor function, language and communication, feeding and swallowing, cognition, and behavioral and emotional function in children following stroke. In addition, children who have a stroke and associated disabilities incur a lifelong impact on their daily function, education, social interactions, and eventual work environment, which may have significant psychological and financial implications for the child and his or her family. Please see Section III for further discussion of these important considerations.

Impact of Stroke on Functional Prognosis

Many children who incur a stroke will have long-lasting or permanent neurological deficits. They may present with a myriad of sequelae that affect their mobility, independence in activities of daily living, and ability to learn, including seizures, spasticity, dystonia, motor dyskinesias, fine and gross motor impairments, progressive contractures, sensory impairment, neglect, swallowing dysfunction, speech and language impairment, behavioral disorders, visual impairment, and cognitive dysfunction. The Pediatric National Institutes of Health Stroke Scale (PedNIHSS) can be used to quantitate stroke severity.[4] As a result, it can be helpful in prognostication. A low PedNIHSS is a reliable predictor for eventual resolution of neurological deficits or mild residual deficits associated with ischemic strokes. Hemorrhagic strokes result in the highest mortality in the acute phase with an in-hospital mortality of up to 6% to 9%. Larger volume hemorrhages correlate with worse 30-day outcomes.[5]

Medical Management and Surveillance Poststroke

Following medical stabilization after an acute stroke, it is imperative to perform ongoing assessments for signs and symptoms of seizure activity, increased intracranial pressure with hydrocephalus, and new focal neurological deficits. There should also be constant vigilance for any subsequent decline in respiratory status. New-onset headaches, seizures, or focal neurological deficits should prompt consideration of a recurrent stroke and requires immediate evaluation.

In children with neurological deficits, which include swallowing difficulties, careful attention to prevention of aspiration is critical for prevention of further respiratory compromise and aspiration pneumonia. Formal evaluation and management by a speech and language pathologist is indicated to help identify the extent and severity of the swallowing dysfunction and appropriate conservative measures for addressing the swallowing impairment. In addition, some children may require initial feeding via a nasogastric tube and avoidance of food by mouth until their swallowing and oromotor function recovers sufficiently to initiate oral feeding. In situations where it is anticipated that a child will be unable to consume food or drink by mouth for a protracted period (3 months or more), placement of a gastrointestinal tube (GT) may be indicated. In the latter case, an upper gastrointestinal series is performed to ensure that there are no abnormalities that may be a contraindication to placement of a GT. Formal assessment of a child's swallowing function via a modified barium swallow study and a flexible endoscopic evaluation may be indicated. The child may subsequently require a slowly progressive increase in the texture of his or her food and the consistency of his or her liquids as he or she recovers his or her swallowing function.

Prevention of Medical Complications

The interprofessional rehabilitation team can be instrumental in continuing or implementing measures to prevent potential poststroke complications, such as aspiration pneumonia, joint contractures, pressure sores, deep vein thrombosis, pulmonary emboli, sleep disturbances, sleep apnea, seizures, constipation, disuse atrophy, deconditioning, and falls. Rehabilitation therapists can initiate early range-of-motion and progressive mobility exercises; provide activities to enhance balance, coordination, and endurance; and promote the recovery of premorbid activity of daily living skills. The physiatrist can be helpful in recommending the timely prescription of assistive devices, adaptive equipment, and static and dynamic orthotics to stabilize an extremity and/or facilitate functional mobility. In addition, the physiatrist may perform chemodenervation in selected muscles and/or order antispasticity medications to address functionally limiting or painful spasticity, prevent joint contractures, ease the burden on the caregiver, and facilitate progressive mobility. Ideally, the prevention of medical complications begins immediately after a patient incurs a stroke and continues as the patient transitions to a postacute care setting.

As a general principle, it is important to minimize the use of medications that may adversely affect a child's mental status to the lowest dose necessary for achieving effective results, particularly in patients who have incurred a stroke with associated mental status changes. Neuroleptics, benzodiazepines, and barbiturates may impair a child's mental alertness and endurance and, thus, his or her ability to participate in his or her rehabilitation therapies and his or her functional progress; therefore, they should be avoided unless absolutely necessary.

Prevention of Joint Contractures

Consider use of a multipodus boot on the affected paretic limb when in bed or ankle stretch splints and range-of-motion exercises on the affected limb to prevent progressive ankle plantarflexion contracture formation. Upper extremity resting and/or dynamic splints coupled with range-of-motion exercises to prevent contractures at the elbow, wrist, and fingers; knee immobilizers to prevent knee joint contractures; a hip abductor wedge to address excessive hip adductor tone; and ankle–foot orthotics to facilitate ambulation may also be indicated depending on the extent and severity of the child's deficits. Functional electrical stimulation of selected muscle groups may be indicated in patients with significant weakness to facilitate improved strength and functional movement. Weight-supported ambulation and selective use of assistive devices such as a rolling walker, lofstrand crutches, or canes may be indicated depending on the patient's clinical deficits and functional progression.

Prevention of Shoulder Pain and Subluxation

Pain in the shoulder and other joints after a stroke is not uncommon and may require local modalities such as ice application, moist heat, gently progressive range-of-motion exercises, proper positioning, and judicious use of pain medications, such as acetaminophen and nonsteroidal anti-inflammatory medications, if not contraindicated. When a patient presents with significant shoulder subluxation, he or she may benefit from kinesiotaping or rigid taping of the shoulder, which may help to minimize the subluxation and also help alleviate the mechanical strain and associated pain at the shoulder. He or she may also benefit from periodic use of a shoulder sling. Prolonged use of a sling, however, may promote shoulder adduction contracture formation and inhibits swing of the affected arm during ambulation.

Prevention of Pressure Sores

Careful skin inspection and periodic weight-bearing relief in the bed (turning the patient side to side every 2 hours) and in a wheelchair (weight shifting at least every 15 minutes) may be necessary to prevent pressure ulcers, particularly in the sacral, hip, and posterior heel areas. Wheelchair cushions and specialty beds with mattresses designed to minimize focal pressures and provide more even weight distribution may also be helpful in preventing pressure ulcers in children, particularly those with more severe weakness secondary to a stroke.

Identification and Management of Depression and Anxiety

Although sometimes overlooked, some children experience significant depression and anxiety associated with their deficits and the extensive medical management required in their acute and subacute stages. Early attention to providing psychological support for counseling and to assist with coping strategies may be necessary. In some cases of severe depression or more serious psychiatric disturbances, it may be necessary to include the consultative expertise of a psychiatrist for selective treatment with antidepressant or antianxiety medication.

In the adult population, fluoxetine has been prescribed to enhance motor recovery following a stroke. In a double-blind, placebo-controlled trial, patients ranging from 18 to 85 years of age who had experienced ischemic stroke complicated by hemiplegia or hemiparesis were randomly assigned fluoxetine. Early prescription of fluoxetine enhanced motor recovery after 3 months.[6] Although the specific mechanism for its clinical efficacy remains obscure, it is postulated that fluoxetine may have a role in modulating spontaneous brain plasticity. These results, however, have not been reproduced in the pediatric population to date.[6]

Management of Spasticity

Spasticity is the consequence of an imbalance between the afferent excitatory and descending inhibitory pathways after a central nervous system insult, such as a brain injury, brain tumor, or stroke. The management of spasticity in the stroke patient may be implemented as soon as hypertonia begins to emerge. Proper positioning, passive range of motion, and selective splinting may be helpful in preventing progressive contracture formation as the patient's tone increases. Depending on the patient's cognitive and behavioral status, the presence of other medical comorbidities, the patient's metabolic and nutritional status, and the degree of his or her hypertonia, a patient may be a potential candidate for oral antispasticity medications such as baclofen, tizanidine, diazepam, or clonidine. Baclofen is a gamma-aminobutyric acid (GABA) analog that binds to GABA-B receptors. It inhibits the release of excitatory neurotransmitters from presynaptic terminals synapsing on alpha motor neurons. Diazepam is a benzodiazepine that binds to the GABA-A receptor. It facilitates GABA-A–mediated inhibition at the brain and postsynaptic effects at the spinal cord level. Tizanidine is an imidazole derivative that acts centrally as an alpha-2 agonist by facilitating presynaptic inhibition though the alpha-adrenergic receptors. Clonidine is a potent antihypertensive agent and a centrally acting alpha-2 agonist. It has been demonstrated to reduce hypertonicity in patients incurring brain insults. Although these medications can be effective in reducing spasticity, their use can be limited by their potential concomitant side effects such as somnolence, drowsiness, and cognitive and psychomotor impairment. In addition, particularly in the case of diazepam, they may cause respiratory depression. If any one of the latter antispasticity medications are implemented, it is important to obtain baseline liver function studies because they can also cause transaminitis and eventual liver dysfunction if not closely monitored and adjusted as clinically appropriate. Dantrolene is a potential alternative oral antispasticity medication that typically causes less mental status impairment than baclofen, tizanidine, or diazepam. Dantrolene acts peripherally by inhibiting the excitation-contraction coupling of muscle fibers by blocking the release of calcium from the sarcoplasmic reticulum, which inhibits muscle contraction. However, it, too, can cause transaminitis and potentially life-threatening hepatotoxicity. Therefore, careful monitoring of liver function studies at periodic intervals is imperative when prescribing dantrolene.[7]

Botulinum toxin (Botox) injections provide an additional or alternative intervention to the aforementioned oral antispasticity medications. Although Botox injections are off-label for treatment of spasticity in patients less than 18 years of age, they provide a potential additional or alternative intervention to the aforementioned oral antispasticity medications. Multiple studies attest to the efficacy of Botox injections in reducing functionally limiting hypertonicity in stroke.[8-11] Botox is produced by the anaerobic bacterium *Clostridium botulinum*. It can effectively block neurotransmission at the neuromuscular junction, resulting in weakness of the muscle injected and thus an attenuation of the hypertonicity affecting that particular muscle. It specifically acts to inhibit the release of acetylcholine from the cholinergic neurons at peripheral neuromuscular junctions.[12] Electrical stimulation via an electromyography needle may be used to confirm needle placement in the appropriate muscle prior to administration of Botox. Side effects include injection site discomfort, flu-like symptoms, and excessive weakness of the affected muscles. The therapeutic effect can be manifest within 72 hours after the injection, with peak effect typically occurring by 2 weeks after the injection. The effect ranges from 3 to 6 months in duration. As resistance to Botox, and thus attenuation of its affect, may occur as a consequence of antibody development and neutralization of the toxin, injections should not be given more frequently than every 3 months.[13] As Botox can be selectively injected into target muscles, it has the advantage of causing a reduction in muscle hypertonicity in specific muscles while avoiding the systemic effects of oral antispasticity medications, such as impairment of a patient's mental status, diffuse weakness, and, in the case of baclofen, potential lowering of a patient's seizure threshold.

Neuroplasticity

Neuroplasticity is the proposed mechanism by which we adapt to changes, learn and retain new facts, and develop new skills. This mechanism can also be operative following brain insult, such as a stroke, which implies the brain has an intrinsic adaptive ability to remodel itself following injury. It offers the injured brain the potential for variable degrees of functional recovery. This recovery in the chronic stage of stroke is felt by some to be predominantly due to reorganization of the damaged hemisphere.[14]

Several principles are thought to underlie neuroplasticity. One includes the principle that body parts compete for representation in the brain, and the area of representation increases or decreases based on its use. Plasticity is thought to assist in the restoration of cortical representation.[15,16]

Another principle recognizes that mechanisms involved in neuroplasticity can be facilitated by intensive rehabilitation, and the earlier and more intensive the therapy, the better the outcome.[17] Examples of intensive rehabilitation include constraint-induced movement therapy and bilateral upper extremity intensive training.[18-23]

Other potentially promising interventions under research study that utilize the proposed principles of neuroplasticity include prolonged sensory nerve stimulation of the motor cortex via transcutaneous electrical stimulation to increase excitability of the latter area, neuromuscular stimulation, robotic training, and virtual reality training.[24-27] Please see Chapter 7 for further discussion.

Despite the aforementioned promising interventions, the specific mechanisms of neuroplasticity have not been fully or clearly elucidated to date. More definitive understanding of the mechanisms involved in neuroplastic changes following brain injury is necessary for guiding and justifying selected forms of intervention, including the type, dose, and intensity of rehabilitation therapies, and may also prove helpful in both diagnosis and prognostication.

Future research focus in this area has promise for identifying novel approaches to enhancing and sustaining functional outcomes in pediatric patients who incur a stroke.

Contractures and Gait Dysfunction

Orthotics may be prescribed early in the patient's course if clinically indicated. Orthotics are typically prescribed when a patient's hypertonia causes muscle imbalance, static and dynamic misalignment of the extremities, joint instability, and potential for joint contracture formation. If the lower extremities are affected, foot, ankle, and/or knee orthotics may be indicated to address both joint instability and gait dysfunction. The muscle imbalance may occur in either the upper or lower extremities. This typically occurs unilaterally in patients experiencing a stroke; however, in patients with multiple strokes or recurrent strokes, they may experience hypertonia, static and dynamic extremity misalignment, and contracture formation bilaterally.

Static orthotics such as resting hand/wrist splints are designed to prevent progressive contracture formation, but do not provide further stretch of the muscles acting at the joint; thus, as an isolated treatment, the static orthotics do not increase the range of motion at a contracted joint. Use of the latter orthotics must be coupled with physical and occupational therapy range-of-motion exercises, serial casting, antispasticity medication, and/or dynamic splinting to achieve improved range of motion at an affected joint. When the tone is mild to moderate, passive and active range-of-motion exercises and orthotics may be sufficient to facilitate function and prevent progressive contractures. When the hypertonia is moderate to severe, however, patients may require Botox injections of selected hypertonic muscles followed by serial casting, in turn followed by prescription of dynamic extension or flexion orthotics for the upper or lower extremities for daytime use and night stretch splints for night wear to tolerance. The latter measures may be coupled with the prescription of an appropriate antispasticity medication.

Dynamic extension or flexion orthotic splints are designed to provide variable degrees of tension counter to the direction of contracture formation. The latter splints are designed to provide continuous, but tolerable, stretch of contracted muscles. They can be used during the day or overnight depending on the patient's clinical presentation and needs. The tension pressure of the dynamic splints can be progressively increased to the patient's tolerance to incrementally improve range of motion at a selected joint. Upper extremity dynamic splints are available for patients with elbow and wrist contractures. Lower extremity dynamic splints are available for patients with knee and ankle contractures. Whenever upper or lower extremity splints are applied, it is important that the skin be assessed on a regular basis to monitor for any evidence of skin irritation or pressure sore development. If the latter occurs, the splint may need readjustment or replacement. Patients with bilateral strokes may demonstrate scissoring of their lower extremities due to hip adductor spasticity, particularly with attempted ambulation; this may also hinder the caregiver attempts to provide proper hygiene. Botox injections of their hip adductors coupled with range-of-motion exercises, as well as a hip abduction wedge, may be helpful in minimizing this functionally limiting problem.

Equinovarus posturing at the ankle–foot complex is the most common deformity experienced in patients who incur a stroke.[28] The ankle–foot orthosis (AFO) is commonly prescribed to address gait dysfunction in patients with hemiparesis secondary to a stroke. An AFO may be prescribed to provide stability, block abnormal motion at a joint, counter deforming forces, compensate for weakness, and/or facilitate movement to normalize the gait pattern, increase stride length and speed, prevent progressive contractures, minimize potential for falls, and reduce energy expenditure. Some physical therapists and physicians, however, are resistant to prescription of AFOs for fear it will cause disuse atrophy and further ankle dorsiflexion weakness, particularly solid ankle orthoses. However, regular active ankle range-of-motion exercises without the orthosis and timely discontinuation of the orthotic when the patient has progressed sufficiently enough to consistently perform antigravity ankle dorsiflexion will minimize the occurrence of disuse atrophy.

AFOs are generally classified as articulated or nonarticulated. The articulated AFOs are fabricated with a hinge or ankle joint. The degree of articulation can be adjusted to meet a patient's specific needs. The permissible motion at the ankle joint can also be adjusted to accommodate a patient's particular needs. Both the articulated and non-articulated AFOs, if properly designed and prescribed for the appropriate clinical indications, can facilitate improved ambulation. In a Cochrane systematic review by Tyson and Kent, they concluded that the overall effect of AFOs on the walking disability (speed), walking impairment (step/stride/length), and balance impairment (weight distribution in standing) was significantly beneficial.[29]

Falls

After a stroke, because children may have impulsivity, poor safety awareness, visual field deficits, neglect, weakness, incoordination, imbalance, and/or hypertonia, they are at particular risk for falls. As such, special attention to preventing falls, including parental education and constant supervision when indicated, should be implemented. In addition, avoidance of overly long clothing over which children may trip, the wear of proper shoes or slippers with traction soles, and repeated reminders that a child is at particular fall risk by the use of wrist bands, door signs, or alerts may help decrease the potential of falls.

FAMILY FOCUS BOX

1. The medical care of a child following a stroke typically begins in the emergency room or an acute care hospital. Some of the care may be provided in an intensive care unit. As a child's medical status stabilizes, the emphasis shifts to rehabilitation. This may occur in an inpatient rehabilitation hospital, outpatient rehabilitation day program, or outpatient or school-based therapies. Ideally, the care of a child following a stroke involves a team of professionals who work together to develop an individualized treatment plan for that child. The eventual goal is the child's return to home and school with whatever supports, equipment, or accommodations are needed to optimize function.

2. A clear understanding of the medical and rehabilitative needs of the patient and the respectful acknowledgment of the family's input are vital to ensuring quality care is provided throughout the continuum of a child's care. Special attention should be directed toward ensuring that the patient and family, wherever practical and appropriate, are allotted opportunities to provide constructive feedback regarding the care provided throughout the continuum of care.

3. Family members are particularly encouraged to participate in family conferences, be present for clinical rounds, and attend, when appropriate, rehabilitation therapies. They are also encouraged to participate in special training sessions, such as training in the proper performance of transfers, nasogastric tube placement, gastrointestinal tube feedings, seizure prophylaxis administration, cardiopulmonary resuscitation, and other training necessary for the safe transition of their child to the home environment.

CASE STUDY

Clinical History in the Acute Care Setting

A 16-year-old, previously healthy female initially presented to the hospital emergency room with a 10/10 frontal headache and subsequent acute onset of left hemiparesis, dysphagia, and dysarthria. An emergent computed tomography (CT) scan of the brain revealed an acute intraparenchymal hemorrhage in the right frontoparietal region. She was subsequently identified per additional cranial studies to have a right arteriovenous malformation rupture resulting in a right frontal intraparenchymal hematoma extending into the third and fourth ventricles with a midline shift toward the left. She therefore underwent a right craniotomy and decompression with evacuation of the hematoma by neurosurgery. Her hospital course was complicated by persistent headaches, fevers, and a ventilator-acquired pneumonia, which required treatment with multiple antibiotics; iron-deficient anemia; and a left occlusive deep vein thrombosis of the innominate, internal jugular, subclavian, axillary, and cephalic veins. After it was determined that the risk of venous stroke outweighed the risk of rebleed, she was started on a low dose of a low-molecular-weight anticoagulant.

Physical medicine and rehabilitation, and physical, occupational, and speech and language therapy consults were ordered early in the patient's acute care course. Physical and occupational therapy began to mobilize the patient as soon as she was medically cleared to do so by her neurosurgeon and initiated efforts to help her restore her ability to perform her activities of daily living, as well as her ability to ambulate. Fall precautions were also implemented early in her course. She was continued on anticoagulation therapy because of her left arm occlusive thrombosis. She underwent a neuro-ophthalmology exam, which excluded a visual field deficit, and an ophthalmology exam, which revealed intact visual acuity and no evidence of papilledema or retinopathy. Her hearing was assessed, and no abnormalities were identified. She had no complaints of pain, but was placed on a mild analgesic for pain relief, as deemed necessary.

The patient's physical exam was consistent with an incomplete left hemiparesis and left hemiplegic gait dysfunction. The physical medicine and rehabilitation (PM&R) consultant in the acute care setting recommended use of a left lower leg multipodus boot and sequential compression devices for both lower extremities for use when in bed and bilateral lower extremity compression hose when up out of bed, as well as progressive mobilization for deep vein thrombosis prophylaxis. A stool softener to prevent significant constipation was recommended and implemented. Rehabilitation therapies, including physical, occupational, and speech and language therapy, were implemented in the acute care setting.

When the patient was noted to be medically stable, clinically capable of tolerating more intensive rehabilitation therapies, no longer required any further diagnostic workup, and had the approval of the parents or guardian for inpatient rehabilitation, the PM&R consultant promptly notified the rehabilitation admission coordinator, who then submitted the information for potential insurance approval. After obtaining insurance approval for inpatient rehabilitation and after ensuring a bed was available on the inpatient rehabilitation unit, the attending physician in the acute care setting promptly completed a discharge summary and discharged the patient from the acute care

(continued)

CASE STUDY (CONTINUED)
setting for subsequent admission to the inpatient rehabilitation unit. Prior to discharge of the patient from the acute setting, a formal handoff of information was exchanged between the acute and postacute nurses and between the acute and postacute care physicians. As this transfer occurred in an academic center, the formal communication of patient information included residents and fellows rotating on the service. This process was implemented per protocol to minimize miscommunication of pertinent clinical, social, and psychological issues, including proper medication reconciliation at the time of discharge from the acute care setting to the postacute care site.

Clinical Care in the Postacute Care Setting

Due to accurate and timely handoff of pertinent patient clinical information, the discharge from acute care and the admission to the inpatient rehabilitation unit occurred in a smooth and efficient manner. The patient showed appreciable functional gains over the course of her inpatient rehabilitation stay, underwent formal documentation of the gains, and was discharged to her home in stable medical condition. Due to residual left-sided neurological deficits in her gross and fine motor coordination, her persistent gait dysfunction, and her speech and language, as well as swallowing impairments, she was admitted for ongoing comprehensive therapies, including physical, occupational, and speech and language therapy, into the day hospital rehabilitation program after obtaining insurance approval. Due to her subsequent functional improvement and her achievement of independence in multiple activities of daily living at the time of discharge from the day hospital setting, she no longer required outpatient physical or occupational therapy, but continued to receive speech and language therapy on an outpatient basis. The patient's primary physician was notified of her admission to the inpatient rehabilitation unit at the time of admission, regarding any significant clinical problems during her inpatient course, and her status at the time of discharge to home, including a discharge summary to help ensure follow up of pertinent clinical issues and outstanding laboratory work ordered while in the inpatient rehabilitation setting. The patient was also set up for a follow-up appointment with the PM&R physician consultant 4 weeks after discharge from the day hospital to ensure the patient complied with her prescribed medications, received the equipment ordered, and followed through with her outpatient speech and language therapy appointments. On her follow-up assessment by the PM&R physician, she was noted to be compliant with her medications, had started her outpatient therapies, and had no interim medical complications or new focal neurological deficits. She had not yet received all the equipment ordered, but it was confirmed that delivery was pending. Both the parents and the patient were pleased with her functional recovery when seen on follow-up 4 weeks after her discharge from the day hospital rehabilitation program (Table 5-8).

SUMMARY

A child who incurs a stroke embarks on a continuum of care of variable complexity. A well-organized and well-coordinated process for incorporating the experience and expertise of multiple health care providers in the child's care from the acute to the postacute care setting will help ensure the patient's safety while simultaneously optimizing the child's functional recovery.

REFERENCES

1. Gresham GE, Duncan PW, Stason WB, et al; Agency for Health Care Policy and Research. Post-stroke rehabilitation (Clinical Practice Guideline, no. 16; publication no. 95-0662). Rockville, MD: U.S. Department of Health and Human Services, Public Health Service. AHCPR, 1995.
2. Veterans Affairs/Department of Defense. Clinical practice guideline for the management of stroke rehabilitation in the primary care setting, Department of Veterans Affairs, Department of Defense, Version 1.1. Prepared by The Management of Stroke Rehabilitation Working Group, February 2003, p 2.
3. Cifu DX, Stewart DG. Factors affecting functional outcome after stroke: a critical review of rehabilitation interventions. *Arch Phys Med Rehabil.* 1999;80(5 Suppl 1):S35-S39.
4. Ichord RN, Bastian R, Abraham L, et al. Interrater reliability of the Pediatric National Institutes of Health Stroke Scale (PedNIHSS) in a multicenter study. *Stroke.* 2011;42(3):613-617.
5. Landi G, D'Angelo A, Boccardi E, et al. Venous thromboembolism in acute stroke. Prognostic importance of hypercoagulability. *Arch Neurol.* 1992;49:279-283.
6. Chollet F, Tardy J, Albucher JF, et al. Fluoxetine for motor recovery after acute ischaemic stroke (FLAME): a randomised placebo-controlled trial. *Lancet Neurol.* 2011;10(2):123-130. doi: 10.1016/S1474-4422(10)70314-8.
7. Hindener SR, Dixon K. Physiologic and clinical monitoring of spastic hypertonia. Spastic hypertonia. *Phys Med Rehabil Clin N Am.* 2001:733-746.
8. Brashear A, Gordon MF, Elovic E, et al; BOTOX Post-Stroke Study Group: a multicenter, double-blind, randomized, placebo-controlled, parallel study of the safety and efficacy of BOTOX (Botulinum Toxin Type A) Purified Neurotoxin in the treatment of focal upper limb spasticity post-stroke. *Neurology.* 2001;56(Suppl 3):A78.
9. Hesse S, Reiter F, Konrad M, et al. Botulinum toxin type A and short term electrical stimulation in the treatment of upper limb flexor spasticity after stroke: a randomized, double-blind, placebo controlled trial. *Clin Rehabil.* 1998;12:381-388.
10. Reiter F, Danni M, Lagalla G, et al. Low-dose botulinum toxin with ankle taping for the treatment of spastic equinovarus foot after stroke. *Arch Phys Med Rehabil.* 1998;79:532-535.
11. Smith SJ, Ellis E, White S, et al. A double-blind placebo-controlled study of botulinum toxin in upper limb spasticity after stroke or head injury. *Clin Rehabil.* 2000;14:5-13.
12. Brin MF. Botulinum toxin: chemistry, pharmacology, toxicity, and immunology. *Muscle Nerve.* 1997;20(Suppl 6):S146-S168.

TABLE 5-8. REHABILITATION AND MEDICAL DIAGNOSES IN THE INPATIENT REHABILITATION SETTING

REHABILITATION DIAGNOSES	MEDICAL DIAGNOSES

1. Left spastic hemiparesis
2. Gait dysfunction
3. Decreased strength
4. Decreased endurance
5. Impaired coordination
6. Impaired static/dynamic balance
7. Impaired activities of daily living skills, improved
8. Impaired cognition
9. Impaired speech and language
10. Impaired swallowing function
	1. Right frontal intraparenchymal hemorrhage secondary to an arteriovenous malformation
	  a. Status post craniotomy and decompression
	  b. Initial dense flaccid left hemiplegia, slowly improving strength and emerging spasticity
	  c. Dysphagia, status post removal of nasogastric tube improved
	  d. Dysarthria, improved
	2. Deep vein thrombosis of left innominate, internal jugular, subclavian, axillary and mid and peripheral cephalic veins, on low molecular weight heparin.
	3. History of ventilator-dependent respiratory failure, status post intubation, status post successful extubation
	4. Iron deficient anemia
	5. Thrombocytosis, likely reactive
	6. Ventilator acquired pneumonia–*staph aureus*, status post antibiotic treatment
	7. Left shoulder subluxation
	8. Vitamin D deficiency

Clinical example of the rehabilitation and medical diagnoses in a patient presenting with a hemorrhagic stroke.

13. Hindener SR, Dixon K. Physiologic and clinical monitoring of spastic hypertonia. Spastic hypertonia. *Phys Med Rehabil Clin N Am.* 2001: 733-746.
14. Hallet M. Plasticity of the human motor cortex and recovery from stroke. *Brain Res Rev.* 2001;36(2-3):169-174.
15. Hallett M. Guest editorial. Neuroplasticity and rehabilitation. *J Rehabil Res Dev.* 2005;42(4):17-22.
16. Nudo RJ. Functional and structural plasticity in motor cortex: implications for stroke recovery. *Phy Med Rehabil Clin N Am.* 2003;14(1 Suppl):S57-S76.
17. Taub E, Morris DM. Constraint-induced movement therapy to enhance recovery after stroke. *Curr Atheroscler Rep.* 2001;3(4):279-286.
18. Taub E, Uswatte G, Pidikiti R. Constraint-induced movement therapy: a new family of techniques with broad application to physical rehabilitation—a clinical review. *J Rehabil Res Dev.* 1999;36:237-251.
19. Gillick B, Zirpel L. Clinical implications of basic research. Neuroplasticity: an appreciation from synapse to system. *Arch Phys Med Rehabil.* 2012;93:1846-1854.
20. Case-Smith J, DeLuca SC, Stevenson R, Ramey SL. Multicenter randomized controlled trial of pediatric constraint-induced movement therapy: 6-month follow-up. *Am J Occup Ther.* 2012;66:15-23.
21. Gillick BT, Koppes A. Gross motor outcomes in children with hemiparesis involved in a modified constraint-induced therapy program. *J Pediatr Rehabil Med.* 2010;3:171-175.
22. Zipp GP, Winning S. Effects of constrain-induced movement therapy on gait, balance, and functional locomotor mobility. *Pediatr Phys Ther.* 2012;24:64-68.
23. Gordon AM, Hung Y, Brandao M, et al. Bimanual training and constraint-induced movement therapy in children with hemiplegic cerebral palsy: a randomized trial. *Neurorehabil Neural.* 2011;25:692-702.
24. Ridding MC, McKay DR, Thompson PD, Miles TS. Changes in corticomotor representations induced by prolonged peripheral nerve stimulation in humans. *Clin Neurophysiol.* 2001;112(8):1461-1469.
25. Cauraugh J, Light K, Kim S, Thigpen M, Behrman A. Chronic motor dysfunction after stroke: recovering wrist and finger extension by electromyography-triggered neuromuscular stimulation. *Stroke.* 2003;31(6):1360-1364.
26. Volpe BT, Ferraro M, Krebs HI, Hogan N. Robotics in the rehabilitation treatment of patients with stroke. *Curr Atheroscler Rep.* 2002;4(4):270-276.
27. You SH, Jang SH, Kim YH, et al. Virtual reality-induced cortical reorganization and associated locomotor recovery in chronic stroke: an experimenter-blind randomized study. *Stroke.* 2005;36(6):1166-1171.
28. Fennell CW, Yang AN, Elson D. Orthoses for brain-injured patients. In: Goldberg B, Hsu J, eds. *Atlas of Orthoses and Assistive Devices,* 3rd ed. St Louis, MO: Mosby; 1997:379-389.
29. Tyson SF, Kent RM. Orthotic devices after stroke and other non-progressive brain lesions. *Cochrane Database Syst Rev.* 2009;(1):CD003694.

SUGGESTED READINGS

Bowers RJ. Non-articulated ankle-foot orthoses. In: Condie E, Campbell J, Martina J, eds. *Report of a Consensus Conference on the Orthotic Management of Stroke Patients.* Copenhagen, Denmark: International Society for Prosthetics and Orthotics; 2004:87-94.

Brady K, Garcia T. Constraint-induced movement therapy (CIMT): pediatric applications. *Dev Disabil Res Rev.* 2009;16(2):102-111.

Englemann KA, Jordan C. Outcome measures used in pediatric stroke studies: a systematic review. *Arch Neurol.* 2012;69(1):23-27.

Ganesan F, Kirkham FJ (eds.). *Stroke and Cerebrovascular Disease in Childhood.* London, United Kingdom: MacKeith Press for the International Child Neurology Association; 2011.

Hoy DJ, Reinthal MA. Articulated ankle foot orthoses designs. In: Condie E, Campbell J, Martina J, eds. *Report of a Consensus Conference on the Orthotic Management of Stroke Patients.* Copenhagen, Denmark: International Society for Prosthetics and Orthotics; 2004:95-111.

Hurvitz E, Beale L, Ried S, Nelson V. Functional outcome of pediatric stroke survivors. *Pediatr Rehabil.* 1999;3(2):43-51.

Hurvitz E, Warschausky S, Berg M, Tsai S. Long-term functional outcome of pediatric stroke survivors. *Top Stroke Rehabil.* 2004;11(2):51-59.

Miller EL, Murray L, Richards L, et al. Comprehensive overview of nursing and interdisciplinary rehabilitation care of the stroke patient: a scientific statement from the American Heart Association. *Stroke.* 2010;41(10):2402-2448.

Olsen T. Stroke—Understanding the problem. In: Condie E, Campbell J, Martina J, eds. *Report of a Consensus Conference on the Orthotic Management of Stroke Patients.* Copenhagen, Denmark: International Society for Prosthetics and Orthotics; 2004:37-44.

Roach ES, Golomb MR, Adams R, et al. Management of stroke in infants and children: a scientific statement from a Special Writing Group of the American Heart Association Stroke Council and the Council on Cardiovascular Disease in the Young. *Stroke.* 2008;39(9):2644-2691.

Robinson KR. Self-directed physiatric education program in physical medicine and rehabilitation: foreword: pediatric rehabilitation. *PMR.* 2010;2(3):S1-S2.

Stein J, Harvey RL, Winstein CJ, Zorowitz R, Wittenberg, GF (eds.). *Stroke Recovery and Rehabilitation,* 2nd ed. New York, NY: Demos Medical Publishing, LLC; 2015.

II

Optimizing Functional Outcomes After Pediatric Stroke

Examination and Evaluation of Neuromotor Function in Children With Stroke

Heather L. Atkinson, PT, DPT, NCS and Susan V. Duff, EdD, MPT, OTR/L, CHT

Neural recovery patterns that unfold after perinatal and childhood stroke can differ based on the child's age at the time of occurrence and associated neuroplasticity. The outcome may be further influenced by the location and size of the stroke. Some children develop significant impairments that contribute to long-lasting disability, whereas others exhibit subtle signs of dysfunction. This chapter will review the key features of examination and evaluation of neuromotor function within the framework of the International Classification of Functioning, Disability and Health of Children and Youth (ICF-CY)[1] as applied to infants and children who have sustained perinatal or childhood stroke. The ICF-CY provides a useful framework to organize examination data into the domains of impairment, activity, and participation. Through careful assessment, clinicians can ascertain the extent of impairments and the influence they may have on activity and participation.

EXAMINATION

History/Interview

Information on history is gathered from a chart review and interview with the client and family. From the chart the clinician can obtain details of the injury with initial and recent findings from neurological examinations and medical tests (ie, imaging, laboratory studies). A list of comorbidities, current medications, and allergies can also be acquired. The interview helps to clarify the medical history and provides information on the social history,

prior/current rehabilitation services, available equipment/orthoses, and previous level of function. The clinician can discuss overarching client and family goals and determine the specific learning style and needs of both.

General Appearance and Presentation

Assessment of the client's appearance, including the presence of medical accessories, physical posture, and skin condition, can begin in the interview. Medical accessories such as lines and tubes indicate the acuity of the current situation and the need for further investigation regarding the purpose and time course for use. The observation allows the clinician to gauge the client's current level of awareness and the ability to engage in reciprocal interaction or conversation. Posture at rest and intentional movement can be screened for subtle asymmetries and movement quality. Specific concerns found during the observation can be formally assessed.

Impairment Measures

Physical Function

Components of physical function that should be assessed include passive range-of-motion (PROM), muscle strength, and muscle tone. PROM gathered with goniometry[2] precedes other measures because grading is often dependent on the findings. Gross strength assessments can be followed up with manual muscle tests[3] or handheld dynamometry.[4] Grip and pinch dynamometry can be used to document hand strength.[5,6] For very young children or those unable

Atkinson HL, Nixon-Cave K, Smith SE, eds.
*Pediatric Stroke Rehabilitation: An Interprofessional and
Collaborative Approach* (pp 91-112).© 2018 Taylor & Francis Group.

TABLE 6-1. MODIFIED ASHWORTH SCALE[7]	
0	No increase in muscle tone
1	Slight increase in muscle tone, manifested by a catch and release or by minimal resistance at the end of ROM when the affected part(s) is (are) moved in flexion or extension
1+	Slight increase in muscle tone, manifested by a catch followed by minimal resistance through the remainder of ROM, but the affected part(s) is (are) easily moved
2	More marked increase in muscle tone through most of ROM, but the affected part(s) is (are) easily moved
3	Considerable increases in muscle tone, passive ROM difficult
4	Affected part(s) is (are) rigid in flexion or extension

to follow strength test instructions, clinicians observe and note the child's ability to move with gravity minimized, against gravity, and/or with the resistance of body weight or toys and common objects. Muscle tone is objectively assessed with a standard measure such as the Modified Ashworth Scale (MAS)[7] or the Modified Tardieu Scale (MTS).[8-10] The MAS grades muscle tone as the resistance of muscle to passive stretch on a 6-point ordinal scale from 0 to 4. The authors[7] added a 1+ score to the original scale to indicate the presence of increased tone after an initial catch. The MTS is a measure of spasticity made through the assessment of resistance to passive movement at slow and fast speeds.[8] Sufficient reliability and validity have been established for adult stroke using the MAS[11-14] and the MTS.[15-18] The MAS and MTS have been recommended for use by the Stroke Taskforce of the American Physical Therapy Association. Tables 6-1 and 6-2 outline the MAS and MTS scales.

Movement Analysis

After strength, ROM, and muscle tone are assessed, the clinician can begin to analyze the available movement. One priority is to determine if the individual has isolated joint movement or tends to move the joints of the upper or lower limbs together in a synergy pattern. Two scales that can be used to perform this assessment are the Brunnstrom Stages of Recovery[19-20] and the Selective Control Assessment of the Lower Extremity.[21] Another priority is to determine if the individual shows signs of ataxia or dystonia.[22]

The Brunnstrom Stages of Recovery[19-20] can be used to assess selective movement. The stages are as follows: 1) complete flaccidity without myotactic reflexes; 2) no active movement, yet hyperreflexive myotactic reflexes with decorticate/decerebrate posturing or mild resistance to PROM; 3) active synergistic movement with <50% full PROM in at least one plane of movement for one joint; 4) active synergistic movement >50% of full PROM in at least one plane of movement for one joint; 5) active movement >50% full PROM with less synergistic pattern noted in at least 2 joints; and 6) individual joint movement

proximally and distally within functional limits with trace or no synergistic movement.

Eileen Fowler and her colleagues at the University of Southern California designed the Selective Control Assessment of the Lower Extremity.[21] This tool is intended for use in children with cerebral palsy to assess selective motor control. Although this scale has not been validated in children poststroke, it is a good reference for the assessment of hemiplegia. The scale scores lower extremity movement on a 3-point scale: normal=2 points; impaired=1 point; and unable=0 points. Hip motion is assessed in sidelying, whereas the remaining motions are assessed in sitting: knee extension and flexion, ankle dorsiflexion and plantarflexion, subtalar inversion and eversion, toe flexion and extension. All motions are to be performed to a verbal cadence in a reciprocating pattern. Wagner and colleagues have recently designed a similar tool, Selective Control of the Upper Extremity Scale,[23] for use with children with unilateral cerebral palsy. Reliability and content/construct validity are supported for this tool.

As a clinician conducts an assessment of selective motor control, he or she should consider the following: 1) Can the patient elicit movement within a synergy pattern or association reactions? Is there isolated joint motion? 2) How is the patient able to move with consideration of his or her other impairments? For example, he or she may have scored a 3 on the MAS in the ankle plantarflexors but still have sufficient strength to dorsiflex against that tone to achieve 0 degrees of dorsiflexion, which affords them more mobility and efficiency during movement.

Posture

Postural asymmetry at rest and during select movements is common in persons with hemiplegia. Atypical trunk and extremity posturing can be the result of weakness and muscle imbalances, but may also be due to perceptual changes and altered sensory feedback. One motor action that occurs frequently is when persons lean heavily on the more affected hip, exhibiting trunk elongation on the unaffected side and trunk shortening on the affected side. This

TABLE 6-2. MODIFIED TARDIEU SCALE[8]					
QUALITY OF MUSCLE REACTION (X)		ANGLE OF MUSCLE REACTION (Y)		VELOCITY OF STRETCH	
0	No resistance throughout the course of passive movement	Measured relative to the position of minimal stretch of the muscle (corresponding to angle zero) for all joints except hip where it is relative to the resting anatomical position	V1	As slow as possible (slower than the natural drop of the limb segment under gravity)
1	Slight resistance throughout the course of passive movement; no clear catch at a precise angle	Angle of muscle reaction (Y) should be measured by universal goniometry	V2	Speed of the limb segment falling under gravity
2	Clear catch at a precise angle, interrupting the passive movement, followed by release		V3	As fast as possible (faster than rate of the natural drop of the limb segment under gravity)
3	Fatigable clonus (> 10 s when maintaining the pressure) at a precise angle			
4	Infatigable clonus (> 10 s when maintaining the pressure) at a precise angle			
5	Joint immovable			

has been classified as *pusher syndrome*[24] wherein persons push away from the less-affected side. These individuals often have an impaired perception of the body's orientation to gravity such that the longitudinal axis of the body is shifted to the affected side in sitting and standing.

Assessment of trunk alignment can be accomplished using a plumb line or central mark of vertical in sitting or standing. In the anterior/posterior position asymmetries can be noted, such as unilateral scapular elevation with or without trunk elongation, head or trunk tilt to one side, and height of the anterior superior iliac spine. From a lateral view one can assess for the presence of forward head posture, kyphosis, or anterior/internally rotated positioning of the humeral head. It is also important to assess for torticollis and head preference at rest as noted when the infant or child tends to posture toward the right or left side. Further assessment of muscular and soft tissue tightness can follow visual inspection. Head preference may be the result of prolonged positioning in one direction or stem from visual or sensory deficits. A visual and manual assessment of skull shape should follow because children with a strong head preference to one side are at risk for deformational plagiocephaly.

Sensibility

Sensibility, or the perception and recognition of a stimulus,[25] plays an important role in motor control. Sensation is the stimulus for spinal reflexive action and modulation of the motor activity associated with central pattern generators. Sensory information is essential for motor function and in particular tasks that incorporate manual dexterity.[26-29] Diminished somatosensation has been found to be associated with functional outcome in adults poststroke.[30-34]

A recent study of 50 adults poststroke found approximately 50% of participants with deficits in tactile discrimination.[34] Given the relationship between sensibility and motor function, it is essential that sensibility tests are conducted poststroke.

Sensibility tests can be divided into 3 test categories: threshold, discrimination, and function. The most common threshold test is the Semmes Weinstein Monofilament test.[35] Moving and static 2-point discrimination are the most widely used discrimination tests.[36] Haptic sensibility or stereognosis is a good measure of function. One standard test of function is the Moberg Pick-up test. Please see the American Society of Hand Therapists' *Clinical Assessment Recommendations*, 3rd edition[37] and a chapter by Bell-Krotoski[35] for details on administration and interpretation of these sensibility tests.

Visual Function

A gross assessment of visual skills that begins during the observation can be validated with formal testing. The clinician can make a gross assessment of visual attention and scanning ability during the interview. Formal visual assessment includes documentation of the ability to fixate on a target followed by horizontal, vertical, and circular tracking, making note of whether the child moves the eyes only, the head only, or employs both during these tasks. Older children can be assessed in a similar manner. However, assessment of the school-aged child must include the functional skill of near and far visual scanning and copying.

Visual-Motor and Visual-Perceptual Function

Standardized tests of visual perception are useful to assess status and change with intervention. A common tool to assess visual-motor function is the Beery-Buktenica Developmental Test of Visual-Motor Integration, 6th edition.[38] It is standardized for persons aged 2 to 99 years with new normative data for ages 2 to 18 years. The primary test item has a design-copy format with supplemental visual-perceptual and visual-motor subtests. It takes 10 to 15 minutes or less to administer. Another common test of visual function is the Motor Free Visual Perceptual Test-4 (MVPT-4).[39] The MVPT-4 has normative data for ages 4 to 80 and takes about 20 to 25 minutes to conduct. This motor-free tool provides an assessment of visual discrimination, spatial relationships, visual memory, figure-ground, and visual closure. Another tool is the Test of Visual-Perceptual Skills, 3rd edition.[40] This nonmotor tool covers 7 perceptual areas. It is standardized for children 4 to 18.11 years of age and takes about 30 to 40 minutes to administer.

Cognition

A general cognitive screen can be conducted during the initial interview. Young infants and toddlers should also be assessed for visual regard and the ability to follow directions. If they are old enough, they can be tested for alertness and orientation to person, place, and time. Formal testing can be done to assess status and change with intervention.

A common standardized assessment tool used to examine cognitive skills in young children is the Bayley Scales of Infant and Toddler Development, 3rd edition.[41] The Wechsler Preschool and Primary Scale of Intelligence, 3rd edition[42] is often used to examine cognition in children aged 2.5 to 7 years, 3 months, and the Wechsler Intelligence Scale for Children, 4th edition[43] for those aged 6 to 16 years. Another useful tool is the Kaufman Brief Intelligence Test, 2nd edition[44] standardized for ages 4 to 90 years. Please refer to Chapter 9 for a detailed review of cognitive outcome measures.

Activity Measures

Physical Activity Levels

Assessment of physical activity levels is often done with interviews or questionnaires. More recently therapists have been taking advantage of technology to assess activity levels in typical and atypical populations using simple wearable devices such as pedometers[45] or the Fitbit (www.fitbit. com).[46] More sophisticated devices such as the StepWatch

(https://modushealth.com) or APDM sensors (www.apdm. com) provide more detailed information. Bjornson et al[47] found the StepWatch to provide excellent accuracy and precision during gait in typically developing children and more recently used it to examine gait intensity in children with cerebral palsy.[48] The Opal APDM sensors have been used to examine the amount of infant arm and leg movement.[49,50] Expansion of this form of technology to foster tracking of physical activity is expected.

Functional Mobility

This category includes an assessment of bed mobility, transfers, and gait. During gait assessment common deviations can be recorded. Performance on alternative modes of ambulation such as stair climbing can also be examined (Figure 6-1). As appropriate, the efficiency of walking and running ability can be tested using a stopwatch within a measured area. A formal test of walking speed and capacity can be done using the 6-minute walk test (6MWT).[51] Reference values are available from healthy children 7 to 11 years of age. In addition, clinicians can utilize the Energy Expenditure Index (EEI) by taking the child's heart rate before and after a walking test such as the 6MWT. The EEI is calculated by subtracting the resting heart rate from the walking heart rate and dividing by walking speed (meters/minute). The index gives an indication of energy expenditure and has been validated for use in typical children and adolescents[52] as well as children with cerebral palsy.[53]

A quick assessment of anticipatory standing balance, gait control, and motor function within a typical activity is the Timed "Up & Go" Test (TUG).[54] The standard TUG has been validated in children with tetraplegia or diplegia from 2 to 18 years of age.[55] The modified TUG has been validated for use with typically developing children 3 to 9 years of age and children with disabilities from 3 to 19 years of age.[54] The modified TUG for children requires that a child rises from a seat without arms, stand momentarily, walk 3 meters, touch a target on the wall, turn, return to the same seat, and sit down. Timing for the modified TUG begins as the child leaves the chair and ends when the child's bottom touches the chair seat. Qualitative instructions such as "walk as fast as you can" are not used in the modified TUG.

Gait Analysis

Gait in children with hemiparesis may be slow and asymmetric with limits in selective motor control, diminished equilibrium responses, and decreased weight bearing on the more affected limb. Common gait deviations in children with hemiplegia that may present alone or in combination include 1) equinus foot, 2) equinus foot and genu recurvatum, 3) in-toeing, 4) excess hip flexion, and 5) crouch.[56,57] Other common deviations include compensations for foot drop, which may include decreased heel strike or toes first/foot flat for initial contact, steppage pattern, hip hiking or circumduction during swing, or external rotation of the lower extremity. Position of the pelvis and ability to push off on the affected limb should be observed. Step asymmetry during typical and fast walking should be noted. Postural alignment of the foot and ankle complex as well as the entire lower quarter, spine, and upper extremity should be assessed. All gait kinematics including joint angles and timing components should be evaluated, and gait analysis should be done with and without orthoses and shoes to be complete. Gait analysis can include observational examination of the qualitative features of gait, and can also be supplemented with an outcome measure such as the Dynamic Gait Index (DGI)[58,59] or with comprehensive measurement through an instrumented device such as the GAITRite system.[60,61]

The DGI assesses the ability for one to balance while walking on level and unlevel ground when external demands are present. The following items receive a score on a 4-point scale: 1) steady-state walking, 2) walking with changing speeds, 3) walking with head turns both horizontally and vertically, 4) walking while stepping over and around obstacles, 5) pivoting while walking, and 6) stair climbing. The 4-point scale includes 3 = no gait dysfunction, 2 = minimal impairment, 1 = moderate impairment, and 0 = severe impairment. The test takes about 10 minutes to administer. The DGI has been investigated for use with children with various conditions,[58,59] but has not yet been validated for use in children poststroke.

The GAITRite system can capture spatial and temporal parameters such as velocity, step/stride length, base of support, step/stride time, swing/stance time, single/double support times, and toe-in/-out angle.[60,61] The instrumented GAITRite system can be used to examine gait parameters at a single point in time or in response to intervention in children with hemiparesis.[62]

Activities of Daily Living

A general screen of activities of daily living (ADLs) can be accomplished through an interview with the client or parent. A more objective measure of ability can be obtained through alternative scales such as the Functional Independence Measure for Children (WeeFIM)[63] or the Functional Independence Measures (FIM).[64] Both tools are designed to determine the severity of child or adolescent disability, the measurement of caregiver assistance needed to perform functional activities, and the outcome from rehabilitation. The WeeFIM is standardized for children without disabilities aged 6 months to 8 years and for children with developmental disabilities aged 6 months to 12 years. It includes 18 items classified into Motor and Cognition categories. The Motor category is divided into domains: Motor; Self-care (eating, grooming, bathing, dressing, toileting); Sphincter control (bladder and bowel management); transfers (chair, wheelchair, toilet, tub, and shower); and locomotion (wheelchair/crawl, stairs). The cognitive category is divided into communication

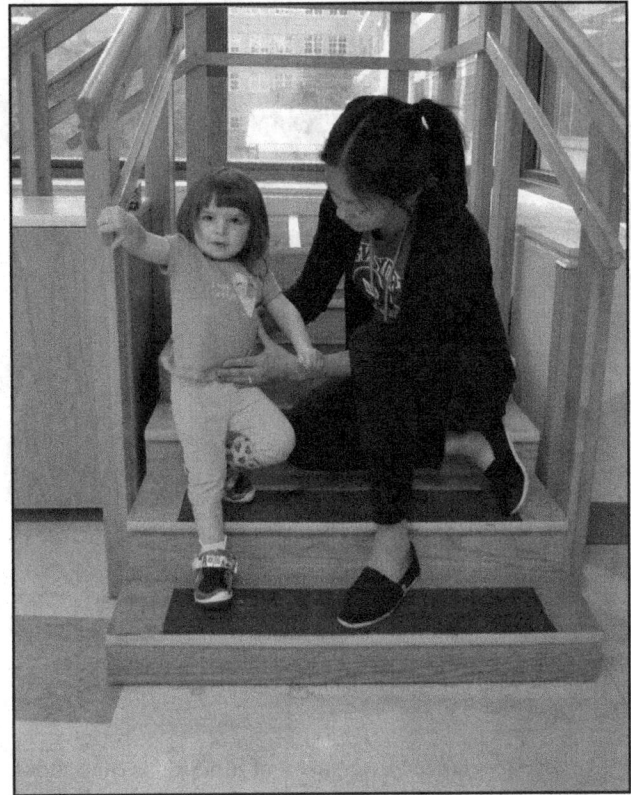

Figure 6-1. The therapist evaluates the child's mobility on the stairs.

(comprehension, expression) and social cognition (social interaction, problem solving, memory). The FIM is standardized for ages 7 to adulthood. It measures mobility in the home and community environment as well as self-care, sphincter control, transfers, locomotion, communication, and social cognition.

A formal tool of functional mobility and ADL function is the Pediatric Evaluation of Disability Inventory (PEDI).[65] This tool is standardized for children 6 months to 7.6 years. The purpose of this tool is to determine functional capabilities and performance, monitor progress in functional skill performance, and evaluate rehabilitative program outcome in children with disabilities. It is divided into three subtests in the functional skill scale: self-care: eating, grooming, dressing, bathing, toileting; mobility: transfers, indoors and outdoors mobility; and Social function: communication, social interaction, household and community tasks. Environmental modification and amount of caregiver assistance are systematically recorded in the Modification Scale and Caregiver Assistance Scale. The PEDI has been modified for use on the computer into the PEDI-Computer Adaptive Test (PEDI-CAT).[66] This modified tool has four content domains: daily activities, mobility, social/cognitive, and responsibility. It has been standardized for use with parents of typically developing children and parents of children and adolescents with disabilities age 0 to 21 years. The 10-item and 15-item versions of the PEDI-CAT have been shown to be accurate and precise assessments of daily performance.

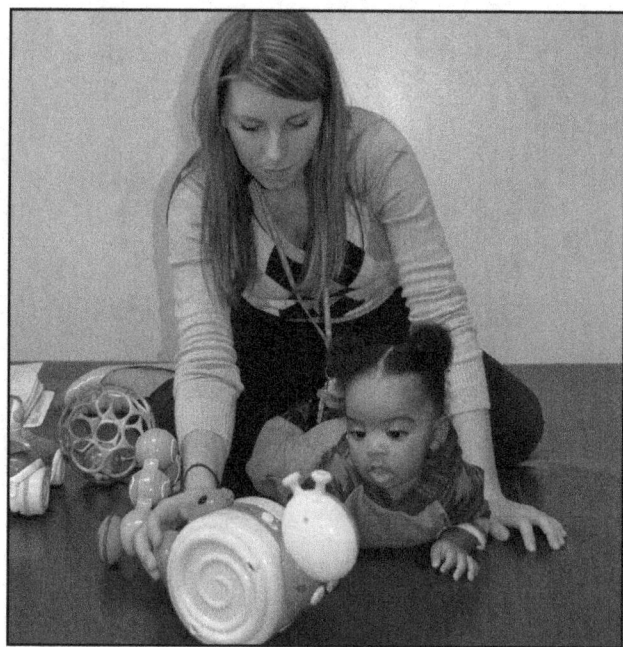

Figure 6-2. The clinician uses a variety of age-appropriate toys to observe and elicit movements during the exam.

A more specialized assessment of function is the School Function Assessment.[67] The purpose of this tool is to assess and monitor student performance of functional tasks in the context of the school environment. It can also be used to guide program planning. This tool is standardized for children from kindergarten to sixth grade. The 3 scales of assessment are participation, task supports, and activity performance.

Gross Motor Skills

Observational checklists or formal assessments can be used to examine gross motor skills. Therapists will use developmental toys to observe or elicit movement (Figure 6-2). Although many developmental tests are available, we will provide examples of assessments that we have found useful. For the young infant, the Test of Infant Motor Performance[68] provides a standardized measure of posture and selective control of movement. It is standardized for infants 32 weeks preterm to the postconceptual age of 4 months post-term. From birth to 18 months, the Alberta Infant Motor Scale provides the clinician with a gross screen of motor skills.[69] This norm-referenced measure of motor development has been found to be reliable and to have concurrent and predictive validity.[70] The Peabody Developmental Motor Scales-2[71] is a gross and fine-motor assessment standardized for use with children from birth to 5 years of age. This assessment has been shown to be reliable and sensitive to change in children with cerebral palsy.[72]

The Gross Motor Function Measure-66 (GMFM-66)[73] is designed to examine current level of motor function and evaluate change in gross motor function in children with cerebral palsy. The test is appropriate for children whose motor skills are at or below those of a 5-year-old child without any motor disability. The tool consists of 66 gross motor items from 5 dimensions: 1) lying and rolling; 2) sitting; 3) crawling and kneeling; 4) standing; and 5) walking, running, and jumping. Items were selected to represent those typically performed by children by age 5. This tool takes about 45 to 60 minutes to administer. The GMFM-66 is a useful tool for children with hemiplegia, as it tests both the left and right sides on various skills.

Balance

The examination of static and dynamic balance is essential. After a gross assessment formal testing can be done with tools such as the Pediatric Balance Scale.[74-76] The Pediatric Balance Scale is a criterion-referenced 14-item measure that examines functional balance in the context of everyday tasks. Each balance item is scored on a scale of 0 to 4, with and without vision, for a maximum of 56 points. Other useful tools that may require further validation in pediatric stroke include the Functional Reach Test[77] and the High-Level Mobility Assessment Tool.[78] In addition, some clinicians may have access to technology such as computerized posturography, which can give objective data on a child's ability to integrate the visual, vestibular, and somatosensory systems of balance. Therapists also observe how the child responds to both static and dynamic balance activities (Figures 6-3 and 6-4).

Coordination

There are two popular assessments of motor coordination. One is the Bruininks-Oseretsky Test of Motor Proficiency, 2nd edition.[79] It is a widely used assessment of gross and fine-motor coordination and is standardized for use with children ages 4.5 to 14.5 years. This tool provides an assessment of the following areas: balance, strength, coordination, running speed and agility, upper limb coordination (ball skills), dexterity, fine motor control, and visual-motor skills. Another tool is the Movement Assessment Battery for Children, 2nd edition (Movement ABC-2).[80] The Movement ABC-2 is an assessment of motor coordination standardized for children 3 to 16.11 years of age.[80] This tool has normative data from the United Kingdom. It contains 8 tasks for 3 age groups (3 to 6 years, 7 to 10 years, and 11 to 16 years) examining manual dexterity, ball skills, and static/dynamic balance. The Movement ABC-2 also has a checklist for use with children 5 to 12 years to assess movement during everyday tasks.

Prehension

Prehension involves the behaviors of visual regard or locating a target, reach, grasp, manipulation, and release.[81] Therefore, a thorough prehensile assessment should involve

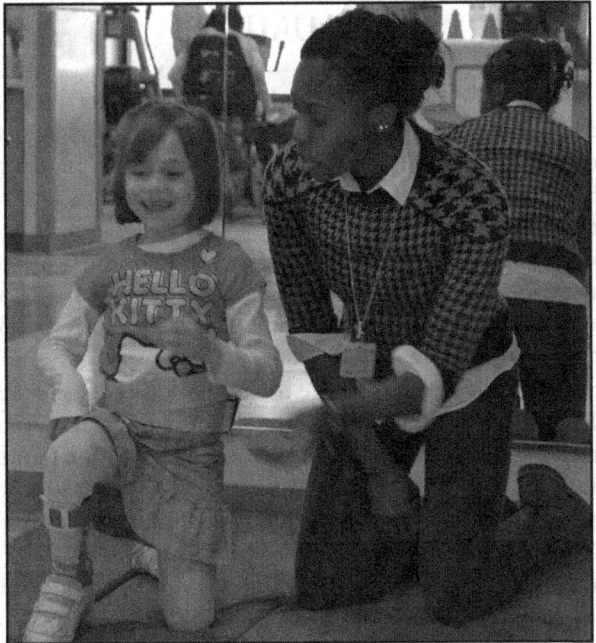

Figure 6-3. The therapist evaluates how a child can maintain a variety of static balance postures.

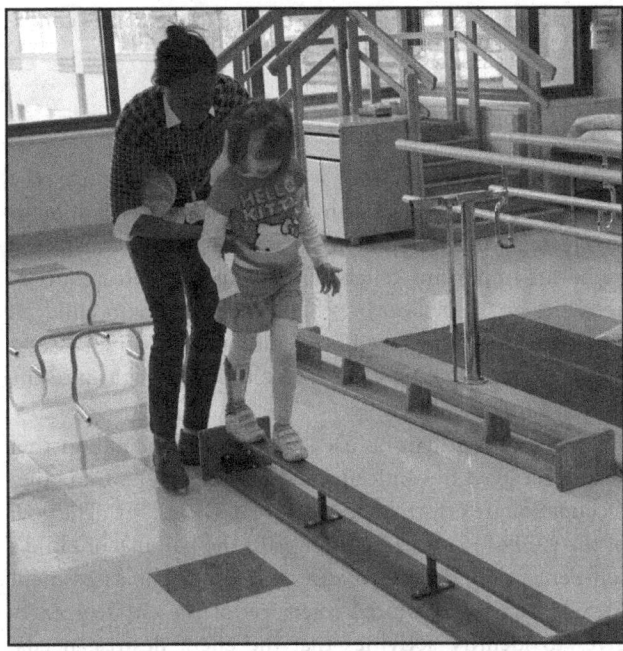

Figure 6-4. The clinician examines dynamic balance during a challenging gross motor task.

all components and is best done with videotaping. Visual regard requires examination of visual attention, perception, and central and peripheral vision. If vision is diminished, auditory or somatosensory cues can be used to locate a target. An examination of intentional reach or reach-to-grasp behaviors can be unimanual or bimanual. Components include the hand path, speed, and extent of the reach. During reaching, the clinician can ascertain whether the child preshapes the hand sufficiently to the shape and size of the target object. Examination of grip and pinch begins with an assessment of the available prehension patterns. Gross grasp patterns include the cylindrical, spherical, and hook grasp. Pinch patterns include a lateral pinch, pad-to-pad pinch, and tip-to-tip pinch. A frequently used pinch pattern is the 3-jaw chuck or 3-fingered pinch. During grasp, the clinician can closely observe the grasp points in which the thumb and fingers oppose the object to stabilize it within the hand. An assessment of manipulation can include the ability to regulate fingertip forces when grasping and lifting an object[81] or the ability to display in-hand manipulation.[82] In-hand manipulation is the ability to move objects within one hand and includes the components of translation, shift, and rotation. Finally, object release or the gradation of pressure relief is assessed with regard to ability and ease of movement. Other features of prehension that can be assessed include interlimb coordination and motor lateralization or hand preference/dominance.

The Manual Ability Classification Scale (MACS)[83] allows the clinician to classify the hand function of children with cerebral palsy 4 to 18 years of age. Information to determine classification can be obtained through observation or verbal descriptions from parents, teachers, and the child. The 5 levels of self-initiated ability on the MACS are classified as follows:

- Level I—handles most objects easily and successfully
- Level II—handles most objects but with somewhat reduced ability and/or speed
- Level III—handles objects with difficulty and requires help preparing and/or modifying activities
- Level IV—handles a limited selection of easily managed objects in adapted situations
- Level V—cannot handle objects and has severely limited ability to perform simple actions

Classification using the MACS has been found to be stable over time and to have predictive value.[84]

Cardiopulmonary Screen

During an initial cardiopulmonary assessment, vital signs should be checked along with signs of respiratory distress, breathing patterns, and chest auscultation.[85] Vitals can be taken at rest, during, and after select activity.[86] Further review of comorbidities such as congenital heart defects and sickle cell anemia should be done.[80] A timed walking test such as the 6MWT (reviewed earlier) can be done while monitoring vital signs, breathing patterns, and oxygen saturation. If indicated the child can be referred for more extensive exercise testing on a treadmill or bicycle ergometer so that an electrocardiogram and measures of oxygen consumption can be obtained. The ongoing assessment of cardiopulmonary status can determine the child's tolerance to select activities and change in the child's condition as treatment progresses.[85]

Participation Measures

As children move from infancy to preschool age, the focus can begin to include an assessment of participation or involvement in life situations.[87] Participation is considered to be an important rehabilitation outcome. Recreational activities and social outings build competency in children and help them connect with the community. Formal assessments of participation can provide unique insight into the overall care of children.

One tool that can be used to assess participation that is well received by clinicians and families is the Canadian Occupational Performance Measure (COPM).[88,89] The goal of the COPM is to detect changes in the parent's or child's self-perception of performance over time. The assessment includes a semistructured interview of the child or caregiver to identify activities that the client desires, needs, or is expected to perform across the domains of self-care, productivity, and leisure. Then goals in one or all of the performance domains are set up by the child or parent and clinician. Satisfaction and performance of activities identified by the child and family as an important part of daily life are rated. The COPM can be used to assess outcome from intervention.

Two other tools that are companion measures of participation are the Children's Assessment of Participation and Enjoyment (CAPE) and the Preferences for Activities of Children (PAC).[90] The CAPE is a questionnaire with 55 items that examines how children participate in activities outside of school. The CAPE makes an assessment of diversity, intensity, and enjoyment of activities while also considering the context for them. The PAC examines the preferences children have for each of the activities. It takes 30 to 45 minutes to administer the CAPE and 15 to 20 minutes to finish the PAC. Reliability and validity of the 2 measures have been established.[90]

Another useful tool to assess participation is the Pediatric Quality of Life Inventory version 4.0 (PedsQL 4.0).[91] The purpose of this tool is to measure health-related quality of life in children and adolescents aged 2 to 18 years. The 23-item tool measures the core dimensions of health from the World Health Organization (WHO); physical, emotional, and social functioning; and school functioning. There are child self-report forms for children aged 5 years and older and parent proxy forms for children 2 to 18 years of age. Diagnostic modules are available for children and adolescents with asthma, rheumatology, diabetes, cancer, and cardiac conditions. The PEDS QL 4.0 has established reliability and validity.[91]

EVALUATION

The ICF-CY as set forth by the WHO[1] provides a useful framework to synthesize the examination findings. As discussed earlier in this text, the ICF-CY serves as a model of ability rather than disability and shifts the emphasis toward the positive attributes of the whole person.[1] Physical and occupational therapists can use the ICF-CY framework to organize and prioritize the patient's abilities and problems in relation to the patient and family goals and corresponding evidence-based interventions.

The case study and Figure 6-8 at the end of the chapter illustrate how a clinician used the ICF-CY to organize and prioritize examination findings. As depicted in the figure, the ICF-CY can help to categorize, prioritize, and integrate the many factors in a child's life and can ultimately drive clinical decisions around care. Atkinson and Nixon-Cave[92] developed a tool to facilitate clinical reflection and decision making: the Physical Therapy Clinical Reasoning and Reflection Tool (PT-CRT). Some of the reflection points suggested by the authors during the evaluative process are illustrated in Box 6-1. For a child poststroke, these questions can help illuminate a diagnosis, prognosis, and goals and plan of care.

Diagnosis

It is in the scope of practice for both physical and occupational therapists to make diagnoses based on their evaluation.[86] According to Rogers and Holm,[93] diagnostic reasoning is a process that describes a child's problems within the realm of functional and occupational performance limitations. In the *Guide to Physical Therapist Practice 3.0*,[94] the American Physical Therapy Association describes diagnosis as follows: "Although physicians typically use labels that identify disease, disorder, or condition at the level of the cell, tissue, organ, or system, physical therapists use labels that identify the *impact of a condition on function at the level of the system (especially the movement system) and at the level of the whole person.*"

Thus, it is crucial for clinicians to reflect on the underlying pathology and/or medical condition as well as the clinical presentation and examination findings when determining a diagnosis or diagnoses. For children who have experienced a stroke, physical and occupational therapy diagnoses will vary based on the clinical sequelae from the site of the lesion as well as other secondary effects or concurrent medical diagnoses or conditions. For instance, the diagnostic labels for a child with a congenital heart defect and arterial ischemic stroke in the left middle cerebral artery distribution will be very different from the diagnostic labels for a child with a hemorrhage in the cerebellum due to an arterial venous malformation. Please refer to the

Box 6-1

The following is an excerpt from PT-CRT,[92] which describes examples of questions to probe clinical reasoning and reflection during the evaluative process:

- How did you determine your diagnosis? What about this patient suggested your diagnosis?
- How did your examination findings support or negate your initial hypothesis?
- What is your appraisal of the most important issues to work on?
- How do these relate to the patient's goals and identified issues?
- What factors might support or interfere with the patient's prognosis?
- How might other factors such as bodily functions and environmental and societal factors affect the patient?
- What is your rationale for the prognosis, and what are the positive and negative prognostic indicators?
- How will you go about developing a therapeutic relationship?
- How might any cultural factors influence your care of the patient?
- What are your considerations for behavior, motivation, and readiness?
- How can you determine capacity for progress toward goals?

case study at the end of this chapter for further examples in identifying diagnoses.

As with any age or medical diagnosis, using the ICF-CY as a framework to delineate therapeutic diagnoses is helpful to ensure the clinician is placing ample priority on the various levels of health with the potential to be affected by intervention, including impairments, activity limitations, and participation restrictions. As discussed previously, a myriad of factors can contribute to a child's physical presentation, which necessitates an individualized approach to examination and evaluation.

Prognosis

After determining a diagnosis, the therapist considers both positive and negative prognostic indicators that help give clues into that child's overall functional potential and capacity to achieve goals within the desired timeframe. These indicators are multifaceted and embody all aspects of the child's life. By using the ICF-CY as described earlier, the clinician can weigh the various factors to consider an overall prognosis.

Although generating a prognosis is individualized to each patient, there are many common elements for children with stroke that a clinician is often prompted to consider. These include:

- What are the characteristics of the lesion?
  - □ Which areas of the brain were affected? What is known about common sequelae after stroke in these areas? Was it cortical or subcortical?

Unilateral or bilateral? Left or right? What was the size of the lesion? Was it ischemic or hemorrhagic? Was it focal or diffuse?

- What is the clinical presentation?
  - □ Is there weakness? Is there some ability to recruit affected muscle groups? Is there spasticity or flaccidity? What type of movement control is present (isolated movement versus synergies)? Are there ROM restrictions? Are there movement disorders such as dystonia or ataxia?
- What was the age of onset?
  - □ Did the stroke occur prenatally, perinatally, or sometime in childhood? If in childhood, what was the child's level of function before the stroke?
- What is the time since injury?
  - □ Is this child in the acute, subacute, or chronic phase?
  - □ What has the child's progress been like since injury? What type of therapy has the child received thus far, and what has the child's response been?
  - □ Have there been any barriers to recovery such as medical instability or sedating medications?
- What is the child's functioning in other developmental domains?
  - □ How is the child functioning from a language, cognitive, visual-perception, and behavioral standpoint?

    ☐ What is the typically developing presentation in these areas for the child's age, and what, if any, effect did the stroke have?

- What are the other conditions/comorbidities?
- What is the child's level of motivation?
- How is the family's level of support?
- What is the child's access to rehabilitation services?

Although this list is not exhaustive and no question signifies a black-and-white answer, as a gestalt they can provide clues as to an individual's overall capacity to achieve goals. Please see Chapter 7 for further discussion on many of the areas listed earlier.

Goals and Plan of Care

Goal writing is a complex collaborative process that is essentially the synthesis of evaluation findings, including diagnosis and prognosis, as well as the goals and desires of the child and family. Family-centered care necessitates that children and family are key members in the formulation of therapy goals.

The Institute for Patient- and Family-Centered Care (IPFCC) considers patient- and family-centered care as an overall philosophy of practice (please see Section III of this text for further detail).[95] The IPFCC suggests that the unique support that only the family can provide is of integral importance in optimizing health care, and it is critical for providers to involve families in decision making.[95] Although family-centered care is often heralded as a trademark of effective health care delivery, much is still left to be desired, as many clinicians are in need of better ways to integrate the principles of family-centered care into all facets of care.[96,97] For physical and occupational therapists, collaborating with the family from the initial examination through goal setting and establishment of a plan of care can foster this necessary cooperative partnership. Through shared decision making, therapists can ensure that they are providing the most effective and valuable care possible.

Setting goals for a pediatric client with a new neurological insult can be a nebulous endeavor as clinicians can find themselves trying to differentiate between recovery and development. It is a complicated and thought-provoking process to attempt to parcel out what might be expected from natural recovery, natural development, and the effects of any potential intervention. Consider the following scenarios:

1. A 12-month-old with new onset of stroke is admitted to inpatient rehabilitation for hemiplegia. This child was previously creeping and cruising but not yet walking and could easily reach to grasp toys. Considering that the child is in the acute recovery phase and might expect some degree of natural recovery in the early months, the family and team might set goals for the child to return to cruising but also to walk independently. Even though his right arm is more affected, they may also promote reach-to-grasp skills in that limb. Setting these ambitious yet developmentally appropriate goals would focus therapy sessions and challenge both the child and the family to work toward optimal recovery.

2. A 30-month-old with hemiplegia due to perinatal stroke has been receiving early intervention (EI) and outpatient physical therapy once/week each week since age 12 months. This child is ambulating independently with an ankle–foot orthosis (AFO), ascending and descending steps with one rail using a step-toe pattern, and not yet jumping. At the EI re-evaluation, the EI physical therapist and the family decide to continue physical therapy service to continue work on goals listed on the individualized family service plan (see Chapter 12). At the outpatient re-evaluation, however, the family and therapist decide to discontinue, or "take a break," from services. Although more developmental goals could be written (ascending and descending steps using a reciprocal pattern, jumping), outpatient progress has slowed dramatically. The family also wishes to pursue speech language pathology services, and having one less appointment each week would be helpful to their family life. The family agrees to continue EI physical therapy but to discontinue outpatient physical therapy, with future follow-up if new needs arise.

3. A 7-year-old with left hemiplegia due to perinatal stroke receives school-based physical therapy once/month and occupational therapy once/week. He has not received outpatient physical therapy or occupational therapy since age 3. He recently received Botox injections due to decreased ankle and wrist ROM. At his outpatient physical therapy evaluation, the therapist discusses family goals and recommends therapy 3 times/week for 12 weeks. This intensive burst of service is intended to improve his ankle ROM, to strengthen his left ankle dorsiflexion so that he can actively dorsiflex against gravity, orthotic re-evaluation, and gait training. At his outpatient occupational therapy evaluation, his clinician recommends 3 times/week for 12 weeks to work on increasing wrist ROM and strength, fostering neuromuscular re-education in the affected musculature and expanding prehensile skill needed for function.

These examples illustrate how the confounding factors of development and acute recovery may influence potential progress as well as goal writing. As described in Chapter 12, the educational and medical model of therapy service delivery will have different influences on setting goals. Thus, any physical or occupational therapist working with

---

BOX 6-2

The following is an excerpt from PT-CRT,[92] which describes examples of questions to probe clinical reasoning and reflection during the re-evaluation:

- Evaluate the effectiveness of your interventions. Do you need to modify anything?
- What have you learned about the patient/caregiver that you did not know before?
- Using the ICF, how does this patient's progress toward goals compare with that of other patients with a similar diagnosis?
- Is there anything that you overlooked, misinterpreted, or over- or undervalued, and what might you do differently? Will this address any potential errors you have made?
- How has your interaction with the patient/caregiver changed?
- How has your therapeutic relationship changed?
- How might any new factors affect the patient outcome?
- How do the characteristics of the patient's progress affect your goals, prognosis, and anticipated outcome?
- How can you determine the patient's views (satisfaction/frustration) about his or her progress toward goals? How might that affect your plan of care?
- How has physical therapy affected the patient's life?

---

a child who has had a stroke has an important role in defining realistic yet ambitious goals, specific to that particular child that integrates not only evaluation findings but the patient and family goals as well.

Developing a plan of care reflective of the evaluation is detailed in Chapter 7. A good plan of care for a child with a stroke will have the following qualities:

- Evidence-based
- Promote optimal recovery or functional attainment in accordance with goals
- Age-appropriate
- Motivating/meaningful for the child
- Creative
- Efficient
- Valuable
- Easy for family to carry over into daily life
- Incorporate child and family interests

In addition, a good plan of care will continually progress and challenge the child for optimal attainment of goals. Clinicians must be flexible and adaptable to reflect upon which interventions are not working well, which need to be modified, and which need to be progressed. It is critical for clinicians to maintain safety in care yet remain one step ahead of the child's progress so as to continually challenge functional performance to the highest potential.

Re-Evaluation

Re-evaluation is the episodic reassessment of the child's status that occurs at intervals appropriate to both the child's progress and setting of care. A child in the acute or subacute phase of recovery will require at least a partial re-evaluation of status, goals, and intervention plan at almost every encounter, whereas a child in the chronic phase will likely need re-evaluation on a weekly, monthly, or even an annual basis, depending on the setting, level of service, and child's needs. Atkinson and Nixon-Cave[92] suggest some reflective questions to consider during a formal or informal re-evaluation (Box 6-2).

For a child poststroke, frequent re-evaluation is needed to assess the evolution of neurological recovery and potential secondary complications. Furthermore, growth and development present a unique and dynamic influence on stroke rehabilitation, as can concurrent conditions. Changes in status can take many different directions, even in the chronic phase of recovery. Careful re-evaluation is necessary to judge progress toward goals, modify goals as needed, and consider optimal intervention.

In addition to the questions posed in Box 6-2, specific considerations for the re-evaluation of a child with stroke include the following:

- Growth and development
  - Has the child experienced a recent growth spurt? What is its influence on muscle length, spasticity, muscle strength, muscle activation, gait mechanics, and functional ability? Has the neuromuscular balance around the joint been altered in some way? How?
  - How are the fit and function of adaptive equipment, splints, and orthotics?
  - Has the child reached a stage of cognitive/emotional readiness to be able to focus more on voluntary muscle activation in therapy?
  - Does the child have different motivation or different goals for therapy?
- Concurrent conditions
  - What is the influence of any concurrent condition with the child's level of impairment and functioning? Concurrent conditions that may be present in children with stroke that may have an effect on the re-evaluation include the following:
    - Cardiopulmonary conditions and congenital heart defects
    - Disorders of the blood such as sickle cell disease
    - Disorders of the blood vessels
    - Developmental syndromes
    - Cancer
    - Metabolic disorders
    - Vision or hearing problems
  - Are there any pending surgeries that may have an effect on function?
  - How is the child's function being affected by current medications?
- Neurological and/or functional recovery
  - Is the child experiencing changes in movement ability? Is the child able to move in a synergistic pattern when he or she was not able to before? Is he or she able to move with more isolated control?
  - How do gains in neurological recovery or skills in function set the stage for further goals?
  - Is progress slowing, or is the child experiencing an increase in skill in a different area?

For children with neuromuscular changes such as hemiplegia, frequent assessment is necessary to evaluate how all of the previous factors are affecting the child's body structures, functions, and activities in the context of physical impairment. Consider the following scenario. A 7-year-old child with left spastic hemiplegia due to a right middle cerebral artery infarction sustained at age 5 presents to an occupational therapist and a physical therapist with left arm weakness, limited prehensile patterns, increased toe drag on the left side, and increased tripping at home. Occupational therapy re-examination reveals that the child often displays a left wrist drop during reach-to-grasp movements and a tendency to have objects slip from his grasp. Physical therapy re-examination reveals that the child's articulating AFO is not fitting properly and his heel does not maintain contact within the device. Although his previous left ankle dorsiflexion was within normal limits 3 months ago (10 degrees for R1 and 20 degrees for R2 with the knee extended), he is now −10 degrees for R1 and 5 degrees for R2. His spasticity also appears increased in his left gastrocnemius (was previously MAS 1+, now is at 3). The clinician surmises that the child's change in gait function is directly related to the child's change in muscle balance around the left ankle. These changes in limb function could be due to growth or other factors that could influence strength and spasticity, such as a reduction in neural representation or changes in muscle integrity due to the time poststroke and pharmacological intervention. The occupational therapist and physical therapist discuss changes in limb motion and function. Together they decide to address these primary problem areas through a revised intervention plan and refer the child to his rehabilitation medicine physician for lower limb spasticity management.

Concurrent conditions may also have a dynamic influence on the child's response to intervention. For example, a child undergoing chemotherapy or radiation due to an oncological process may have varying ability to participate depending on medication side effects such as fatigue and nausea. A child with sickle cell disease could have new issues arise if he or she develops a pain crisis in a joint. Children with congenital heart defects may have limited endurance depending on current cardiopulmonary function.

For children in the acute or subacute phase of recovery from stroke, almost daily re-evaluation is needed to determine changes in movement ability as well as to provide ongoing communication with the family and team regarding the evolution of the stroke's effects on the child's impairments and activity abilities and limitations. Physical and occupational therapists are experts in strategies to facilitate and elicit movement. Once muscle activity is observed through the course of re-evaluation, interventions can be put into place that capitalize on muscle activation and focus on maximizing isolated control. Dynamic muscular control may change on a daily basis, and the entire interprofessional team must have regular discussions about how those changes are affecting the child's functional recovery. Also, the physical and occupational therapist should keep in mind that medications that are started or weaned could affect the neuromuscular system, and their

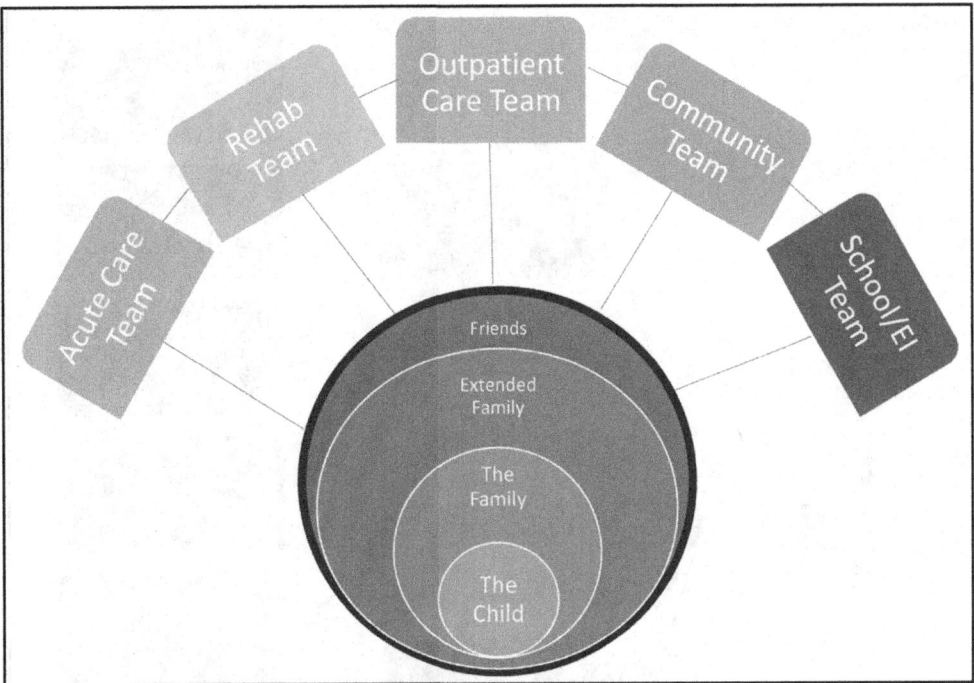

Figure 6-5. Interprofessional team members across the continuum of care.

ongoing assessment of the patient's abilities and challenges are crucial to the medical team's decision making as the entire team strives to help the child optimize function.

Communication and Coordination of Care

Physical and occupational therapists regularly communicate with one another regarding a child's care, as well as with varied members of the interprofessional team. Communication regarding progress, the need for referrals, and education is common. Also, as discussed throughout this book, all members of the interprofessional team have an important opportunity to carry over goals and interventions from the various disciplines to help support maximal outcome. For example, a physical therapist may incorporate a cognitive linguistic activity while a child is ambulating on a treadmill, or a nurse may encourage use of the affected upper extremity during morning ADLs. Depending on the setting, professionals from various teams may interface with the child and family to ensure safe and optimal coordination of care (Figure 6-5).

Many interprofessional teams care for a child with stroke at various stages of recovery across the lifespan. Team members from acute care, rehabilitation, and outpatient may consist of physicians (both attending and consulting services), nursing, physical and occupational therapy, speech and language pathology, psychology, neuropsychology, child life, art and music therapy, education, social work, and case management. The community team may consist of the primary care physician, insurance company/third-party

payers, equipment/orthotic vendors, community resource coordinators, charities, religious organizations, and online support communities. For infants and young children, the EI team may consist of a service coordinator, educators, and other allied health professionals. For older children, the school team may consist of the district administrative team, the principal, the educators and special educators, teaching aides, the school psychologist, school nurse, and school therapy staff such as physical, occupational, and vision therapy, and speech and language pathology.

The family consists of immediate caregivers and various extended supports. All team members should recognize the family as the one constant in the child's life that transcends all teams. Thus, teams should work closely with families to help them prioritize which services they should focus on, as well as when it would be beneficial to take a break. Although well-intentioned, recommending more therapy than a family can handle may be counterproductive and lead to burnout for both the child and family. It is crucial for all caregivers to remember that the child with a stroke is a child first, and although it can be extremely helpful to intensify service when the child is on the cusp of achieving a new skill, it is also very important to allow the child the freedom to "be a kid." Please see Chapter 5 for further discussion on the continuum of care and Chapter 11 for further discussion about the role of the family.

Discharge Planning

Planning for discharge or transition to the next setting often begins at the first visit or soon after through

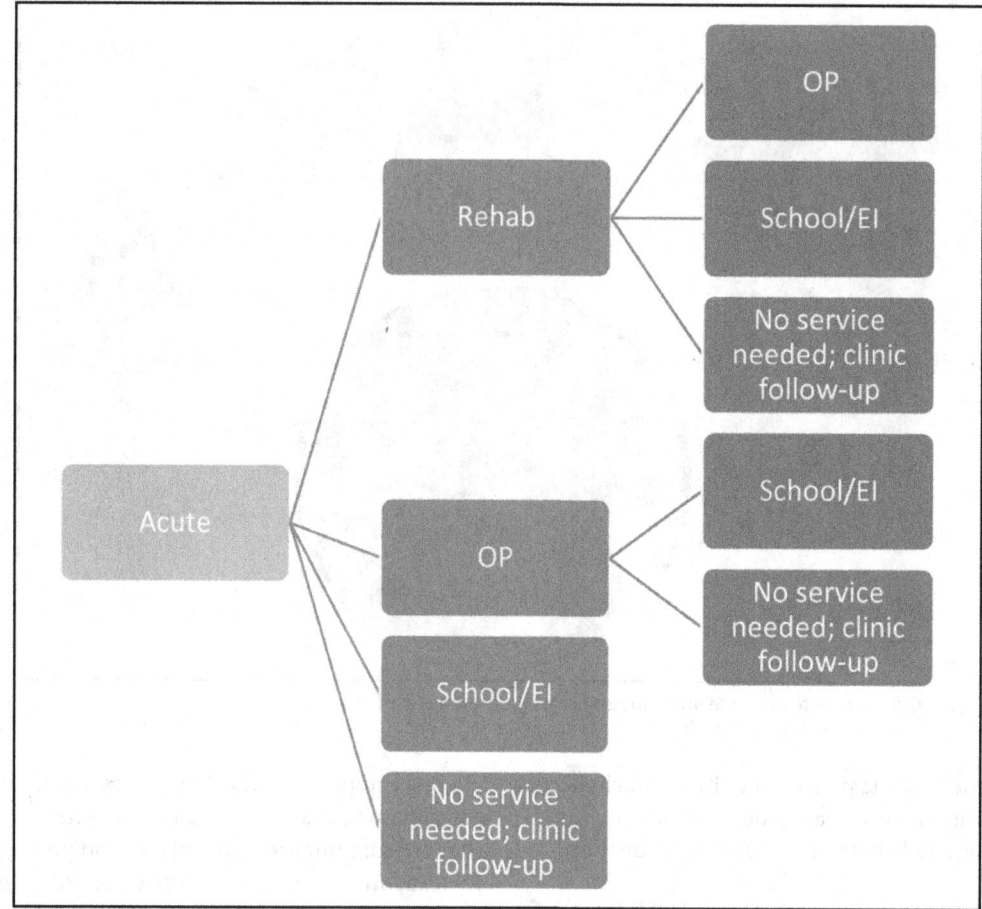

Figure 6-6. One example of a child's progression in the continuum of rehabilitative care, considered as part of the discharge planning process. Services used are dependent on goals, needs, access, and resources. Outpatient and school-based services may complement each other, as they are addressing different goals (medical vs educational model of care). A child may enter the continuum at any point. OP = outpatient

collaborative goal writing. Therapists in various settings have some common and some unique considerations.

Continuation of Rehabilitative Services

If the clinician is working with the child in the medical model of care, he or she must determine what, if any, services are needed in the next stage of recovery. This determination is based on needs, access, and resources, as well as current status. The clinician works in concert with the family and the interprofessional team to facilitate transition to the next setting for the child. For a child with a new onset of hemiplegia due to stroke, a typical progression may be from acute care to inpatient rehabilitation, then to a combination of outpatient rehabilitation and/or school-based therapy (Figure 6-6). If a child's medically based rehabilitation goals are met, he or she may continue with school therapy alone if educationally based goals continue to be present. Often, however, if a child is able to fully access his or her educational experience from a physical perspective, therapy in the school setting may be discontinued or decreased to a consultative basis. Infants and very young children with

stroke will typically be discharged directly to home after the acute hospitalization. Therapy is most often provided through the EI system so that the child can recover and progressively learn in his or her natural environment (see Chapter 12 for details). At times, families may pursue outpatient therapy in addition to EI as an adjunct if additional therapy may help the child achieve his or her goals. In these cases, it is crucial for the outpatient and EI provider to communicate well to effectively coordinate care.

Because the child is constantly growing and developing, therapy needs may periodically arise. Thus, it is critical to have episodic follow up. Ideally, follow up should occur in an interprofessional clinic setting where various disciplines may re-evaluate the child and update home programs. At these visits, suggestions for ongoing services may be provided, or the child could be referred back to therapy for specific needs and goals.

In essence, the rehabilitative continuum of care for a child with stroke is dynamic, and a child may enter the continuum at any point, whether he or she is in the acute, subacute, or chronic phase of recovery.

Equipment/Orthoses/Splints

Physical and occupational therapists routinely prescribe adaptive equipment and aids, as well as orthoses and splints, to help maximize functional independence (please see Chapter 7 for further detail). Clinicians often trial temporary devices, orthoses, and splints, especially when the child is making numerous changes in growth and function. The question as to when definitive equipment should be ordered is a clinical decision that depends on where the child is in the process of recovery, how long it might take to secure the device or equipment, and short-and long-term goals. For example, a child with new-onset hemiplegia may be admitted to inpatient rehabilitation needing a wheelchair, walker, wrist orthosis, and solid AFO, but after a few weeks of rehabilitation that same child may be walking without an assistive device and with a lower profile orthotic such as a posterior leaf-spring orthosis. Also, he or she may no longer require wrist support. Sound clinical decisions can help optimize resource utilization.

Home, School, and Community Evaluation

Evaluation of the child's destination living environment is a key component of discharge planning. Ideally, the clinician travels to the child's home to plan with the child's caregivers the optimal home setup for safety and function. It is even more advantageous if the child can attend this visit so the clinician can assess the child's functioning in a real-world environment. A home visit enhances the therapist's knowledge on how to best simulate training environments during therapy sessions to maximize the carryover of goals. Sometimes, medically based physical and occupational therapists have the opportunity to visit the child's school. If the child attends a public school, they may be able to meet and collaborate with the onsite school therapy team. If the child attends a private school, they will have to work with the family, teacher, and principal to explore any needed accommodations. Please see Chapter 12 for a detailed discussion of potential school accommodations. On occasion, physical and occupational therapists may be invited to speak to the child's class before he or she returns to school. Explaining physical differences to the child's classmates and discussing generalities of rehabilitation may help the child integrate back with peers.

Finally, evaluation of the child's function in the community and incorporating community reintegration training into the therapy plan is of critical importance. A child may walk well within the safe pristine corridors of a hospital environment, but it is important to ascertain his or her mobility and function in real-world situations such as crossing the street, getting onto a bus, or making a purchase at a store. Evaluation of function in the community should be individualized to the child's personal needs and situation (Box 6-3). Outcome measures such as the Community Mobility Assessment[98] and the Community Balance and

---

Box 6-3

Mobility
- Uneven terrain (sidewalks, grass, curbs)
- Crossing the street
- Maneuvering in crowds or stores
- Following directions
- Boarding/unboarding a bus or other public transportation as needed for that child
- Playground safety
- Endurance

Activities of Daily Living
- Route finding
- Safety awareness
- Safe interaction with adults and peers
- Age-appropriate money management for financial transactions
- Toileting management in public restrooms
- Community leisure activity
- Managing a backpack or school books
- Managing outdoor clothing and rain and snow gear

Mobility Scale[99] can be used to evaluate the performance of children and adolescents with acquired brain injury within the community. These assessments provide an objective tool to assess and determine progress toward goals.

School Recommendations

Physical and occupational therapists may play a role in transition to school after a stroke and work closely with the family and the school team to develop an educational plan that will help maximize the child's access to his or her education (Box 6-4). Please see Chapter 12 for details regarding common recommendations for educational environments from a physical or occupational therapy perspective.

Child and Family Education

Physical and occupational therapists integrate child and family education into all aspects of care (Figure 6-7). Clinicians should talk with the family about the child's preferred learning style and seek to provide ongoing education throughout the episode of care. Education may be around exercises, positioning, equipment management, safe guarding techniques, understanding of diagnosis, future considerations, and advocacy. See Box 6-5 for considerations of culturally competent family education.

Box 6-4

Coordination of School-Based and Medically Based Therapy Services
School-based therapy and medically based therapy serve different needs of the child. For a school-aged child, school-based services are driven by the individualized education program and are designed to help the child access his or her education (see Chapter 12). Medically based therapy is episodic in nature, usually commencing when the child is demonstrating a new need due to a change in medical status or functional ability, and is driven by the goals set forth by the child, family, and therapist. Coordination between medically and school-based services is important to ensure that they are complementary rather than contradictory to each other. Decisions around special equipment and splinting should be made in conjunction with one another with permission and input from the family.

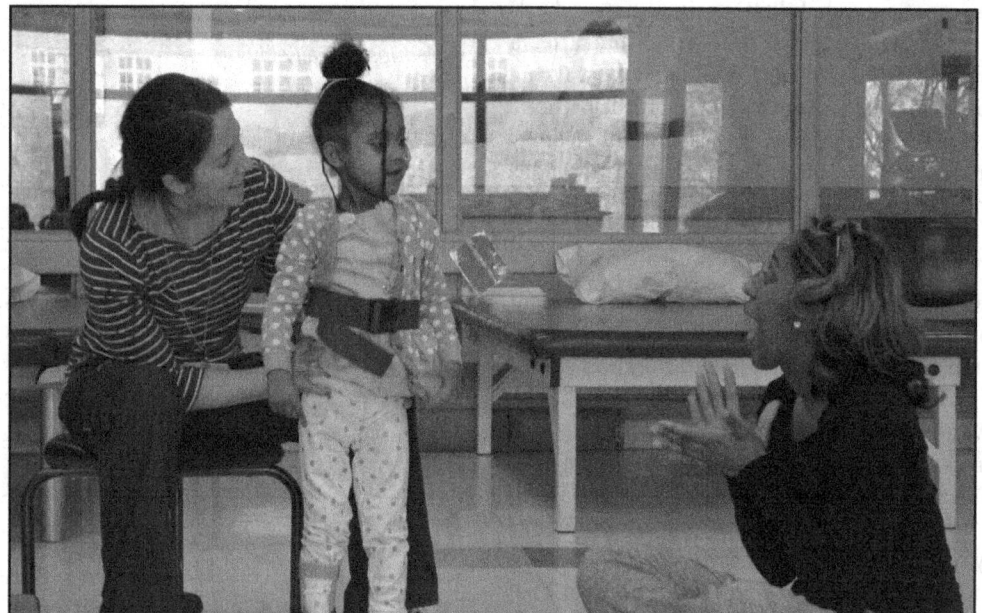

Figure 6-7. During the exam, the caregiver can perform many critical roles: partner, collaborator, motivator, and cheerleader.

Lifelong Follow-up

Although lifelong follow up is covered in detail in Chapters 5 and 13, some discussion is warranted here. Physical and occupational therapists should ensure that a child with a stroke has planned intervals of re-evaluation with a provider who is knowledgeable in poststroke rehabilitation and can refer the child for additional services when needed. As previously discussed, children with stroke can experience declines in function or even demonstrate new capacities for improved function. Depending on access to services, the provider making these referrals for additional physical and occupational therapy may be a rehabilitation physician, a neurologist, a primary care physician, the school therapy team, or even the family themselves. Re-evaluation of rehabilitation needs may take place every few months, every 6 months, or annually.

BOX 6-5
CULTURALLY COMPETENT FAMILY EDUCATION AND CARE

Physical and occupational therapists must strive to provide culturally sensitive education to both the child and the family throughout the episode of care. Developing an understanding of how one's culture relates to expectations and the response to illness or disability is crucial in developing a therapeutic relationship.[100] Providing culturally competent intervention in health care necessitates a process of cultural desire, awareness, knowledge, and skill and should be included in a clinician's ongoing course of lifelong learning.[100]

FAMILY FOCUS BOX

The Role of Physical and Occupational Therapy

1. Physical therapists are experts in the movement system and can help your child move in the best way possible to maximize his or her functional potential.

2. Occupational therapists are experts in maximizing function and participation in ADLs and leisure tasks, which often involve visual perception and cognitive skills.

3. Physical therapy tends to focus on gross motor skills (large body movements) and occupational therapy tends to focus on fine motor skills (small body movements), but there can be overlap.

4. Physical and occupational therapists often collaborate with each other. For very young children under the age of 6 or 7 months, both disciplines tend to work on developmental skills, and it is not uncommon for a child to receive care from only one discipline. Around 6 or 7 months, however, children begin to experience more differentiation in skill development, and it is typically at that age when both disciplines may be quite helpful, depending on the child's individual needs.

5. Your child's therapist will ask you and your child what your goals for therapy are and will help set objectives to be achieved in therapy.

6. Therapists should recognize that you know your child best and your input is invaluable to help motivate your child to participate fully in therapy sessions. Be sure to make the therapist aware of activities that your child enjoys.

7. Children need practice and carryover in real-life environments in order to make a lasting change. Ask your therapist for activities or exercises that you and your child can do at home, and ask how you might be able to make them more challenging as your child masters new skills.

8. Let your therapists know if there are any other care providers in the child's life with whom it would be helpful to discuss your child's care.

9. Your therapy team can help you determine which services will help meet your child's needs best. This may be either school/EI therapy or outpatient therapy, a combination of the two, or even a break from therapy so your child can focus on other community activities.

CASE STUDY

An 8-year-old boy with right hemiplegia due to arterial ischemic stroke of the left middle cerebral artery sustained during the perinatal period is referred to outpatient physical and occupational therapy 2 weeks after receiving Botox injections to his right upper and lower extremity (right brachioradialis, biceps brachii, gastrocnemius, hamstrings). His stated goals for occupational therapy include increasing his ability to use his right hand and arm to manage his clothes and fasteners (particularly don and zip his coat and tie his shoelaces). His goal for physical therapy is to "walk faster without a limp."

The occupational and physical therapists complete their respective exams, using some of the tests and measures discussed. They each use the ICF-CY to organize and prioritize examination findings (see Figure 6-8). After considering how the various factors influence each other, the clinicians circled the areas that were of critical importance to help the child meet his goals and identified the following rehabilitation diagnoses:

- Right spastic hemiplegia due to stroke; decreased strength of the right upper and lower extremity, PROM of the right upper and lower extremity, selective motor control of the right upper and lower extremity, functional mobility, balance, gross motor skills, ADLs, and participation in age-appropriate sports and individual leisure activities.

- Visual field cut affecting his performance of ADLs and leisure.

- Sufficient cognition to engage in educational and leisure activities.

- Well-motivated and energetic.

Using the ICF-CY, the therapists identified the positive prognostic indicators of a high level of motivation, very engaged family, and some minimal ability to move the affected side, as well as the potential negative prognostic indicators of increased spasticity through his right side, family stress, and time since initial lesion. Taken all together and integrated with current knowledge of stroke recovery in response to targeted therapeutic intervention, the therapists may postulate that the child has a good prognosis to achieve his therapy goals. Progress toward those goals will help inform the prognosis for any further advanced goals in the future.

Both the occupational and physical therapist develop a plan of care to achieve the child's goals based on the child's/family's preferences, as well as the principles of neurorecovery outlined in Chapter 7.

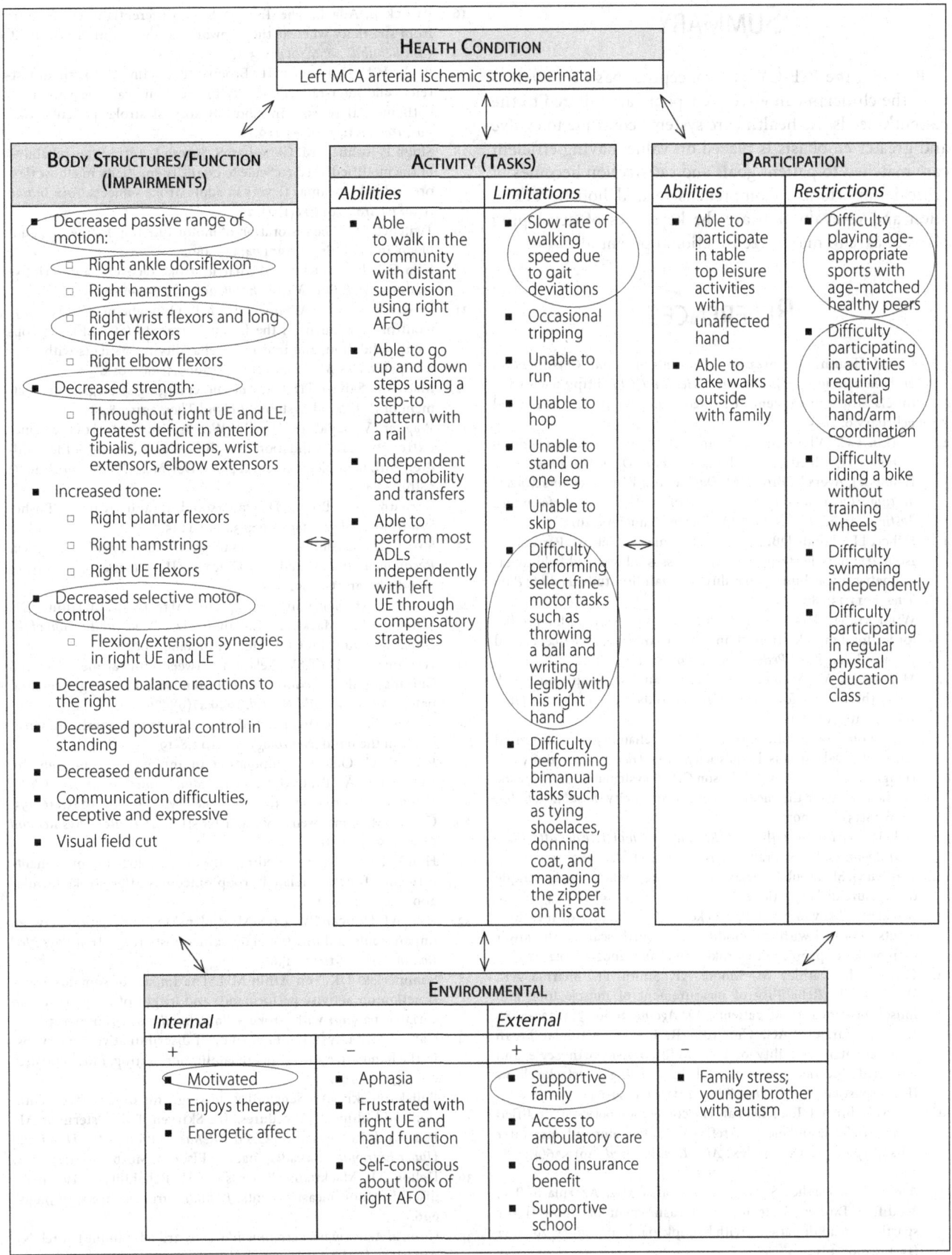

Figure 6-8. This diagram illustrates how to use the ICF-CY to organize and prioritize examination findings. After considering how the various factors influenced each other, the clinician circled the areas that were of critical importance to help the child meet his goals. UE=upper extremity; LE=lower extremity; MCA=middle cerebral artery.

SUMMARY

By using the ICF-CY as a conceptual basis for evaluation, the clinician can effectively plan care tailored to the patient's needs. As health care systems continue to evolve and greater emphasis is placed on value, having efficient care matched to patient goals and satisfaction becomes of critical importance. Comprehensive and holistic evaluation and re-evaluation are the keystones of developing plans of care to maximize functional potential.

REFERENCES

1. World Health Organization. *The International Classification of Functioning, Disability, and Health (ICF)*. http://www.who.int/classifications/icf/en/. Updated January 27, 207. Accessed February 6, 2015.
2. Norkin CC, White DJ. *Measurement of Joint Motion: Guide to Goniometry*, 4th ed. Philadelphia, PA: F. A. Davis Co, 2009.
3. Hislop HJ, Avers D, Brown M. *Daniels and Worthingham's Muscle Testing: Techniques of Manual Examination and Performance Testing*, 9th ed. St. Louis, MO: Elsevier-Saunders, 2013.
4. Hébert LJ, Maltais DB, Lepage C, Saulnier J, Créte M, Perrom M. Isometric muscle strength in youth assessed by hand-held dynamometry: a feasibility, reliability, and validity study. *Pediatr Phys Ther*. 2011;23:289-299.
5. Wind AE, Helders PJ, Engelbert RHH. Is grip strength a predictor for total muscle strength in healthy children, adolescence and young adults? *Eur J Pediatr*. 2010;169:281-287.
6. Mathiowetz V, Wiemer DM, Federman SM. Grip and pinch strength: norms for 6- to 19-year olds. *Am J Occup Ther*. 1986;40(10):705-711.
7. Bohannon RW, Smith MB. Interrater reliability of a modified Ashworth scale of muscle spasticity. *Phys Ther*. 1987;67:206-207.
8. Haugh AB, Pandyan AD, Johnson GR. A systematic review of the Tardieu scale for the measurement of spasticity. *Disabil Rehabil*. 2006;28(15):899-907.
9. Held JP, Pierrot-Deseilligny E. *Reeducation mortrice des affections neurologiques*. Paris, France: J. B. Balliere et fils; 1969.
10. Tardieu G, Shentoub S, Delarue R. A la recherche d'une technique de measure de la spasticite. *Rev Neurol (Paris)*. 1954;91:143-144.
11. Blackburn M, van Vliet P, Mockett SP. Reliability of measurements obtained with the modified Ashworth scale in the lower extremities of people with stroke. *Phys Ther*. 2002;82(1):25.
12. Gregson J, Leathley M, Moore AP, Smith TL, Sharma AK, Watkins CL. Reliability of measurement of muscle tone and muscle power in stroke patients. *Age Ageing*. 2000;29(3):223-228.
13. Kaya T, Karatepe AG, Gunaydin R, Koc A, Altundal Ercan U. Inter-rater reliability of the Modified Ashworth Scale and modified Modified Ashworth Scale in assessing poststroke elbow flexor spasticity. *Int J Rehabil Res*. 2011;34(1):59-64.
14. Min JH, Shin Y-I, Joa KL, et al. The correlation between Modified Ashworth Scale and biceps T-reflex and inter-rater and intra-rater reliability of biceps T-reflex. *Ann Rehabil Med*. 2012;36(4):538-543.
15. Ansari NN, Naghdi S, Hasson S, Azarsa MH, Azarnia S. The Modified Tardieu Scale for the measurement of elbow flexor spasticity in adult patients with hemiplegia. *Brain Injury*. 2008;22(13-14):1007-1012.
16. Patrick E, Ada L. The Tardieu Scale differentiates contracture from spasticity whereas the Ashworth Scale is confounded by it. *Clin Rehabil*. 2006;20(2):173-182.
17. Paulis WD, Horemans HL, Brouwer BS, Stam HJ. Excellent test-retest and inter-rater reliability for Tardieu Scale measurements with inertial sensors in elbow flexors of stroke patients. *Gait Posture*. 2011;33(2):185-189.
18. Singh P, Joshua AM, Ganeshan S, Suresh S. Intra-rater reliability of the modified Tardieu Scale to quantify spasticity in elbow flexors and ankle plantar flexors in adult stroke subjects. *Ann Indian Acad Neurol*. 2011;14(1):23-26.
19. Twitchell TC. The restoration of motor function following hemiplegia in man. *Brain*. 1951;74:443-480.
20. Kim C-T, Han J, Kim H. Pediatric stroke recovery: a descriptive analysis. *Arch Phys Med Rehabil*. 2009;90:657-662.
21. Fowler E, Staudt LA, Greenburg MB, Oppenheim WL. Selective Control Assessment of the Lower Extremity (SCALE): development, validation, and interrater reliability for patients with cerebral palsy. *Dev Med Child Neurol*. 2009;51:607-614.
22. Matteo B, Sanger TD. Current and emerging strategies for treatment of childhood dystonia. *J Hand Ther*. 2015;28:185-194.
23. Wagner LV, Davids JR, Hardin JW. Selective Control of the Upper Extremity Scale: validation of a clinical assessment tool for children with hemiplegic cerebral palsy. *Dev Med Child Neurol*. 2016;58(6):612-617.
24. Karnath H-O, Broetz D. Understanding and treating "Pusher Syndrome." *Phys Ther*. 2003;83:1119-1125.
25. Stone JH. Sensibility. In: Casanova J, ed. *Clinical Assessment Recommendations*, 2nd ed. Chicago, IL: American Society of Hand Therapists; 1992:71-84.
26. Callahan AD. Sensibility testing: clinical methods. In: Hunter JM, Schneider LH, Mackin EJ, Callahan AD, eds. *Rehabilitation of the Hand*. St. Louis, MO: CV Mosby; 1990:600-602.
27. Gordon AM, Duff SV. Relation between clinical measures and fine manipulative control in children with hemiplegic cerebral palsy. *Dev Med Child Neurol*. 1999;41(9):586-591.
28. Moberg E. Criticism and study of methods for examining sensibility in the hand. *Neurology*. 1962;12:8-19.
29. Pehoski C. Object manipulation in infants and children. In: Henderson A, Pehoski C, eds. *Hand Function in the Child: Foundations for Remediation*. St. Louis, MO: Mosby. 1995:136-153.
30. Carey LM. Somatosensory loss after stroke. *Crit Rev Phys Rehabil Med*. 1995;7:51-91.
31. Han L, Law-Gibson D, Reding M. Key neurological impairments influence function-related group outcomes after stroke. *Stroke*. 2002;33:1920-1924.
32. Patel AT, Duncan PW, Lai S-M, Studenski S. The relation between impairments and functional outcomes poststroke. *Arch Phys Med Rehabil*. 2000;81:1357-1363.
33. Sommerfeld DK, von Arbin MH. The impact of somatosensory function on activity performance and length of hospital stay in geriatric patients with stroke. *Clin Rehabil*. 2004;18:149-155.
34. Carey LM, Matyas TA. Frequency of discriminative sensory loss in the hand after stroke in a rehabilitation setting. *J Rehabil Med*. 2011;43:257-263.
35. Bell-Krotoski JA. Sensibility testing: history, instrumentation, and clinical procedures. In: Skirven TM, Osterman AL, Fedorcyzk JM, Amadio PC, eds. *Rehabilitation of the Hand and Upper Extremity*. Philadelphia, PA: Elsevier-Mosby. 2011:132-151.
36. Dellon AL, Mackinnon SE, Crosby PM. Reliability of two-point discrimination measurements. *J Hand Surg Am*. 1987;12(5):693-696.
37. *Clinical Assessment Recommendations*, 3rd ed. Mount Laurel, NJ: American Society of Hand Therapists; 2015.

38. Beery KE, Buktenica NA, Beery NA. *Beery-Buktenica Developmental Test of Visual-Motor Integration,* 6th ed. San Antonio, TX: Pearson Education Inc; 2010.

39. Colarusso RP, Hammill DD. *Motor-Free Visual Perception Test-4.* Torrance, CA: WPS Publishing. 2015.

40. Martin NA. *Test of Visual-Motor Skills,* 3rd ed. Torrance, CA: WPS Publishing; 2006.

41. Bayley N. *Bayley Scales of Infant and Toddler Development Technical Manual,* 3rd ed. San Antonio, TX: Harcourt Assessment; 2006.

42. Wechsler D. *Manual for the Wechsler Preschool and Primary Scale of Intelligence* (WPPSI-III), 3rd ed. San Antonio, TX: The Psychological Corporation; 2002.

43. Wechsler D. *Administration and Scoring Manual for the Wechsler Intelligence Scale for Children,* 4th ed. San Antonio, TX: The Psychological Corporation; 2003.

44. Kaufman AS, Kaufman NL. *Kaufman Assessment Battery for Children Manual,* 2nd ed. Circle Pines, MN: AGS; 2004.

45. Hazell TJ, Ellery CV, Cohen TR, Vanstone CA, Rodd CJ, Weiler HA. Assessment of pedometer accuracy in capturing habitual types of physical activities in overweight and obese children. *Pediatr Res.* 2016;80(5):686-692.

46. Hooke MC, Gilchrist L, Tanner L, Hart N, Withycombe JS. Use of a fitness tracker to promote physical activity in children with acute lymphoblastic leukemia. *Pediatr Blood Cancer.* 2016;63(4):684-689.

47. Bjornson KF, Yung D, Jacques K, Burr RL, Christakis D. StepWatch stride counting: accuracy, precision, and prediction of energy expenditure in children. *J Pediatr Rehabil Med.* 2012;5(1):7-14.

48. Bjornson KF, Zhou C, Stevenson R, Christakis D, Song K. Walking activity patterns in youth with cerebral palsy and youth developing typically. *Disabil Rehabil.* 2014;36(15):1279-1284.

49. Duff SV, Sargent B, Kutch JJ, Berggren J, Fetters L. Self-generated feedback to increase muscle activation in children. Poster presentation at the Society for Neuroscience (SFN) Annual Meeting. Chicago, IL, October 2015.

50. Smith BA, Trujillo-Priego IA, Lane CJ, Finley JM, Horak FB. Daily quantity of infant leg movement: wearable sensor algorithm and relationship to walking onset. *Sensors (Basel).* 2015;15(8):19006-19020.

51. Klepper SE, Muir N. Reference values on the 6-Minute Walk Test for children living in the United States. *Pediatr Phys Ther.* 2011;23:32-40.

52. Rose J, Gamble JG, Lee J, Lee R, Haskell WL. The energy expenditure index: a method to quantitate and compare walking energy expenditure for children and adolescents. *J Pediatr Orthop.* 1991;11(5):571-578.

53. Rose J, Gamble JG, Burgos A, Medeiros J, Haskell WL. Energy Expenditure Index of walking for normal children and for children with cerebral palsy. *Dev Med Child Neurol.* 1990;32(4):333-340.

54. Williams EN, Carroll SG, Reddinhough DS, Phillips BA, Galea MP. Investigation of the Timed 'Up & Go' test in children. *Dev Med Child Neurol.* 2007;47(8):518-524.

55. Chrysagis N, Skordilis EK, Koutsouki D. Validity and clinical utility of functional assessments in children with cerebral palsy. *Arch Phys Med Rehabil.* 2014;95:369-374.

56. Dana R, Antonescu D. Cerebral palsy gait, clinical importance. *Maedica (Buchar).* 2013;8(4):388-393.

57. Wren TAL, Rethlefsen S, Kay RM. Prevalence of specific gait abnormalities in children with cerebral palsy: influence of cerebral palsy subtype, age and previous surgery. *J Ped Ortho.* 2005;25(1):79-83.

58. Janky KL, Givens D. Vestibular, visual acuity, and balance outcomes in children with cochlear implants: a preliminary report. *Ear Hear.* 2015;36(6):e364-e372.

59. Lubetzky-Vilnai A, Jirikowic TL, McCoy SW. Investigation of the Dynamic Gait Index in children: a pilot study. *Pediatr Phys Ther.* 2011;23(3):268-273.

60. Dusing SC, Thorpe DE. A normative sample of temporal and spatial gait parameters in children using the GAITRite® electronic walkway. *Gait Posture.* 2007;25(1):135-139.

61. van Uden CJT, Besser MP. Test-retest reliability of temporal and spatial gait characteristics measures with an instrumented system (GAITRite®). *BMC Musculoskelet Disord.* 2004;5:13.

62. Coker P, Karakostas T, Dodds C, Hsiang S. Gait characteristics of children with hemiplegic cerebral palsy before and after constraint-induced movement therapy. *Disabil Rehabil.* 2010;32(5):402-408.

63. Granger CV, McCabe MA. *Pediatric Functional Independence Measure* (Wee-FIM). Amherst, NY: Uniform Data System for Medical Rehabilitation; 1990.

64. Dodds T, Andrew DP, Martin WC, Stolov WC, Deyo RA. A validation of the Functional Independence Measurement and its performance among rehabilitation inpatients. *Arch Phys Med Rehabil.* 1993;74 (5):531-536.

65. Haley SM. *Pediatric Evaluation of Disability Inventory (PEDI): Development, Standardization and Administration Manual.* PEDI Research Group; 1992.

66. Haley SM, Coster WJ, Dumas HM, et al. Accuracy and precision of the Pediatric Evaluation of Disability Inventory computer-adaptive tests (PEDI-CAT). *Dev Med Child Neurol.* 2011;53(12):1100-1106.

67. Coster W, Deeney T, Haltiwanger J, Haley S. *School Function Assessment (SFA).* San Antonio, TX: The Psychological Corporation; 1998.

68. Campbell SK, Kolobe THA, Wright BD, Linacre JM. Validity of the Test of Infant Motor Performance for prediction of 6-, 9- and 12- month scores on the Alberta Infant Motor Scale. *Dev Med Child Neurol.* 2002;44(4):263-272.

69. Piper MC, Darrah J. *Alberta Infant Motor Scale (AIMS).* Philadelphia, PA: Saunders; 1994.

70. Piper MC, Pinnell LE, Darrah J, Maquire T, Byrne PJ. Construction and validation of the Alberta Infant Motor Scale. *Can J Public Health.* 1992;83:S46-S50.

71. Fewell RR, Folio MR. *Peabody Developmental Motor Scales.* Austin, TX: Pro-Ed; 2000.

72. Wang H-H, Liao H-F, Hsieh C-L. Reliability, sensitivity to change, and responsiveness of the Peabody Developmental Motor Scales-Second Edition for children with cerebral palsy. *Phys Ther.* 2006;86:1351-1359.

73. Russell DJ, Leung KM, Rosenbaum PL. Accessibility and perceived clinical utility of the GMFM-66: evaluating therapists' judgments of a computer-based scoring program. *Phys Occup Ther Pediatr.* 2003;23(2):45-58.

74. Chen C, Shen I, Chen C, et al. Validity, responsiveness, minimal detectable change, and minimal clinically important change of pediatric balance scale in children with cerebral palsy. *Res Dev Disabil.* 2012;34:916-922.

75. Franjoine MR, Gunther JS, Taylor MJ. Pediatric balance scale: a modified version of the Berg balance scale for the school-age child with mild to moderate motor impairment. *Pediatr Phys Ther.* 2003;15(2):114-128.

76. Franjoine MR, Darr N, Held S, Kott K, Young BL. The performance of children developing typically on the Pediatric Balance Scale. *Pediatr Phys Ther.* 2010;22(4):350-359.

77. Katz-Leurer M, Fishe I, Need M, Schwartz I, Carmeli E. Reliability and validity of the modified functional reach test at the sub-acute stage post-stroke. *Disabil Rehabil.* 2009;31(3):243-248.

78. Williams G, Hill B, Pallant JF, Greenwood K. Internal validity of the revised HiMAT for people with neurological conditions. *Clin Rehabil.* 2012;26(8):741-747.

79. Bruininks RH, Bruininks BD. *Bruininks-Oseretsky Test of Motor Proficiency (BOT™-2)*, 2nd ed. Toronto, ON, Canada: Pearson Education Inc; 2005.

80. Barnett A, Henderson SE, Sugden DA. *Movement Assessment Battery for Children (Movement ABC-2)*, 2nd ed. San Antonio, TX: Pearson Education Inc; 2007.

81. Duff SV. Prehension. In: Cech D, Martin S, eds. *Functional Movement Development Across the Life Span*, 3rd ed. Philadelphia, PA: WB Saunders; 2011.

82. Exner C. Clinical interpretation of in-hand manipulation in young children: translational movements. *Am J Occup Ther.* 1997;51(9):729-732.

83. Eliasson AC, Krumlinde-Sundholm L, Rösblad Bet al. The Manual Ability Classification System (MACS) for children with cerebral palsy: scale development and evidence of validity and reliability. *Dev Med Child Neurol.* 2006;48(07):549-554.

84. Öhrvall AM, Krumlinde-Sundholm L, Eliasson AC. The stability of the Manual Ability Classification System. *Dev Med Child Neurol.* 2014;56(2):913-918.

85. Gould A. Cardiopulmonary evaluation of the infant, toddler, child, and adolescent. *Ped Phys Ther.* 1991;3(1):9-13.

86. Urbina E, Albert B, Flynn J, et al. Ambulatory blood pressure monitoring in children and adolescents: recommendations for stand and assessment. *Hypertension.* 2008;52:433-451.

87. Roach ES, Golomb MR, Adams R, et al. Management of stroke in infants and children. *Stroke.* 2008;39:2644-2691.

88. Law M, Anaby D, Imms C, Teplilck R, Turner L. Improving the participation of youth with physical disabilities in community activities: an interrupted time series design. *Aust Occup Ther J.* 2015;62(2):105-115.

89. Law M, Polatajko H, Pollock N, et al. *The Canadian Occupational Performance Measure.* Ottawa, ON, Canada: CAOT Publications ACE; 1998.

90. King G, Law M, King S, et al. *Children's Assessment of Participation and Enjoyment (CAPE) and Preferences for Activities of Children (PAC).* San Antonio, TX: Harcourt Assessment, Inc.; 2004.

91. Varni JW, Seid M, Kurtin PS. PedsQL 4.0: reliability and validity of the Pediatric Quality of Life Inventory version 4.0 generic core scales in healthy and patient populations. *Med Care.* 2001;39(8):800-812.

92. Atkinson HL, Nixon-Cave K. A tool for clinical reasoning and reflection using the International Classification of Functioning, Disability and Health (ICF) framework and patient management model. *Phys Ther.* 2011;91(3):416-430.

93. Rogers JC, Holm MB. Occupational therapy diagnostic reasoning: a component of clinical reasoning. *Am J Occup Ther.* 1991;45(11):1045-1053.

94. American Physical Therapy Association. *Guide to Physical Therapist Practice 3.0.* http://guidetoptpractice.apta.org. Accessed March 24, 2016.

95. Institute for Patient- and Family-Centered Care. Patient- and Family-Centered Care. www.ipfcc.org/about/pfcc.html. Accessed April 13, 2017.

96. Kuo DZ, Houtrow AJ, Arango P, Kuhlthau KA, Simmons JM, Neff JM. Family-centered care: current applications and future directions in pediatric health care. *Matern Child Health J.* 2012;16(2):297-305.

97. Kuhlthau KA, Bloom S, Van Cleave J, et al. Evidence for family-centered care for children with special health care needs: a systematic review. *Academic Pediatrics.* 2011;11(2):136-143.

98. Moody KD, Wright FV, Brewer KM, Geisler PE. Community mobility assessment for adolescents with an acquired brain injury: preliminary inter-rater reliability study. *Dev Neurorehabil.* 2007;10(3):205-211.

99. Wright FV, Ryan J, Brewer K. Reliability of the Community Balance and Mobility Scale (CB&M) in high-functioning school-aged children and adolescents who have an acquired brain injury. *Brain Injury.* 2010;24(13-14):1585-1594.

100. Spearing EM. Providing family-centered care in pediatric physical therapy. In: Tecklin JS, ed. *Pediatric Physical Therapy*, 5th ed. Baltimore, MD: Lippincott Williams & Wilkins; 2015:1-14.

SUGGESTED READINGS

American Physical Therapy Association. *Guide to Physical Therapist Practice 3.0.* http://guidetoptpractice.apta.org. Accessed March 24, 2016.

de Campos AC, Kukke SN, Hallett M, Alter KE, Damiano DL. Characteristics of bilateral hand function in individuals with unilateral dystonia due to perinatal stroke: sensory and motor aspects. *J Child Neurol.* 2014;29(5):623-632.

Duff SV. Prehension. In: Cech D, Martin S, eds. *Functional Movement: Development Across the Life Span*, 3rd ed. Philadelphia, PA: WB Saunders; 2011.

Duff SV. Functional development. In: Abzug JM, Kozin SH, Zlotolow DA, eds. *The Pediatric Upper Extremity.* Philadelphia, PA: Springer; 2015:25-36.

Gordon AM, Duff SV. Relation between clinical measures and fine manipulative control in children with hemiplegic cerebral palsy. *Dev Med Child Neurol.* 1999;41(9):586-591.

Koenraads Y, Porro GL, Braun KP, Groenendaal F, de Vries LS, van der Aa NE. Prediction of visual field defects in newborn infants with perinatal arterial ischemic stroke using early MRI and DTI-based tractography of the optic radiation. *Eur J Paediatr Neurol.* 2016;20(2):309-318.

Krumlinde-Sundholm L, Ek L, Eliasson AC. What assessments evaluate use of hands in infants? A literature review. *Dev Med Child Neurol.* 2015;57(Suppl 2):37-41.

Lynch JK. Epidemiology and classification of perinatal stroke. *Semin Fetal Neonatal Med.* 2009;14(5):245-249.

Moyer, PA. *Guide to Occupational Therapy Practice.* American Occupational Therapy Association, Inc; 2007.

Öhrvall AM, Krumlinde-Sundholm L, Eliasson AC. Exploration of the relationship between the Manual Ability Classification System and hand-function measures of capacity and performance. *Disabil Rehabil.* 2013;35(11):913-918.

Öhrvall AM, Krumlinde-Sundholm L, Eliasson AC. The stability of the Manual Ability Classification System over time. *Dev Med Child Neurol.* 2014;56(2):185-189.

Rosenbaum P, Eliasson AC, Hidecker MJ, Palisano RJ. Classification in childhood disability: focusing on function in the 21st century. *J Child Neurol.* 2014;29(8):1036-1045.

Sainburg RL, Duff SV. Does motor lateralization have implications for stroke rehabilitation? *J Rehabil Res Dev.* 2006;43(3):311-222.

Shumway-Cook A, Woollacott MH. *Motor Control: Theory and Practical Applications*, 5th ed. Baltimore, MD: Lippincott Williams & Wilkins.; 2016

Spearing EM. Providing family-centered care in pediatric physical therapy. In: Tecklin JS, ed. *Pediatric Physical Therapy*, 5th ed. Baltimore, MD: Lippincott Williams & Wilkins; 2015:1-14.

7

Intervention for Functional Motor Skills in Children With Stroke

Heather L. Atkinson, PT, DPT, NCS; Mardee Greenham, PhD;
Anna Cooper, BOT, GC Paediatric OT; and Anne Gordon, PhD, MSc, BAppSc

Over the last few decades, animal and human research has illuminated the fact that the brain has an extraordinary capability to reorganize itself after injury, if provided with the proper stimulus.[1] This creates great opportunity and challenge to physical and occupational therapists to maximize outcomes when providing care to children with stroke. Clinicians must balance and integrate many complex concepts when formulating an intervention plan, including the following:

- What interventions are best suited to the child's and family's goals?

- What interventions will be most effective for this particular child?

- What interventions will have a lasting effect and carryover to support participation in daily life activities?

In addition, clinicians must consider how to balance rehabilitation strategies aimed at recovery of lost neurological function and promotion of new and emerging skills that are developmentally appropriate for the child and those aimed toward compensatory techniques that can focus on functional independence using existing abilities.

This chapter will aim to review models of recovery in human stroke; clinical implications; therapeutic strategies to enhance recovery; adaptive techniques to promote function, balancing recovery, habilitation, and compensation in clinical practice; and considerations for various settings.

CLINICAL DECISION MAKING AND THE PLAN OF CARE

Clinical decision making (CDM) is a complex process used to make judgments around clinical care and to select the best interventions for a patient. It includes the initial generation of treatment strategies based on evidence, theory, and patient goals and the ability to modify the plan of care based on changes in the patient. Several models for CDM exist that can facilitate clinicians in choosing the right strategies at the right time. As previously discussed in Chapter 6, the International Classification System of Functioning, Disability and Health for Children and Youth (ICF-CY)[2] is a framework that describes the functioning of a child in terms of body structures and functions, activity and participation, and the interrelationship between these domains (see Chapter 6 for details). It is a holistic framework that highlights the impact of environmental and personal variables on a child's health. It can guide clinicians in the evaluation process, which ultimately guides the selection of interventions within the plan of care. During the evaluation, the clinician integrates the various levels of the ICF-CY and formulates goals and a plan of care that reflect the patient's needs, goals, and priorities. Participation as described by the ICF-CY is a person's involvement in life situations.[2] Children need to be active participants in therapeutic intervention and goal setting where and when possible to maximize success.

Atkinson HL, Nixon-Cave K, Smith SE, eds.
Pediatric Stroke Rehabilitation: An Interprofessional and
Collaborative Approach (pp 113-134). © 2018 Taylor & Francis Group.

Clinical reflection is an important part of the CDM process. The Physical Therapy Clinical Reasoning and Reflection Tool (PT-CRT)[3] offers questions that rehabilitation professionals can ask to probe clinical reasoning and reflection while assessing, formulating the plan of care, and selecting interventions (Box 7-1). These questions are important to consider when working with a child who has had a stroke and his or her family, and will be important to reflect upon in selecting intervention approaches.

Continuous reflection, using the ICF-CY framework, and considering the clinical reasoning questions illustrated in Box 7-1 support the provision of family-centered care. Therapists can look for opportunities for shared decision making throughout the episode of care. Shared decision making integrates the best evidence, professional expertise, and patient values.[4-6] It is central to family-centered care and increases patient/caregiver satisfaction with care, improves adherence to treatment, and can improve outcomes and lower cost of care.[4-6] Although most of the recent literature in shared decision making has been in medical care, the principles can translate to rehabilitation. By educating patients and families about their condition, possible options for treatment, and facilitating their decision making about their choice of treatment, therapists can seek to improve patient outcomes through collaboration (Figure 7-1).

Another key component of clinical decision making is the integration of evidence. Although a full discussion of evidence-based practice is beyond the scope of this chapter, some general concepts are worth mentioning. As most pediatric therapists recognize, children are not simply "tiny adults" that will have the same response to interventions provided to adults. The relative paucity of pediatric rehabilitation literature when compared to adults can cause frustration when attempting to select the best intervention. Clinicians can supplement the evidence gleaned from the pediatric stroke literature with allied research in adult stroke, cerebral palsy, and other neurological conditions. Furthermore, several clinical practice guidelines have been published in recent years that can help guide clinicians when interpreting evidence and considering recommendations for treatment. Personalized goal setting is a key element to any intervention program to evaluate the effect of a chosen modality, intensity, and dose of intervention.

- Clinical practice guidelines for rehabilitation:

  □ Childhood stroke: In 2017 the Paediatric Stroke Working Group from the Royal College of Paediatrics and Child Health (United Kingdom) published a revised version of *Stroke in Childhood: Clinical Guidelines for Diagnosis, Management, and Rehabilitation*.[7] To date, this is the only published clinical guideline that includes rehabilitation as part of comprehensive care for children

who have had an ischemic or haemorrhagic stroke. It addresses the concepts of motor and sensory impairment and highlights interventions with evidence to support their use in this population.

  □ Adult stroke: Several clinical guidelines have been published for adult stroke, with recommendations spanning initial diagnosis through long-term rehabilitation. The most recent clinical guideline for the rehabilitation of adult stroke as of the writing of this text is the 2014 guideline from the Royal Dutch Society for Physical Therapy.[8] This guideline is written specifically for physical therapists treating adult survivors of stroke. It reviews the evidence and provides recommendations for many specific interventions used in neurorehabilitation, including various forms of treadmill training, constraint-induced therapy (CIT), neuromuscular electrical stimulation, virtual reality, aerobic exercise, strength training, and more.[8]

  □ Cerebral palsy: Recent systematic review papers focusing on interventions primarily for children with cerebral palsy have been published. Novak and colleagues published a systematic review of the evidence on interventions for children with cerebral palsy and developed guidelines using a *traffic light system* approach.[9] The authors categorized various interventions commonly used by therapists working with children with cerebral palsy into red (not effective), yellow (inconclusive evidence), and green (effective). Two reviews undertaken by Sakzewski et al focusing on interventions for children with unilateral motor dysfunction can provide useful guidance for clinicians in scrutinizing the evidence base.[10,11]

Ultimately, physical and occupational therapists must select the best intervention strategy to achieve the desired goal in the most efficient manner. By drawing upon the evidence, collaborating with their patients and caregivers, and considering all of the factors discussed thus far, clinicians can individualize treatment to work toward each child's maximum potential. Using the ICF-CY framework and CDM strategies, clinicians can prioritize interventions to achieve functional goals based on the child's primary problem areas. Take, for example, the case presented in Chapter 6: an 8-year-old child with right hemiplegia who sustained an arterial ischemic stroke (AIS) of the left middle cerebral artery during the perinatal period. Figure 6-8 in Chapter 6 depicts how the ICF-CY can be used as a tool to prioritize the primary areas to work on in the context of the child's goals. It also integrates other important contextual factors that may have a direct influence on a child's response to therapy. So, in using this example, the physical and

Box 7-1

The following is an excerpt from the PT-CRT,[3] which describes examples of questions to stimulate clinical reasoning and reflection while formulating intervention plans:

- How have you incorporated the patient's and family's goals?
- How do the goals reflect your examination and evaluation (ICF framework)?
- How did you determine the physical therapy prescription or plan of care (frequency, intensity, anticipated length of service)?
- How do key elements of the physical therapy plan of care relate back to the primary diagnosis?
- How do the patient's personal and environmental factors affect the physical therapy plan of care?
- Discuss your overall physical therapy approach or strategies (eg, motor learning, strengthening).
  - How will you modify principles for this patient?
  - Are there specific aspects about this particular patient to keep in mind?
  - How does your approach relate to theory and current evidence?
- As you designed your intervention plan, how did you select specific strategies?
- What is your rationale for those intervention strategies?
- How do the interventions relate to the primary problem areas identified using the ICF?
- How might you need to modify your interventions for this particular patient and caregiver? What are your criteria for doing so?
- What are the coordination-of-care aspects?
- What are the communication needs with other team members?
- What are the documentation aspects?
- How will you ensure safety?
- Patient/caregiver education:
  - What are your overall strategies for teaching?
  - Describe learning styles/barriers and any possible accommodations for the patient and caregiver.
  - How can you ensure understanding and buy-in?
  - What communication strategies (verbal and nonverbal) will be most successful?

occupational therapists identified the following areas as the primary areas to work on:

- Impairments of body structures and functions:
  - Decreased passive range of motion of the right dorsiflexors
  - Decreased strength
  - Decreased selective motor control of right lower limb and upper limb
  - Decreased walking speed
  - Limitations in isolated finger and thumb movements
  - Altered sensation of right upper limb

- Activity limitations and participation restrictions:
  - Decreased ability to participate with peers in sports activities
  - Difficulty managing small fastenings when getting dressed (buttons, laces, zips), affecting the ability to get dressed before school and manage independently when changing for physical education class in school
  - Unable to manage a knife and fork independently and reliant on help to cut up food, both at home and at school lunch time

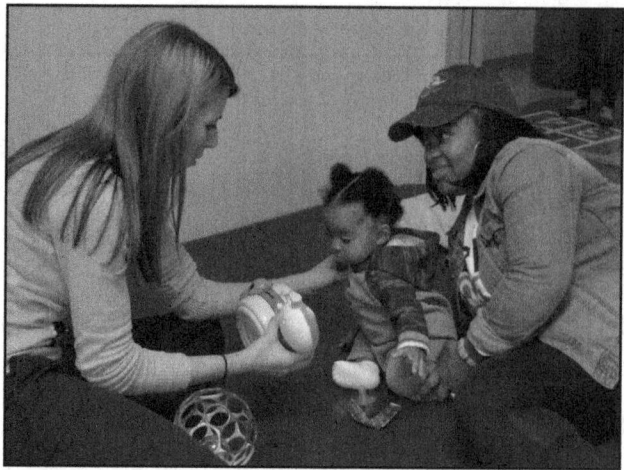

Figure 7-1. The clinician collaborates with the caregiver during treatment, and they work together to help optimize movement for the child.

- Child and parent priorities:
  - The child wanted as much as possible to keep up with his friends at school and found dressing for physical education class challenging; plus, he was becoming more conscious of looking different when walking
  - The parents wanted their child to continue to develop independence skills and support his self-esteem.

The clinicians recognized that the child's high level of motivation and supportive family would be positive factors in helping the child to achieve goals. The child's cognitive abilities, interests, social and emotional skills, and lifestyle are also key components to consider. The reader should keep this case in mind through the following sections and consider which interventions he or she might choose for this child.

MODELS OF RECOVERY

Before reviewing various strategies used in neurorehabilitation, the following is an overview of current models of neuroplasticity in response to brain injury. An understanding of the changes at the level of the brain that may underpin the observable changes seen in response to intervention is important for therapists to consider in their practice.

Neuroplasticity

Neuroplasticity refers to the brain's capacity to change in response to a range of experiences, including sensory stimuli, stress, and injury.[12] Decades of neuroscience research have suggested several core principles of neuroplasticity that have significant implications for rehabilitation (Table 7-1).[13] These principles, when integrated into a rehabilitation program, may offer the optimal experience through which to induce brain changes on a cortical level. These

principles include specificity and salience of training, repetition, and intensity, among others.[13] Physical and occupational therapists can incorporate these principles with the aim of generating experience-dependent plastic changes that may translate into lasting functional and meaningful clinical improvement. The evidence for these principles is changing and evolving rapidly, and the relative impact of one or more of these in influencing intervention outcomes in children in the context of a developing brain is not yet clear. Clinicians should be mindful of the complexity of factors that may mediate or moderate intervention outcomes.

Cortical Reorganization in Animals

Early indications of neuroplasticity in animals emerged with Margaret Kennard's work in the 1930s and 1940s. She found that unilateral motor cortex lesions in infant monkeys resulted in milder impairments than the same lesions in adults,[14-16] which she suggested were the result of cortical reorganization of function, possibly due to the intense development occurring in the immature brain.[16] Similar results have been found in later animal studies with cats and rats.[17-19] Although the scientific community is still developing a better understating of critical periods of brain development and how earlier is not necessarily better for outcome after lesions, Kennard's work helped propel the idea that the brain is capable of change.

Building on these early paradigms of neuroplasticity, Edward Taub, a behavioral psychologist, observed that monkeys who had a surgically induced lesion causing deafferentation and sensory loss to one upper extremity behaved as though they also experienced a motor loss, and he coined the term *learned nonuse*, which describes an intricate pattern of behavior and loss of movement.[1,20] The phenomenon of learned nonuse is not solely attributed to the lesion, as motor ability is technically unaffected; rather, it is due to a learned suppression of movement.[1,20] Furthermore, when these deafferented monkeys had a constraint on the unaffected upper extremity, they were quickly motivated to use their affected upper extremity to retrieve food and water, unlike their unconstrained counterparts.[1,20] Twelve years after Taub's behavioral observations of these monkeys, Pons et al[21] performed somatosensory cortical mapping of these same animals and observed massive cortical reorganization previously unseen. Further landmark animal work by Nudo and colleagues[22] discovered that the same phenomenon happened when the animals received a lesion to the motor cortex, causing a true hemiplegia. The monkeys in the constraint group were said to undergo rehabilitation by forcing the affected upper extremity to retrieve food and water.[22] Through intracortical microstimulation mapping of the motor context, the investigators discovered that the monkeys who underwent the rehabilitation and experienced clinical improvement also exhibited a highly reorganized cortex.[22] Mapping demonstrated that areas

TABLE 7-1. PRINCIPLES OF EXPERIENCE-DEPENDENT NEUROPLASTICITY OUTLINED BY KLEIM AND JONES	
1. Use it or lose it	Failure to drive specific brain functions can lead to functional degradation (also known as *learned nonuse*, or in the case of children, *developmental disregard*).
2. Use it and improve it	Training that drives a specific brain function can lead to an enhancement of that function.
3. Specificity	The nature of the training experience dictates the nature of the plasticity.
4. Repetition matters	Induction of plasticity requires sufficient repetition.
5. Intensity matters	Induction of plasticity requires sufficient training intensity.
6. Time matters	Different forms of plasticity occur at different times during training.
7. Salience matters	The training experience must be sufficiently salient to induce plasticity (the motivation of the individual child/young person, the task, and the context are key components of the intervention to maximize engagement, repetition, and long-term outcome).
8. Age matters	Training-induced plasticity may occur more readily in younger brains; however, emerging evidence from outcome studies in traumatic brain-injured populations suggest there is not a linear relationship between age at injury and outcome, and this continues to be an area of investigation.
9. Transference	Plasticity in response to one training experience can enhance the acquisition of similar behaviors.
10. Interference	Plasticity in response to one experience can interfere with the acquisition of other behaviors.

Adapted from Kleim JA, Jones TA. Principles of experience-dependent neural plasticity: implications for rehabilitation after brain damage. *J Speech Lang Hear Res.* 2008;51(1):225-239.

adjacent to the lesion were newly responsible for motor movements, suggesting the groundbreaking revelation that constraint intervention influenced reorganization of the motor cortex after injury.[22] This important animal work set the stage for the advent of applying these principles to humans, which ultimately created a massive paradigm shift in neurorehabilitation. Clinicians, previously focusing on compensatory strategies for patients with hemiplegia, were now inspired to consider strategies that might induce recovery of function.

Cortical Reorganization in Humans

Soon after these seminal works in animals, investigators began applying the principles of CIT in human subjects. Liepert and colleagues[23] studied 13 adults with chronic stroke who underwent a 12-day course of CIT that incorporated the principles of task specificity, repetition, and intensity. The subjects experienced a significant improvement in function of the paretic limb that was associated with a corresponding enlargement in motor output of the affected hemisphere as seen with transcranial magnetic stimulation.[23] This article gained widespread media attention and influenced the next decade of rehabilitation research for human stroke.

Since that time, over 150 papers on adults and over 70 papers on children have been published regarding CIT with consensus guidelines published for translation in pediatric practice for children with hemiplegic cerebral palsy. Questions remain, however, regarding optimal timing, dosage, and intensity, and some of these will be discussed later in this chapter. However, the broad positive response of the CIT literature, including modified models for children and young people, has helped support the concept of working toward neuroplasticity in rehabilitative training. Furthermore, other treatment strategies for people with stroke, including treadmill training, virtual reality, and robotics, draw upon the CIT literature and how that specific intervention adapted the core principles of neuroplasticity into a rehabilitation program.

PEDIATRIC CONSIDERATIONS FOR NEUROPLASTICITY AND RECOVERY

In clinical practice there is wide variation in how children present and the challenges they encounter following a stroke, even those with similar lesion sizes and locations, age at injury, and response to intervention. When designing a treatment program, physical and occupational therapists must consider the many variables important for the individual, including their family and social and educational environment. Although the focus of a given intervention may be on gross or fine motor function, the marker of success will be whether the gains translate into everyday life for the individual concerned. It is hypothesized that a number of key features may contribute to functional plasticity and intervention outcomes for children who have had a stroke, and these are outlined next.

Location and Size of Lesion

As with adults, lesion location is a significant predictor of motor outcome in both neonatal and later acquired pediatric stroke, yet these factors differ for the 2 age-at-onset groups. For example, hemiparesis in the neonatal population is often associated with multiple lesion site locations (basal ganglia, cerebral cortex, and internal capsule), whereas in later-onset stroke, just one or two of these areas can result in hemiparesis.[24-26] Anecdotally, hemidystonia is not an uncommon consequence of stroke in childhood, associated with injury to the basal ganglia. This has yet to be described in detail in the pediatric stroke literature; however, it presents challenges to the rehabilitation clinician in terms of identifying optimal management.

Associations between lesion size and motor outcome have also been reported in the pediatric stroke literature. Studies of neonatal stroke have found lesions involving the main branch of a cerebral artery,[27] greater extent of major cerebral artery involvement,[28] and bilateral lesions[29] to be associated with poorer motor outcomes. Similarly, more extensive brain damage, including bilateral lesions[30] and greater extent of tissue damage,[31] have been found to predict poorer motor outcomes in later acquired pediatric stroke.

Age at Diagnosis

In pediatric stroke, there are 2 distinct populations based on timing of injury: perinatal or neonatal stroke (occurring between the 20th week in utero and the 28th day of life)[32] and childhood stroke, occurring after the first 30 days of life. A proportion of children are not diagnosed at the time of the stroke event and are diagnosed in infancy with a presumed perinatal stroke upon the emergence of movement asymmetries in infancy. Response to intervention and cortical changes after injury are not well understood in the developing brain, and it is possible that the mechanisms vary from that of adults following a stroke. For example, a child who was typically developing and experienced a stroke later in childhood may experience learned nonuse of the affected upper extremity as described in the adult stroke literature, yet that term does not adequately describe a child who is born with hemiplegia. In these cases, the term developmental disregard may be more appropriate.[33] Furthermore, although the concept of cortical reorganization can be applied in childhood stroke, it does not quite fit for infants with stroke, as the motor cortex is anatomically and physiologically atypical from the early days of life. Rather, in the case of perinatal stroke, rehabilitation therapists should consider the concept of influencing maximal ongoing development of a child with an injured brain. The focus for all therapy interventions in children and young people includes a component of habilitation, that is, ongoing development of skills required to live as independent a life as possible, and depending on the age of the child at the time of stroke, there may also be a focus on recovery of lost function (or rehabilitation).

There is a significant difference in the prevalence of motor impairment in neonatal and later acquired pediatric stroke. In AIS, hemiplegia has been reported to affect around one-third of children with acute presentation of perinatal AIS and more than 80% of infants with presumed perinatal AIS,[25,28] whereas in later acquired AIS the prevalence of neuroimpairment is estimated to be three-quarters.[34,35] The severity of motor deficits varies, but most children will gain or regain independent mobility.[29,36,37] Research on motor outcomes following hemorrhagic stroke is limited. One study investigating long-term outcomes of 31 children with later acquired hemorrhagic stroke found that over half had motor impairments.[38] Another study reported similar findings, with motor impairments in 10 of the 21 children.[39] No studies have explored long-term motor outcomes in perinatal hemorrhagic stroke, but one study followed up 37 children at 20 months of age and found 3 had cerebral palsy, 1 had cerebellar ataxia, and 2 had developed hemiplegia.[40] Little is known of the differences in trajectory of recovery from early vs later stroke in infancy and childhood. No studies have detailed fine motor function trajectories following stroke in children.

From a neuroplasticity perspective, it is well accepted that there are critical periods in brain development. Brain maturation is not a linear process, and research has shown that series of growth spurts occur throughout early development.[41] Although these peak periods of brain development are not yet well understood, they are known to be times when neural networks are most sensitive to environmental influences. Injury during these critical periods can have either beneficial or detrimental effects.[42] In normal brain development, synaptic overproduction in the postnatal period is followed by pruning during adolescence.[43] This overproduction of neurons during early brain development in comparison to the mature brain is thought to support the ability for repair following injury. However, insults during these critical periods can also disrupt neuronal development, resulting in the delay of ongoing development or an altered course of development.[42]

Time Since Injury

A few studies have systematically investigated the recovery course following pediatric stroke. The majority of studies vary widely in time since stroke and age at assessment, making comparison difficult. The primary recovery of motor function in adult stroke takes place during the first 3 months, with some additional, but less extensive, improvements made in the subsequent 3 months.[44] In one of the few studies to investigate patterns of recovery poststroke in children, Kim and colleagues[45] found a similar course to adults, with the majority of motor recovery occurring within the first 2 to 3 months. A recent prospective longitudinal study of 50 children with AIS found sensorimotor impairments the most prevalent clinical consequence up to 6 months after diagnosis, particularly children diagnosed in childhood.[46]

Premorbid Abilities

The effect of premorbid functioning on motor recovery has not been explored in the pediatric stroke literature. However, preinjury factors have been found to be important in predicting outcomes following traumatic brain injury (TBI) in children. Pre-existing problems such as a previous brain injury, learning difficulties, premorbid stressors, and neurological and psychiatric problems have been found to be associated with ongoing cognitive and behavioral difficulties post-TBI.[47] Similarly, premorbid adaptive functioning has been reported to predict adaptive and behavioral outcomes in children 5 years post-TBI.[48] Although premorbid functioning seems to be particularly important for outcomes in the cognitive and psychosocial domains, it may also be relevant in predicting motor and physical impairments following pediatric stroke.

Brain Reserve

Brain reserve capacity is a theoretical construct that refers to the threshold level of brain matter such as brain size and synapse count.[49] It proposes that individuals have differing brain reserve capacity, and this reserve mediates reorganization and functional outcome following brain insult. When brain reserve capacity is depleted beyond its threshold, deficits begin to emerge.[50] The literature on brain reserve capacity has largely focused on its implications for cognitive functions, but this construct may also be relevant to motor function. Education and life experience prior to the stroke can affect brain reserve capacity, so it may be that children who have a stroke at a younger age have more reduced brain reserve capacity compared to older children, as they have not had the same opportunities to increase reserve.

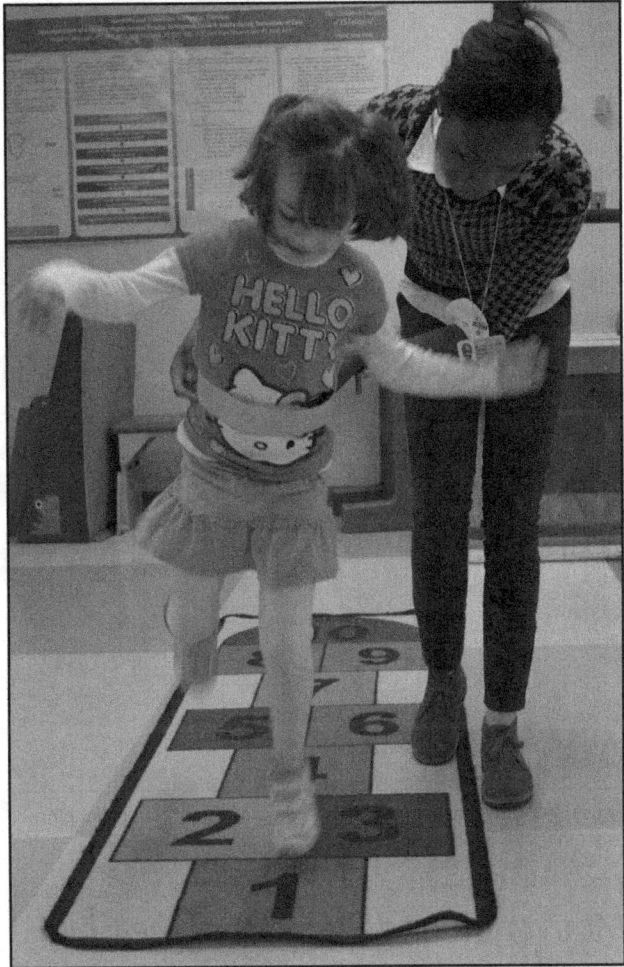

Figure 7-2. Child-directed activities can be therapeutic and rewarding at the end of a session.

Language, Cognition, and Behavior

Pediatric physical and occupational therapists should have a basic knowledge of typical milestones in language and cognitive development, as well as an understanding of typical behaviors for a given age. Language, cognitive, and behavioral impairment can result after stroke (see Chapters 8 through 10), which can affect a child's motivation and ability to participate in physical and occupational therapy activities. Clinicians should work closely with the family and the interprofessional team to develop a thorough understanding of the child's abilities and difficulties in these areas, as well as personal motivators, so as to develop an intervention plan to maximally engage the child in ways appropriate for their developmental level and individual goals (Figures 7-2 and 7-3).

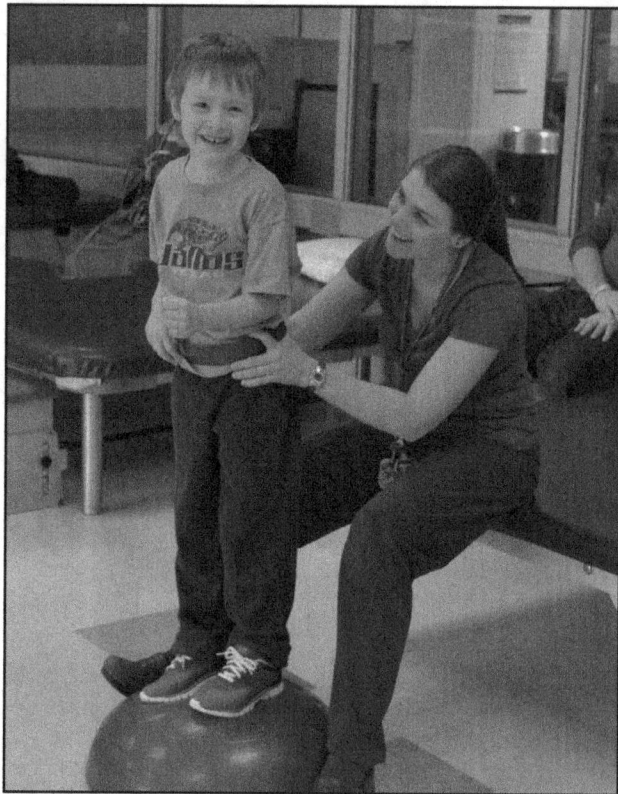

Figure 7-3. Novel activities can provide motivation for challenging or frustrating tasks.

Motivation and Priorities of the Child and Family

The central point in working with children and families following stroke is determining what matters to them at the point in time that you are working with them. It is through harnessing their motivators, interests, and abilities that you can work in partnership to make the greatest difference for the child and transfer your knowledge and skills to empower the child and family for independent living. Spending time undertaking a detailed interview of daily life activities and strengths and weaknesses, as well as partnership working to set goals, will underpin the identification and evaluation of the therapeutic approach taken. The intervention modality, intensity, and dosage will be influenced by this in addition to clinical observations and formal assessments. External factors including the physical and social environment, expectations and health beliefs, school demands, and fatigue can affect therapeutic decision making. Clinical experience also suggests fatigue may be an ongoing issue affecting engagement in therapy, but also requires input to support a young person to participate across home, school, and community environments.

CLINICAL IMPLICATIONS

Intervention principles for stroke rehabilitation have evolved over recent years as evidence for neuroplasticity after injury has emerged. Although the "ingredients" in various protocols vary immensely, most protocols for adults following stroke focus on recovery of function and have at their core some common elements consistent with the neurorehabilitation literature. These common elements include motor learning theory, task-specific training, timing, and the child as an active participant. In working with children and young people, the focus of motor therapies is most importantly a balance of habilitation (ongoing development of skills in line with development), as well as rehabilitation (recovery of skills held prior to the stroke).

Motor Learning

Although a thorough review of motor learning is beyond the scope of this chapter, some points are worth mentioning. The systems model of motor control, first established in the 1960s, suggests that a multitude of body systems interact to produce a motor movement to reach a functional goal, rather than a hierarchical or behavioral sequence of development.[51,52] This theory stimulates therapists to create optimal environments and functional goals while working with a child to promote movement. Over the past few decades, the dynamic systems theory has prevailed as a dominant theory of motor learning, which postulates a complex and dynamic array of influences on neuromaturation.[52] It suggests that development is nonlinear and that the child gains motor skills based on many intrinsic and extrinsic factors.[52] More recently, scientists have recognized both attention and motivation as critical components of motor skill acquisition and have proposed the OPTIMAL (Optimizing Performance Through Intrinsic Motivation and Attention for Learning) theory of motor learning.[53] The OPTIMAL theory brings to the forefront how motivation and attention can affect motor performance and ultimately the development of motor skills.[53]

The principles of motor learning can successfully be applied in pediatrics, and new research is revealing some nuances in how children may learn differently from adults. Like adults, children need task-specific practice at an appropriate level of challenge.[54] Using the concept of the *challenge point* can aid clinicians in developing an intervention strategy that will be at the appropriate level for optimal learning (Box 7-2).[54] In addition, motor skill acquisition is believed to be different in children compared to adults.[54,55] In typically developing children, feedback provided at more regular intervals may lead to earlier learning of a motor skill.[54,55] Longer periods of practice and a slower reduction of feedback in early motor learning may be even more important in children with a new neurological insult.[54,55] As children acquire motor skills, generalization of that skill into functional environments is critical. The features of the environment that can be either barriers or facilitators in therapy include physical, social, and sensory characteristics.

Motor learning shares common elements with several principles of neuroplasticity previously discussed, such as intensity, repetition, and saliency, all of which are important in the clinical application of intervention in stroke recovery and rehabilitation. Several of the specific therapeutic strategies that are discussed in the following section have at their core a foundation rich in motor learning theory, which supports the concept of promoting neuroplasticity. Rehabilitation therapists often use motor learning as a basis when they progress patients from the initial stages of eliciting movement to maximizing neuromotor return and improving selective motor control while concurrently working on optimizing function (Figure 7-4). Progressing intervention in children can be challenging, and therapists must ensure that there is enough intensity to instill change, yet the child must remain safe, be actively engaged, and experience success. By considering important features of various motor learning theories (practice, challenge, feedback, attention, motivation, environmental conditions, generalization), as well as aspects of learning unique to children, clinicians can prepare relevant intervention programs to optimize motor outcomes.

Goal-Directed, Activity-Based Intervention

In developing intervention programs, rehabilitation clinicians should consider the dynamic relationship between the child, the task, and the environment in maximizing the opportunity for learning. The relationship between functional performance and underlying corticospinal tract plasticity is not well understood in the developing brain. It is postulated that a child's active engagement in tasks that

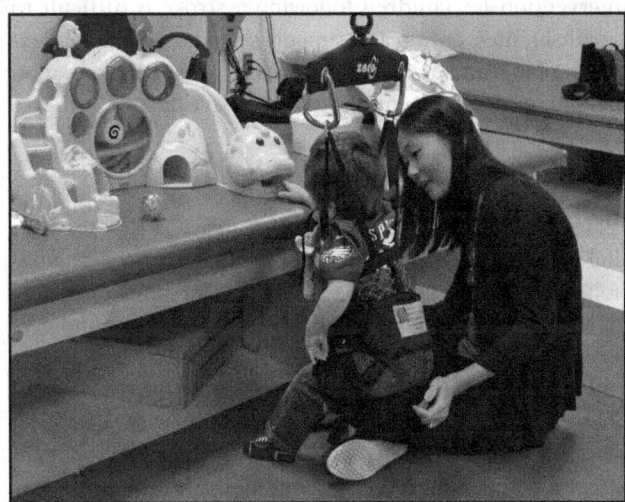

Figure 7-4. The therapist works on repeated sit-to-stand movements, progressively challenging the child by removing body weight support.

are meaningful, motivating, and goal directed offer the opportunity for lasting functional gain.

Task-specific practice will assist with remapping the neural pathways that are required to complete that specific task. For example, hanging a coat on a coat hook incorporates movements of the proximal and distal upper limbs (reaching against gravity, pinching, bimanual coordination) as well as the lower limb (walking, balancing, transferring weight, twisting)—it places a series of motor functions within a context and will be most beneficial if it incorporates a child's own functional goals. Goal-directed training is an activity-based approach that uses client-selected goals, task analysis, and intervention to improve motor function. Goal-directed training theory supports the belief that movement patterns emerge from the interaction between the person's abilities, their environment, and his or her goal.[60]

Timing

As discussed earlier, the trajectory of recovery in children following stroke is not well documented or understood. If they have access to rehabilitation services, many children receive rehabilitation therapies soon after stroke in both the acute and subacute phases of recovery (see Chapter 5). However, cognitive deficits following neonatal stroke have been observed as emerging beyond infancy and in early childhood.[61] This suggests that difficulties may emerge over time and that motor function, along with other developmental abilities, should be closely monitored, particularly at times of transition when environmental and social demands change (ie, starting nursery or school, moving to secondary school or college).

New priorities and challenges, as well as new goals, are likely to emerge over time. Although the optimal timing of intervention for children following a stroke is difficult to establish, intervention and support services need to be flexibly available and delivered on a case-by-case basis based on lifelong needs as the child grows and develops.

The Child as an Active Participant

The Model of Human Occupation provides a framework that portrays the open relationship between how occupation is motivated (*volition*—a child's values and interests), patterned (*habituation*—a child's roles and habits), and performed (a child's performance).[62] It identifies the important role of volition, or what the client *wants* to do, and how that affects a child's performance capacity. Involving the child and the family in the goal-setting process is an integral component in optimizing motor recovery. A study by Webb and Glueckauf[63] explored the outcomes of adults with TBIs in an outpatient rehabilitation setting and found that functional outcomes were better when the participants were involved in the goal-setting process. See Chapter 6 for further discussion on setting meaningful rehabilitation goals for children with stroke.

THERAPEUTIC STRATEGIES TO ENHANCE RECOVERY

Upper Limb Targeted Interventions for Children With Hemiplegia

The majority of studies of pediatric upper limb intervention have included populations of children with varied etiology and timing of brain injury, predominantly children with hemiplegic cerebral palsy. A small number of studies have applied modified constraint therapy to children with hemiparesis following ischemic stroke resulting in functional gains for children with chronic hemiparesis.[64,65] Pediatric studies have used a variety of protocols and inclusion criteria for studies, with promising findings;

although, further studies are needed to determine the optimal model and dosage.[9,66] Modified constraint-induced movement therapy (mCIT) continues to be refined, and studies addressing the outcome of the intervention in combination with botulinum toxin[67] and task-specific training have been reported.[68]

A model of bimanual training is Hand-Arm Bimanual Training (HABIT).[69] HABIT includes structured intensive task practice in bimanual play and functional activities. It was developed utilizing the principles of motor learning (ie, specificity of practice, types of practice, and feedback) and the principles of neuroplasticity (influencing practice-induced brain changes through repetition, motivation, reward, and increasing complexity). Bimanual training delivered in a variety of models has shown emerging evidence as an intervention delivering sustained functional gain, particularly for school-aged children with hemiplegic cerebral palsy.

In recent years there have been rapid developments in the field of upper limb intensive intervention clinical research. The emergence of evidence at the level of randomized controlled trials has explored the differential outcomes between mCIT and bimanual training and the possible inclusion of hybrid models, with all of these intensive approaches showing positive benefits in terms of functional improvement evaluated using a range of methodologies.[70-75]

A meta-analysis undertaken by Sakzewski et al[76] of upper limb therapies for unilateral cerebral palsy concluded there is modest evidence for activity-based, goal-directed interventions but that a therapy block alone is unlikely to lead to sustained changes. Goal-directed occupational therapy home programs, as described by Novak et al,[77] to supplement hands-on therapy were described as having strong evidence of efficacy.

The optimum timing, dose, and impact of repeat episodes of intensive upper limb interventions require ongoing investigation. The key components, as recently described by Sakzewski and colleagues[78] in a review of the field, include collaborative goal setting with the children and families and intensive, repetitive, graded challenging task practice. Intervention selection should consider child and family preferences and circumstances.[79]

Neuromuscular Re-Education

Neuromuscular re-education is broadly defined as the training of the neuromuscular system to regain normal movement after injury. Therapists may work with the child to elicit new movements through a variety of strategies such as facilitation techniques, neuromuscular stimulation, or biofeedback. Once a movement develops, the therapist can create interventions to help the child build upon that movement and develop isolated and graded neuromuscular control in order to complete functional and meaningful tasks.

Strength Training

Strength training can increase the efficiency of motor unit recruitment and lead to a strengthening effect, though more research is needed to explore mechanisms of neural adaptation from strength training in neurological dysfunction.[80,81] For adults with stroke, strengthening protocols may help train remaining motor units to fire in a more organized and successful pattern and may also have an influence on cortical activity.[80] When properly applied, strength training regimens may also improve gait speed and symmetry in adults with stroke.[8] Evidence of efficacy for strength training in children with neurological impairment remains limited.

Despite the lack of guidelines from the literature for strength training in children with stroke, physical and occupational therapists often use strengthening techniques as a vehicle to increase muscle activation and control (Figure 7-5). Ongoing re-evaluation is necessary to ensure the proper challenge point to induce change, as well as carryover into function in order to achieve goals. In upper limb interventions, strength training is often a component of a task-based approach that targets functional goals.

Locomotor Training

All forms of gait training are typically focused on the goal to improve functional mobility through a more efficient gait pattern. After a thorough gait analysis, the clinician determines which impairments in the child's gait will be the priority for treatment based on the child's individual goals. Gait training for children who have had a stroke can take many forms—overground, on a treadmill, with body weight support, or with robotic support. Research in locomotor training has been robust in recent years, and several recent articles serve as good resources.[82-87]

Overground Training

Overground training may be carried out with or without assistive devices or orthotics. For a focus on recovery, physical therapists may emphasize training without these aids, but may need to balance using them at times, as will be discussed later in this chapter. Overground performance and carryover is the ultimate end point. Overground training incorporates motor learning principles of having the participant adapt to changes in the environment through feedback mechanisms and to adjust performance accordingly. Therapists may use facilitatory techniques or visual/auditory cues while in the skill acquisition phase. A study

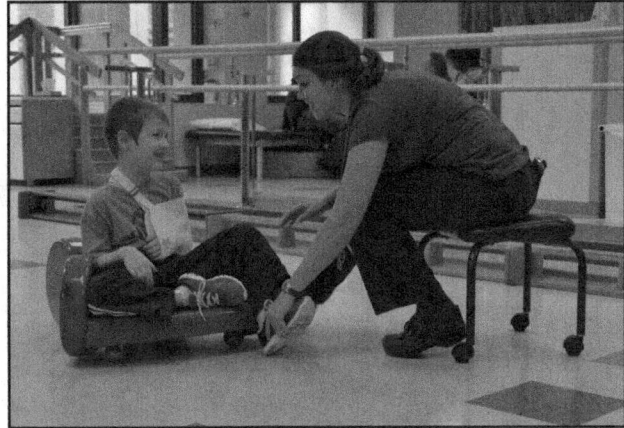

Figure 7-5. Therapists may use a variety of open or closed chain (pictured) exercises to progressively strengthen the affected extremity.

by Hidler and colleagues[88] suggested that overground gait training was superior to robotic treadmill training in adults with subacute stroke and moderate to severe hemiplegia, perhaps because participants had to integrate real-life environmental challenges and adapt appropriately while in the overground condition, rather than relying on a robotic device. It is important to practice overground training in a variety of contexts (uneven terrain, busy environment, differing speeds) to maximize carryover to goals.

Treadmill Training

Step training over a treadmill incorporates the motor learning principles of repetitive practice and allows for a controlled cadence not otherwise available when overground. Therapists may vary treadmill training with the following different components, all of which present with limited evidence for children with stroke:

Body Weight Support

The bulk of body weight support (BWS) literature is in adult neurorehabilitation,[8] but some studies exist in pediatrics, primarily in children with bilateral cerebral palsy.[89-93] Recent reviews of treadmill training with and without partial BWS for children with cerebral palsy concluded that in severely affected children speed and gross motor skills improved.[89] The applicability of this intervention to improve efficiency of gait or functional mobility for children following stroke, where the majority of children gain (or regain) independent ambulation, is unknown.

Robotic Support

Robotic devices offer the advantages of less staff burden when providing facilitatory input, and may allow for increased repetition and intensity in a training program. Although one adult study in subacute stroke found better outcomes with overground training compared to robotic

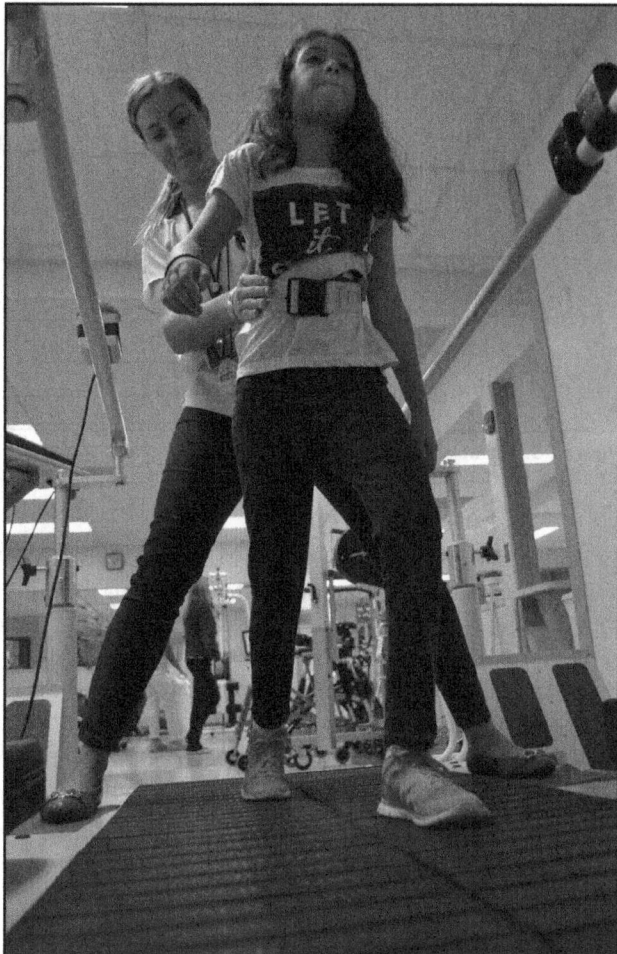

Figure 7-6. Example of asymmetric gait training on a split belt treadmill to work toward a more symmetric and efficient gait pattern.

support on a treadmill,[88] new studies continue to explore the effects that intensive training afforded by robotic support may have for persons with hemiplegia as well as in pediatric neurological populations.[94-96]

Unilateral Training

Evidence is emerging regarding the potential benefits of unilateral step training on a treadmill for adult hemiplegia.[97] This strategy employs having the individual maintain one leg stationary on the immobile edge of the treadmill while the other leg is forced to perform step training on the moving belt. The rationale is that forced use of one side will allow for multiple task-specific repetitions in a massed practice situation. The hemiparetic leg can be either the stepping leg for step practice or the stationary leg for closed-chain strengthening. The stepping leg has been shown to take a longer step length after the training session.[97] Outcomes related to improvements in gait pattern are still unclear, but this approach may have the potential to make changes in certain populations.

Split Belt

Split belt treadmills have two separate belts that can be operated at different speeds for asymmetrical gait training (Figure 7-6). Early evidence indicates that the central nervous system overcompensates for the error experienced while on the treadmill, which may lead to a more symmetrical gait pattern overground.[98,99] The shorter stepping leg is often trained at the faster speed. For an individual with hemiplegia, the affected leg may be the shorter or longer stepping limb. For example, if someone with left hemiplegia has a shorter step length on the left side, that could be due to decreased strength in the hip flexors and impairments in swing phase. Training the left leg faster in that case could help train and strengthen those specific issues. Conversely, another person with left hemiplegia may have a shorter step length on the right side, which could be due to decreased push off and weight bearing on the left side. By training the right side faster in that case, the individual will practice longer step length on the left side and work on those stance phase impairments. Although the intervention shows early promise, more research is needed to understand potential applicability in clinical practice.[98-102]

Virtual Reality

Virtual reality uses technology to simulate environments, activities, and experiences and can take a variety of forms, including 3-D simulation rooms, headwear to simulate a virtual environment, and interface with a computer screen on a table top. The approach aims to individualize the demands of the activity and intensity of task practice, while simultaneously capturing performance and intervention outcome.[103]

Targets for this may include motor or cognitive skills. Virtual reality for upper limb rehabilitation has demonstrated limited evidence but early promise in subjects with acquired brain injury.[104-106] Further research is required to explore translation of changes at the body functions level into activities and participation.

Motor Imagery

Motor imagery as a motor rehabilitation invention is based on mental stimulation theory. This theory suggests that cognitive motor processes (motor imagery, action observation, action verbalization) share similar representations in brain activity as motor execution.[107,108] Modalities that have been used in motor rehabilitation include visualization of self or others and kinesthetic, auditory, or visual imagery of movement. The criteria for selection of candidates based on degree of motor impairment and the effect of cognitive impairment have yet to be clarified and may affect outcome.

Motor in comparison with visual imagery has been shown to influence excitability in cortical motor areas and subcortical areas that are integrated in cerebellothalamocortical loops, as evidenced with functional magnetic resonance imaging and transcranial magnetic stimulation.[107] Activation of the primary motor cortex with motor imagery has been shown in multiple studies, specifically in the adult stroke population.[109-111] For a review see Garrison et al,[112] and for guidance regarding applications in adult clinical practice see Braun et al.[113] Although more research is needed, studies exploring feasibility and potential for children with neurological dysfunction show promise.[114-117]

Mirror Therapy

Mirror therapy involves the use of a visual illusion (through attention to the mirror reflection of the less impaired limb) during bimanual activities.[118] It has been hypothesized that mirror feedback of the less impaired limb may facilitate damaged sensorimotor networks and thus reduce neural drive required for motor performance.[119] Mechanisms underlying this have been hypothesized to include plasticity of the excitatory connections of the primary motor cortex.[120,121]

The majority of research undertaken with adults following stroke or with complex regional pain syndrome is promising, but the methodological quality of published studies is variable. Recent reviews have concluded that further research is required in both adult[122-124] and pediatric populations[76,125] to determine efficacy.

ADAPTIVE TECHNIQUES TO PROMOTE FUNCTION

Although neurorehabilitation often seeks to promote recovery of function and ongoing skill development in accordance with developmental age and abilities there is also a place for adaptive or compensatory strategies to help maximize independence and to achieve a child's goals.

Assistive Devices

Therapists will often trial assistive devices in the early days of rehabilitation poststroke to support gross and fine motor ability. For example, in the early subacute phase of recovery, assistive devices may include a rolling walker, hemiwalker, quad cane, or a single point cane. Depending on the child's abilities, the assistive device is often a bridge to independent ambulation and can help promote safety while working on regaining balance. Although they are less intrusive, unilateral devices can be difficult for some children to learn how to use and can also promote asymmetry of gait. Walkers, although bulkier, may offer the opportunity to gait train more symmetrically until the child is ready to ambulate hands-free. For a child with upper extremity involvement, a forearm platform on a walker can be helpful to support the involved upper extremity if grasp is an issue.

Lower Extremity Orthoses

The field of lower extremity orthotics continues to evolve, and therapists must possess a solid background in the fundamentals of biomechanics and gait analysis in order to prescribe the best device. Some considerations for children with stroke include the following:

Time Since Injury

Before ordering a definitive orthosis, some therapists may have the resources to fabricate temporary low-temperature thermoplastic devices. Children can trial solid ankle–foot orthoses (AFOs), articulating AFOs, or posterior leaf-spring styles as they make changes in the subacute phase of recovery. Clinicians may wish to use a temporary device until recovery progress appears to slow down.

Age and Size of the Child

Younger or smaller children may do well with a lighter or lower-profile orthosis, whereas a larger child/teen or someone prone to excessive spasticity may need a stronger device with a greater amount of contact for it to provide the support needed.

The Least Restrictive Orthotic Device

Recovery purists often advocate for no orthosis at all in order to allow the child maximal practice in moving the joint with every step. However, from a practical standpoint, other clinicians will argue that ambulating with a foot drop or knee hyperextension will lead to decreased safety, potential injury, and potential malalignment in the growing musculoskeletal system due to abnormal forces. To mitigate these 2 viewpoints, therapists would do well to select the least restrictive orthotic device for the child for regular use and consider gait training without the orthosis when in a safe and therapeutic context. Exciting advances in orthotic design are occurring and may benefit children with hemiplegia (Box 7-3).

Neuroprosthesis Considerations

Neuroprostheses such as the Ness system by Bioness and the Walk-Aide system are available to provide wireless electric stimulation to improve foot drop during gait (Figure 7-7). Adults with stroke have demonstrated good short- and long-term outcomes on gait parameters while using the device,[126] but evidence in children is limited. Candidates should have excellent caregiver support and good ability to follow through with their medical team to address dynamic changes such as a growth spurt or change in spasticity or flexibility.

Box 7-3
Examples of Lower Limb Orthotic Devices for Children With Stroke

- Custom or prefabricated shoe insert to control for hindfoot and/or forefoot alignment. These may be used bilaterally or unilaterally.

- Supramalleolar orthosis (SMO): These can be used to control excessive pronation/supination and provide stability in early standing mobility in young children. They are not effective in addressing gastrocnemius spasticity or anterior tibialis weakness.

- Solid molded AFO: Full-support orthosis with full foot plate and full trim lines. Often used in positioning or very early weight bearing in the case of a flaccid extremity.

- Articulating AFO: Articulating AFO to allow for sagittal motion around the ankle. Options include the following:

  □ Free dorsiflexion with plantar flexion stop: Allows tibia to translate over foot in midstance for smoother transition. Allows foot to dorsiflex if child has the ability. Prevents plantar flexion, which can be helpful with excessive gastrocnemius spasticity. Does not allow push off or activation of plantar flexors. Setting plantar flexion stop in a few degrees of dorsiflexion can help prevent knee hyperextension.

  □ Dorsiflexion-assistance hinge with plantar flexion stop: As noted earlier, but assistance hinge can help actively lift foot in swing phase if child presents with weak anterior tibialis or excessive plantar flexor spasticity, which would not allow dorsiflexion in a dynamic situation, such as walking. This feature can help mitigate the issues of circumduction or hip hiking seen with conventional articulating AFOs in these cases. Excessive dorsiflexion assistance can cause steppage pattern.

  □ Free dorsiflexion and plantarflexion with ability to adjust resistance in either direction: This device can be set with dorsiflexion assistance but also allow plantar flexion to allow gastrocnemius activation and push-off.

- Posterior leaf-spring orthosis: Low-profile AFO with trim lines posterior to the malleoli, which provide a lift for foot drop. May be a good choice for children with some dorsiflexion and medial-lateral stability and without excessive spasticity. This device offers the advantage of being less bulky and lightweight. The foot plate may be trimmed to proximal to the metatarsal heads for smoother roll-over and push-off.

- Carbon fiber AFO: Extremely lightweight and energy-storing orthotic that affords lift for foot drop in midswing as well as assisted propulsion in push-off. May be combined with SMO or shoe insert, as there is no contour around the lower foot. May not work well in cases of excessive spasticity. Design does not allow closed chain dorsiflexion.

- AFO set at first resistance: Another philosophy of brace wear includes molding the child at the R1 (for example, setting the AFO in 10 degrees of plantar flexion), accommodating it, and wedging the heel to bring the heel to the ground. This is thought to promote a more typical translation of weight over the foot in midstance. However, the use of these orthotics in children with hemiplegia has not been extensively studied.

- Night splints: Children with spastic hemiplegia may benefit from a night stretching splint for the ankle and/or knee if they are prone to episodes of worsening spasticity and loss of range of motion.

- Dynamic stretching splints: Some children may benefit from either a prefabricated or dynamic stretching splint to manage joints that present with challenging tone or range-of-motion restrictions.

All orthoses should be monitored on a regular basis, as growth, changing abilities, and new goals may prompt modifications or a new device.

Orthoses Prerequisites

The child must have adequate flexibility to not only fit properly into the orthotic, but also to use the orthotic to its maximal benefit. If the child does not have adequate flexibility, other options may need to be considered first, such as serial casting, dynamic splinting, an aggressive stretching program, or a referral to physical medicine and rehabilitation for spasticity management (see Chapter 5 for details).

Upper Extremity Orthoses

Upper extremity orthoses/splints are often broadly classified into 2 categories: static (doesn't move) and dynamic (movable/more functional) (Box 7-4). Static splints serve as a rigid support for optimizing positioning and maintaining joint integrity. They are most often custom-made from thermoplastic material.

Dynamic splints aim to support optimal joint position for functional use. They are primarily used to assist weak or injured muscles and tendons to move in a supported/low-impact/assisted manner. Dynamic or functional splinting may be made from neoprene, Lycra, or a combination of materials to enable a combination of joint or arch support simultaneously with function.

The prescription of an upper extremity orthosis may be indicated depending on the severity of presentation (eg, the presence of or risk of contractures), the significance of impairment of muscle tone (and relationship to function), the area involved (focal or generalized), and whether the child due to his or her health status is at risk (eg, in the acute phase when a child may be in an acute setting and have limited movement). A further consideration is the side effects of any medication that may have been prescribed.

Aims of upper extremity splinting for children with stroke may include the following:

- Minimize deformities
- Increase range of movement
- Protect joint integrity
- Increase functional use of the upper limb
- Restricting unwanted movement around a joint

Despite the common practice of splinting in neurorehabilitation, the evidence to support the use of splinting remains limited, and there is a lack of consensus regarding design and wearing times. In their literature review of the adult stroke population, Lannin and Ada[127] found that evidence did not support splinting to decrease spasticity or reduce contracture development. However, Kanellopoulos et al[128] found that combining splinting with botulinum toxin injections in children with cerebral palsy was effective in both reducing spasticity and improving function. Jackman et al[129] reported some small benefits to the use of splinting alongside therapy. It is important to note that

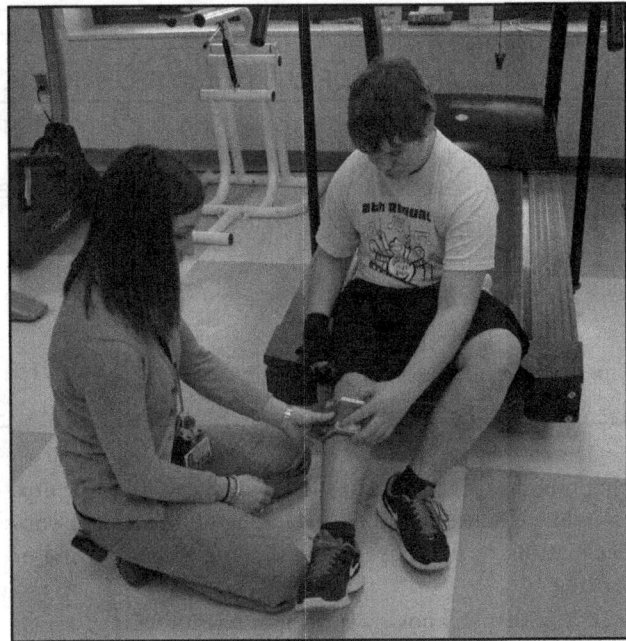

Figure 7-7. Some children may prefer a wireless electrical stimulation device to improve foot drop rather than a conventional orthosis.

these studies were not undertaken with children with acquired brain injury.

The rationale for splinting modalities and regimens may vary depending on the phase of recovery from the stroke. Evidence for specific wearing times of splints is inconclusive at this stage. Due to this uncertainty about splinting, it is important to introduce splints for a short period initially (whether static or dynamic), checking carefully that there are no pressure areas, edema, marks on the skin, or any discomfort or pain. Splinting one part of the body can influence tone or posture in another part of the body, and therefore close monitoring will be required. As the cause of limited range of movement and hypertonicity could be neural (spasticity) or non-neural (shortening of ligament, changes in muscle structures), both aspects need to be considered when splinting.[130] As for other interventions discussed in this chapter, goals should be set for intervention and reviewed to examine effects.

Guidance for therapists in fabricating upper extremity splints can be found in the Suggested Readings section at the end of this chapter.

Adaptive Aids

The prescription of adaptive equipment to support function may be of assistance in the early stages following diagnosis or for long-term use. Examples include beakers with hands to enable self-initiated drinking and cutlery with shaped or larger handles for easier grasp. Other common aids prescribed are adaptions to enable children to complete a bimanual task unimanually; for example, modified

---

Box 7-4
Examples of Upper Limb Orthotic Devices for Children With Stroke

- Custom-made or prefabricated functional splints made from fabric with elastic properties (eg, neoprene). The purpose is to stabilize or position one or more joints or the thumb web space into an optimal position to enable ease of hand function. These may be used bilaterally or unilaterally and are used when the child is actively engaged in tasks (ie, not at rest or when sleeping).

- Static resting hand splints—custom-made or prefabricated. These are most commonly used during the acute and subacute phases of recovery if there is risk of soft tissue contracture due to persistently increased tone or postures that place a joint at risk of stiffness.

- Lycra gauntlet splints—these including full and partial body suits, sleeves, and gloves. The aim is to support the limb or hand into a more functional position and provide sensory feedback.

---

chopping boards to stabilize food while chopping, clamps to stabilize bottles or jars while taking off the lids, or rubber matting to stop paper from slipping while drawing or writing.

Given that technology is such an integral part of learning and communication, adaptive aids for the use of computers and phones are also important to consider. Some examples include the following: repositioning of the mouse and keyboards to alternate sides (note that the left-click and right-click on the mouse need to be swapped through using computer settings if the mouse is moved to the left side), positioning of the screen to maximize functional posture, and lower limb supports such as footstools.

When prescribing equipment or adaptive aids, it is important to do so in the context of a child-centered goal and, where possible, to be graded so that its use can be reduced over time.

Compensatory Strategies

When developing a rehabilitation program for a child following stroke, often a combination of strategies is used. These approaches often integrate maximizing function through rehabilitation (recovery of lost skills or learning and development of new skills) and strategies focusing on compensation for lost or changed abilities. These decisions need to be made carefully through collaboration between the child or family, the treating medical team, and the treating allied health clinicians.

Through clinical experience, it is evident that most children compensate for a lack of movement/function very naturally by completing an action in the easiest way possible, such as using the nonhemiplegic limb to complete a task or completing bimanual tasks unilaterally. Although this can be effective in the short term, unless coupled with appropriate intervention techniques, this has the potential to lead to learned nonuse through the inactivation of use-dependent plasticity.

The following should be taken into consideration when making these decisions about whether to employ compensatory techniques in intervention:

- What was the child's premorbid level of functioning? What is developmentally appropriate? For example, prior to having a stroke, a 12-month-old may or may not have started walking. A 4-year-old may or may not have been getting dressed by him- or herself, and a 5-year-old may or may not be able to ride a bike without training wheels.

- What are the child's and family's goals? Are the child and family motivated to engage in the targeted practice required to affect improvement in this specific task?

- What are the priorities for the child or young person at this point, for example, does the use of aids/equipment help conserve energy and time, enabling getting to school on time and being able to keep up with peers?

- If a compensation approach is used, what may be the cost in short- and long-term function? For example, is the child at risk of muscle shortening or joint contractures by not using his or her affected upper limb?

- Can support such as additional time for examinations or equipment for note taking (eg, a laptop) enable independent function?

- Had the child developed a hand preference at the time of the stroke? Early hand preference usually emerges in the first few years of life but is not well established until about 4 years of age. A child may be more likely to want to use their affected upper limb if premorbidly it was their dominant hand. Alternatively, if their dominant upper limb remains unaffected, the child may not have such strong motivations to use their affected upper limb, and they may naturally employ more compensatory techniques to complete activities of daily living.

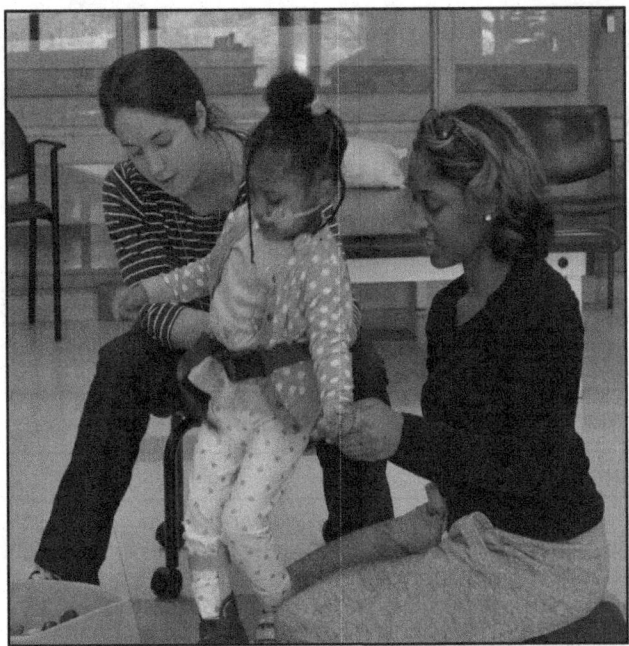

Figure 7-8. Integrating caregivers into all aspects of the intervention program is critical for long-term carryover and success.

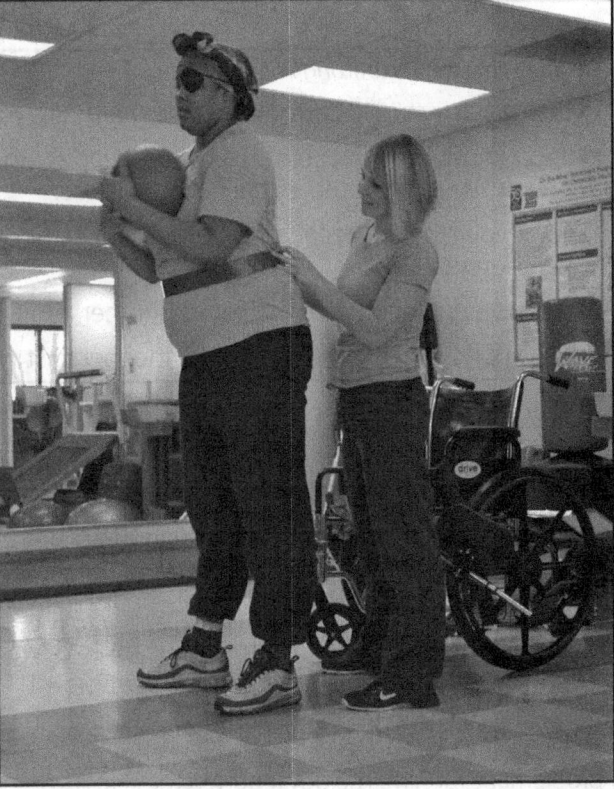

Figure 7-9. The physical therapist is using a weighted ball to carry over the occupational therapy goal of increased use of the affected upper extremity while the patient is working on a dynamic standing balance activity.

CHILD AND FAMILY EDUCATION

A critical piece of therapeutic intervention is the education provided to both the child and family throughout the rehabilitation experience. Providing meaningful and quality education is both an art and a science and can truly make or break the final outcome. Clinicians should strive to involve caregivers throughout the process, from the early days of relearning bed mobility and positioning, to encouraging use of the more affected side in meaningful ways (Figure 7-8). Therapists should also seek to engage in shared decision making with the selection and provision of interventions to work toward optimal family-centered care.

THE INTERPROFESSIONAL TEAM

The best rehabilitative care for stroke necessitates having a well-functioning interprofessional team. By collaborating closely with other professionals, clinicians can help carry over therapeutic strategies from other domains. It is known that repetition and generalization into other contexts help reinforce learning, and by communicating well, therapists

can seek to support the child's holistic goals for recovery. For example, physical and occupational therapists can carry over speech and language activities into their sessions by practicing skills suggested by the speech therapist while doing an activity (eg, having the child name ice cream flavors or pizza toppings while on the treadmill). Likewise, physical and occupational therapists can seek to increase repetition of purposeful movement by having colleagues in nursing or speech therapy encourage active use of the affected side (eg, having the child open and close the therapy door with the affected side, or using both hands to help position a chair at a table). Furthermore, clinicians may wish to cotreat a child when appropriate if the child's performance and learning would be enhanced by having professionals with different perspectives guiding the session. When all team members coordinate goals and communicate strategies to the child's family and to each other, the functional gains for the child are maximized (Figure 7-9).

FAMILY FOCUS BOX

Helpful Hints for Maximizing Therapy

- All therapy should be related to the goals that you, your child, and therapist set at the evaluation.

- You know your child best! Tell your therapist what motivates your child at home and what might help if he or she is frustrated with a new challenge.

- Ask your therapists for activities to help carry over gains at home. Let your therapist know if there are challenges.

- Involve the whole family. Siblings or other family members can be a great motivator.

- As your child nears discharge, ask the therapist when you should return for a re-evaluation.

CASE STUDY

This case study is a continuation of the child presented in Chapter 6. The child is an 8-year-old boy with right hemiplegia due to AIS of the left middle cerebral artery sustained during the perinatal period, who is referred to outpatient physical and occupational therapy 2 weeks after receiving botulinum toxin injections to his right upper and lower extremity (right brachioradialis, biceps brachii, gastrocnemius, hamstrings). His stated goals for occupational therapy include increased ability to use his right upper extremity to manage the zip on his coat and his shoelaces, and his goal for physical therapy is to "walk faster without a limp." Both the occupational and physical therapists collaborated while setting goals and a plan of care in order to carry over and reinforce learning.

Occupational Therapy

The occupational therapist observed the child's function in the 2 bimanual activities he identified as most problematic for him. The boy reported these tasks were particularly difficult when at school when there is pressure on time, and he was aware of being slower than his friends. Through task observation Goal Attainment Scaling (GAS) goals were devised and the tasks video-recorded. Challenging components of functional performance observed included maintaining balance in standing while using 2 hands cooperatively, accurate grasp and release of the edge of the coat or lace, lack of experience of the steps in the process, difficulty actively extending his right wrist and abducting his right thumb to achieve the appropriate grasp, and increased tone of right arm when under time pressure or stressed (associated reactions). Through discussion with the boy and his family, it was agreed to practice at home initially when there was more time. It was agreed that each day both tasks would be performed when appropriate in the usual daily routine and time arranged for focused task practice. A thumb abduction splint that supported the wrist position to neutral and opened the thumb web space was provided. Practice of shoelace tying was prescribed using the shoe on the boy's lap to maximize visual regard and minimize balance demands. A backward chaining approach with the boy performing the final stage of each task was utilized. With confidence and ability to perform the final step, the preceding step of the task was taught using both verbal and demonstration cues. Eventual transition to undertaking the tasks in seated or supported standing (eg, leaning with back to the wall) was found easier by the boy so he could attend to his hands. After 6 weeks of daily practice GAS goals were reviewed and videoed and the boy encouraged to reflect on what changes he found and what strategies worked best for him that he might find helpful for other tasks.

Physical Therapy

In physical therapy, the therapist developed goals with the child and family focused on walking at a fast speed and running. She recommended physical therapy 3 times/week for 8 weeks, with a plan of care that emphasized regaining lost range of motion, strengthening key muscle groups in the right leg, improving active control throughout the gait cycle, and gait training. By using the literature and concepts discussed previously in this chapter, the clinician selected the intervention strategies of strengthening using progressive resistive exercise and neuromuscular re-education, using functional electric stimulation, treadmill training, and overground gait training as well as task-specific practice for running. Although these largely focus on the philosophy of recovery, the clinician also utilized some compensatory strategies by prescribing a new AFO to aid in foot lift during the swing phase and to help maintain optimal postural alignment. In addition, the physical therapist discussed the child's goals with the occupational therapist and integrated increased opportunities for right upper extremity practice into physical therapy sessions. After the completion of the physical therapy course of care, the child and his mother both rated a high level of satisfaction with his goal attainment.

Summary

Recent advances in both animal and human research have suggested that the brain is capable of making adaptive changes after injury with associated improvement in functional ability, if provided with a stimulus capable of inducing clinical change. Although more research is needed to elaborate on the optimal parameters of these interventions, therapists should continue to integrate concepts gleaned from research evidence with the principles of family-centered care to develop an overall approach to stroke rehabilitation. Working as collaborative partners with the child, family, and interprofessional team can help ensure holistic care and meaningful carryover into the child's daily life.

References

1. Taub E, Uswatte G, Elbert T. New treatments in neurorehabilitation founded on basic research. *Nat Rev Neurosci.* 2002;3(3):228-236.

2. World Health Organization. Merger of ICF-CY into ICF. 2012; http://www.who.int/classifications/icf/en/. Updated January 27, 2017. Accessed March 29, 2017.

3. Atkinson HL, Nixon-Cave K. A tool for clinical reasoning and reflection using the international classification of functioning, disability and health (ICF) framework and patient management model. *Phys Ther.* 2011;91(3):416-430.

4. Agency for Health care Research and Quality. The SHARE Approach. http://www.ahrq.gov/professionals/education/curriculum-tools/shareddecisionmaking/index.html. Updated February 2017. Accessed March 22, 2016.

5. Hoffmann TC, Montori VM, Del Mar C. The connection between evidence-based medicine and shared decision making. *JAMA.* 2014;312(13):1295-1296.

6. Stacey D, Legare F, Col NF, et al. Decision aids for people facing health treatment or screening decisions. *Cochrane Database Syst Rev.* 2014;1:CD001431.

7. Paediatric Stroke Working Group, Royal College of Paediatrics and Child Health London. *Stroke in Childhood: Clinical Guidelines for Diagnosis, Management and Rehabilitation.* London, United Kingdom: Royal College of Paediatrics and Child Health London; 2017.

8. Royal Dutch Society for Physical Therapy. KNGF Clinical Practice Guideline for Physical Therapy in Patients with Stroke. http://neurorehab.nl/wp-content/uploads/2012/03/stroke_practice_guidelines_2014.pdf. Accessed April 20, 2017.

9. Novak I, McIntyre S, Morgan C, et al. A systematic review of interventions for children with cerebral palsy: state of the evidence. *Dev Med Child Neurol.* 2013;55(10):885-910.

10. Sakzewski L, Ziviani J, Boyd R. Systematic review and meta-analysis of therapeutic management of upper-limb dysfunction in children with congenital hemiplegia. *Pediatrics.* 2009;123(6):e1111-e1122.

11. Sakzewski L, Ziviani J, Boyd RN. Efficacy of upper limb therapies for unilateral cerebral palsy: a meta-analysis. *Pediatrics.* 2014;133(1):175-204.

12. Kolb B, Mychasiuk R, Gibb R. Brain development, experience, and behavior. *Pediatric Blood Cancer.* 2014;61(10):1720-1723.

13. Kleim JA, Jones TA. Principles of experience-dependent neural plasticity: implications for rehabilitation after brain damage. *J Speech Lang Hear Res.* 2008;51(1):225-239.

14. Kennard M. Reorganization of motor function in the cerebral cortex of monkeys deprived of motor and premotor areas in infancy. *J Neurophysiol.* 1938;1:477-496.

15. Kennard M. Relation of age to motor impairment in man and in subhuman primates. *Arch Neurol Psychiatry.* 1940;44:377-397.

16. Kennard M. Cortical reorganization of motor function. *Arch Neurol Psychiatry.* 1942;48:227-240.

17. Kolb B, Gibb R. Possible anatomical basis of spatial learning after neonatal prefrontal lesions in rats. *Behav Neurosci.* 1993;107(5):799-811.

18. Villablanca J, Carlson-Kuhta P, Schmanke T, Hovda D. A critical maturational period of reduced brain vulnerability to developmental injury. I. Behavioral studies in cats. *Dev Brain Res.* 1998;105(2):309-324.

19. Villablanca J, Hovda D, Jackson G, Infante C. Neurological and behavioral effects of a unilateral frontal cortical lesion in fetal kittens. II. Visual system tests, and proposing an "optimal developmental period" for lesion effects. *Behav Brain Res.* 1993;57(1):79-92.

20. Taub E, Uswatte G, Mark VW, Morris DM. The learned nonuse phenomenon: implications for rehabilitation. *Eura Medicophys.* 2006;42(3):241-256.

21. Pons TP, Garraghty PE, Ommaya AK, Kaas JH, Taub E, Mishkin M. Massive cortical reorganization after sensory deafferentation in adult macaques. *Science.* 1991;252(5014):1857-1860.

22. Nudo RJ, Wise BM, SiFuentes F, Milliken GW. Neural substrates for the effects of rehabilitative training on motor recovery after ischemic infarct. *Science.* 1996;272(5269):1791-1794.

23. Liepert J, Bauder H, Wolfgang HR, Miltner WH, Taub E, Weiller C. Treatment-induced cortical reorganization after stroke in humans. *Stroke.* 2000;31(6):1210-1216.

24. Boardman JP, Ganesan V, Rutherford MA, Saunders DE, Mercuri E, Cowan F. Magnetic resonance image correlates of hemiparesis after neonatal and childhood middle cerebral artery stroke. *Pediatrics.* 2005;115(2):321-326.

25. Mercuri E, Barnett A, Rutherford M, et al. Neonatal cerebral infarction and neuromotor outcome at school age. *Pediatrics.* 2004;113(1):95-100.

26. Mercuri E, Rutherford M, Cowan F, et al. Early prognostic indicators of outcome in infants with neonatal cerebral infarction: a clinical, electroencephalogram, and magnetic resonance imaging study. *Pediatrics.* 1999;103(1):39-46.

27. Mercuri E, Cowan F. Cerebral infarction in the newborn infant: review of the literature and personal experience. *Eur J Paediatr Neurol.* 1999;3(6):255-263.

28. Lee J, Croen LA, Lindan C, et al. Predictors of outcome in perinatal arterial stroke: a population-based study. *Ann Neurol.* 2005;58(2):303-308.

29. Golomb MR, deVeber GA, MacGregor DL, et al. Independent walking after neonatal arterial ischemic stroke and sinovenous thrombosis. *J Child Neurol.* 2003;18:530-536.

30. Kim CT, Han J, Kim H. Pediatric stroke recovery: a descriptive analysis. *Arch Phys Med Rehabil.* 2009;90(4):657-662.

31. Gordon AL, Ganesan V, Towell A, Kirkham FJ. Functional outcome following stroke in children. *J Child Neurol.* 2002;17(6):429-434.

32. Basu A, Graziadio S, Smith M, Clowry GJ, Cioni G, Eyre JA. Developmental plasticity connects visual cortex to motoneurons after stroke. *Ann Neurol.* 2010;67(1):132-136.

33. Deluca SC, Echols K, Law CR, Ramey SL. Intensive pediatric constraint-induced therapy for children with cerebral palsy: randomized, controlled, crossover trial. *J Child Neurol.* 2006;21(11):931-938.

34. deVeber GA, MacGregor D, Curtis R, Mayank S. Neurologic outcome in survivors of childhood arterial ischemic stroke and sinovenous thrombosis. *J Child Neurol.* 2000;15(5):316-324.

35. Salih MA, Abdel-Gader AG, Al-Jarallah AA, Kentab AY, Al-Nasser MN. Outcome of stroke in Saudi children. *Saudi Med J.* 2006;27(Suppl 1):S91-S96.

36. Ganesan V, Hogan A, Shack N, Gordon A, Isaacs E, Kirkham FJ. Outcome after ischaemic stroke in childhood. *Dev Med Child Neurol.* 2000;42(7):455-461.

37. Lanska MJ, Lanska DJ, Horwitz SJ, Aram MA. Presentation, clinical course, and outcome of childhood stroke. *Pediatr Neurol.* 1991;7:333-341.

38. Blom I, De Schryver EL, Kappelle LJ, Rinkel GJ, Jennekens-Schinkel A, Peters AC. Prognosis of haemorrhagic stroke in childhood: a long-term follow-up study. *Dev Med Child Neurol.* 2003;45(4):233-239.

39. Beslow LA, Licht DJ, Smith SE, et al. Predictors of outcome in childhood intracerebral hemorrhage: a prospective consecutive cohort study. *Stroke.* 2010;41(2):313-318.

40. Brouwer AJ, Groenendaal F, Koopman C, Nievelstein RJ, Han SK, de Vries LS. Intracranial hemorrhage in full-term newborns: a hospital-based cohort study. *Neuroradiology.* 2010;52(6):567-576.

41. Kolb B, Cioe J, Whishaw IQ. Is there an optimal age for recovery from motor cortex lesions? I. Behavioral and anatomical sequelae of bilateral motor cortex lesions in rats on postnatal days 1, 10, and in adulthood. *Brain Res.* 2000;882(1-2):62-74.

42. Anderson V, Spencer-Smith M, Wood A. Do children really recover better? Neurobehavioural plasticity after early brain insult. *Brain.* 2011;134(Pt 8):2197-2221.

43. Kolb B, Gibb R, Gorny G. Cortical plasticity and the development of behavior after early frontal cortical injury. *Dev Neuropsychol.* 2000;18(3):423-444.

44. Kelly-Hayes M, Wolf PA, Kase CS, Gresham GE, Kannel WB, D'Agostino RB. Time course of functional recovery after stroke: the Framingham Study. *Neurorehabil Neural Repair.* 1989;3(2):65-70.

45. Kim CT, Han J, Kim H. Pediatric stroke recovery: A descriptive analysis. *Arch Phys Med Rehabil.* 1999;90(4):657-662.

46. Gordon AL, Anderson V, Ditchfield M, et al. Factors associated with six-month outcome of pediatric stroke. *Int J Stroke.* 2015;10(7):1068-1073.

47. Ponsford J, Willmott C, Rothwell A, et al. Cognitive and behavioral outcome following mild traumatic head injury in children. *J Head Trauma Rehabil.* 1999;14(4):360-372.

48. Catroppa C, Anderson VA, Morse SA, Haritou F, Rosenfeld JV. Outcome and predictors of functional recovery 5 years following pediatric traumatic brain injury (TBI). *J Pediatr Psychol.* 2008;33(7):707-718.

49. Satz P. Brain reserve capacity on symptom onset after brain injury: A formulation and review of evidence for threshold theory. *Neuropsychology.* 1993;7(3):273-295.

50. Stern Y. What is cognitive reserve? Theory and research application of the reserve concept. *J Int Neuropsychol Soc.* 2002;8:448-460.

51. Muratori LM, Lamberg EM, Quinn L, Duff SV. Applying principles of motor learning and control to upper extremity rehabilitation. *J Hand Ther.* 2013;26(2):94-102; quiz 103.

52. Aubert E. Motor development in the normal child. In: Tecklin J, ed. *Pediatric Physical Therapy*, 5th ed. Baltimore, MD: Lippincott Williams & Wilkins; 2015:17-67.

53. Wulf G, Lewthwaite R. Optimizing performance through intrinsic motivation and attention for learning: The OPTIMAL theory of motor learning. *Psychon Bull Rev.* 2016;23(5):1382-1414.

54. Sullivan KJ, Kantak SS, Burtner PA. Motor learning in children: feedback effects on skill acquisition. *Phys Ther.* 2008;88(6):720-732.

55. Goh HT, Kantak SS, Sullivan KJ. Movement pattern and parameter learning in children: effects of feedback frequency. *Res Q Exerc Sport.* 2012;83(2):346-352.

56. Guadagnoli MA, Lee TD. Challenge point: a framework for conceptualizing the effects of various practice conditions in motor learning. *J Mot Behav.* 2004;36(2):212-224.

57. Sullivan JE, Crowner BE, Kluding PM, et al. Outcome measures for individuals with stroke: process and recommendations from the American Physical Therapy Association neurology section task force. *Phys Ther.* 2013;93(10):1383-1396.

58. Burtner PA, Leinwand R, Sullivan KJ, Goh HT, Kantak SS. Motor learning in children with hemiplegic cerebral palsy: feedback effects on skill acquisition. *Dev Med Child Neurol.* 2014;56(3):259-266.

59. Pollock CL, Boyd LA, Hunt MA, Garland SJ. Use of the challenge point framework to guide motor learning of stepping reactions for improved balance control in people with stroke: a case series. *Phys Ther.* 2014;94(4):562-570.

60. Mastos M, Miller K, Eliasson AC, Imms C. Goal-directed training: linking theories of treatment to clinical practice for improved functional activities in daily life. *Clin Rehabil.* 2007;21(1):47-55.

61. Westmacott RP, MacGregor DMD, Askalan RMD, deVeber GMD. Late emergence of cognitive deficits after unilateral neonatal stroke. *Stroke.* 2009;40(6):2012-2019.

62. Burke JP, Kielhofner G. A model of human occupation, Part 1. Conceptual framework and content. *Am J Occup Ther.* 1980;34:572-581.

63. Webb PM, Glueckauf RL. The effects of direct involvement in goal setting on rehabilitation outcome for persons with traumatic brain injuries. *Rehabil Psychol.* 1994;39(3):179-188.

64. Taub E, Griffin A, Nick J, Gammons K, Uswatte G, Law CR. Pediatric CI therapy for stroke-induced hemiparesis in young children. *Dev Neurorehabil.* 2007;10(1):3-18.

65. Gordon A, Connelly A, Neville B, et al. Modified constraint-induced movement therapy after childhood stroke. *Dev Med Child Neurol.* 2007;49(1):23-27.

66. Eliasson AC, Krumlinde-Sundholm L, Gordon AM, et al. Guidelines for future research in constraint-induced movement therapy for children with unilateral cerebral palsy: an expert consensus. *Dev Med Child Neurol.* 2014;56(2):126-137.

67. Hoare B, Wallen M, Imms C, Villanueva E, Rawicki H, Carey L. Botulinum toxin A as an adjunct to treatment in the management of the upper limb in children with spastic cerebral palsy (UPDATE) [review]. *Cochrane Database Syst.* 2010;1:CD003469.

68. Aarts P, Jongerius P, Geerdink Y, van Limbeek J, Geurts A. Effectiveness of modified constraint-induced movement therapy in children with unilateral spastic cerebral palsy: a randomized controlled trial. *Neurorehabil Neural Repair.* 2010;24:509-518.

69. Gordon A, Schneider J, Chinnan A, Charles J. Efficacy of a hand-arm bimanual intensive therapy (HABIT) in children with hemiplegic cerebral palsy: a randomized control trial. *Dev Med Child Neurol.* 2007;49:830-838.

70. Boyd R, Sakzewski L, Ziviani J, et al. INCITE: A randomised trial comparing constraint induced movement therapy and bimanual training in children with congenital hemiplegia. *BMC Neurol.* 2010;10:4.

71. Gordon AM. To constrain or not to constrain, and other stories of intensive upper extremity training for children with unilateral cerebral palsy. *Dev Med Child Neurol.* 2011;53(Suppl 4):56-61.

72. Gordon AM, Chinnan A, Gill S, Petra E, Hung YC, Charles J. Both constraint-induced movement therapy and bimanual training lead to improved performance of upper extremity function in children with hemiplegia. *Dev Med Child Neurol.* 2008;50(12):957-958.

73. Gordon AM, Okita SY. Augmenting pediatric constraint-induced movement therapy and bimanual training with video gaming technology. *Technol Disabil*. 2010;22(4):179-191.

74. Hoare BJ, Imms C, Rawicki HB, Carey L. Modified constraint-induced movement therapy or bimanual occupational therapy following injection of botulinum toxin-A to improve bimanual performance in young children with hemiplegic cerebral palsy: A randomised controlled trial methods paper. *BMC Neurology*. 2010;10:58.

75. Sakzewski L, Ziviani J, Abbott DF, Macdonell RAL, Jackson GD, Boyd RN. Equivalent retention of gains at 1 year after training with constraint-induced or bimanual therapy in children with unilateral cerebral palsy. *Neurorehabil Neural Repair*. 2011;25(7):664-671.

76. Sakzewski L, Ziviani J, Boyd RN. Efficacy of upper limb therapies for unilateral cerebral palsy: a meta-analysis. *Pediatrics*. 2014;133(1):e175-e204.

77. Novak I, Cusick A, Lannin N. Occupational therapy home programs for cerebral palsy: double-blind, randomized, controlled trial. *Pediatrics*. 2009;124(4):e606-e614.

78. Sakzewski L, Gordon A, Eliasson A-C. The state of the evidence for intensive upper limb therapy approaches for children with unilateral cerebral palsy. *J Child Neurol*. 2014;29(8):1077-1090.

79. Andersen JC, Majnemer A, O'Grady K, Gordon AM. Intensive upper extremity training for children with hemiplegia: from science to practice. *Semin Pediatr Neurol*. 2013;20(2):100-105.

80. Eng JJ. Strength training in individuals with stroke. *Physiother Can*. 2004;56(4):189-201.

81. Harris JE, Eng JJ. Strength training improves upper-limb function in individuals with stroke: a meta-analysis. *Stroke*. 2010;41(1):136-140.

82. Duncan PW, Sullivan KJ, Behrman AL, et al. Protocol for the Locomotor Experience Applied Post-stroke (LEAPS) trial: a randomized controlled trial. *BMC Neurol*. 2007;7:39.

83. Tilson JK, Sullivan KJ, Cen SY, et al. Meaningful gait speed improvement during the first 60 days poststroke: minimal clinically important difference. *Phys Ther*. 2010;90(2):196-208.

84. Holleran CL, Rodriguez KS, Echauz A, Leech KA, Hornby TG. Potential contributions of training intensity on locomotor performance in individuals with chronic stroke. *J Neurol Phys Ther*. 2015;39(2):95-102.

85. Hornby TG, Moore JL, Lovell L, Roth EJ. Influence of skill and exercise training parameters on locomotor recovery during stroke rehabilitation. *Curr Opin Neurol*. 2016;29(6):677-683.

86. Hornby TG, Straube DS, Kinnaird CR, et al. Importance of specificity, amount, and intensity of locomotor training to improve ambulatory function in patients poststroke. *Top Stroke Rehabil*. 2011;18(4):293-307.

87. Zwicker JG, Mayson TA. Effectiveness of treadmill training in children with motor impairments: an overview of systematic reviews. *Pediatr Phys Ther*. 2010;22(4):361-377.

88. Hidler J, Nichols D, Pelliccio M, et al. Multicenter randomized clinical trial evaluating the effectiveness of the Lokomat in subacute stroke. *Neurorehabil Neural Repair*. 2009;23(1):5-13.

89. Willoughby KL, Dodd KJ, Shields N. A systematic review of the effectiveness of treadmill training for children with cerebral palsy. *Disabil Rehabil*. 2009;31(24):1971-1979.

90. Damiano DL, DeJong SL. A systematic review of the effectiveness of treadmill training and body weight support in pediatric rehabilitation. *JNPT*. 2009;33(1):27.

91. Mattern-Baxter K. Effects of partial body weight supported treadmill training on children with cerebral palsy. *Pediatric Physical Therapy*. 2009;21(1):12.

92. Celestino ML, Gama GL, Barela AM. Gait characteristics of children with cerebral palsy as they walk with body weight unloading on a treadmill and over the ground. *Res Dev Disabil*. 2014;35(12):3624-3631.

93. Chrysagis N, Skordilis EK, Stavrou N, Grammatopoulou E, Koutsouki D. The effect of treadmill training on gross motor function and walking speed in ambulatory adolescents with cerebral palsy: a randomized controlled trial. *Am J Phys Med Rehabil*. 2012;91(9):747-760.

94. Ucar DE, Paker N, Bugdayci D. Lokomat: a therapeutic chance for patients with chronic hemiplegia. *NeuroRehabilitation*. 2014;34(3):447-453.

95. Druzbicki M, Rusek W, Snela S, et al. Functional effects of robotic-assisted locomotor treadmill therapy in children with cerebral palsy. *J Rehabil Med*. 2013;45(4):358-363.

96. Kelley CP, Childress J, Boake C, Noser EA. Over-ground and robotic-assisted locomotor training in adults with chronic stroke: a blinded randomized clinical trial. *Disabil Rehabil Assist Technol*. 2013;8(2):161-168.

97. Kahn JH, Hornby TG. Rapid and long-term adaptations in gait symmetry following unilateral step training in people with hemiparesis. *Phys Ther*. 2009;89(5):474-483.

98. Reisman DS, Bastian AJ, Morton SM. Neurophysiologic and rehabilitation insights from the split-belt and other locomotor adaptation paradigms. *Phys Ther*. 2010;90(2):187-195.

99. Patrick SK, Musselman KE, Tajino J, Ou HC, Bastian AJ, Yang JF. Prior experience but not size of error improves motor learning on the split-belt treadmill in young children. *PLoS One*. 2014;9(3):e93349.

100. Lauziere S, Mieville C, Betschart M, Duclos C, Aissaoui R, Nadeau S. Plantarflexion moment is a contributor to step length after-effect following walking on a split-belt treadmill in individuals with stroke and healthy individuals. *J Rehabil Med*. 2014;46(9):849-857.

101. Tyrell CM, Helm E, Reisman DS. Locomotor adaptation is influenced by the interaction between perturbation and baseline asymmetry after stroke. *J Biomech*. 2015;48(11):2849-2857.

102. Helm EE, Reisman DS. The split-belt walking paradigm: exploring motor learning and spatiotemporal asymmetry poststroke. *Phys Med Rehabil Clin N Am*. 2015;26(4):703-713.

103. Adamovich SV, Fluet GG, Tunik E, Merians AS. Sensorimotor training in virtual reality: a review. *NeuroRehabilitation*. 2009;25(1):29-44.

104. Galvin J, McDonald R, Catroppa C, Anderson V. Does intervention using virtual reality improve upper limb function in children with neurological impairment: a systematic review of the evidence. *Brain Injury*. 2011;25(5):435-442.

105. Mumford N, Wilson PH. Virtual reality in acquired brain injury upper limb rehabilitation: evidence-based evaluation of clinical research. *Brain Injury*. 2009;23(3):179-191.

106. Parsons TD, Rizzo AA, Rogers S, York P. Virtual reality in paediatric rehabilitation: a review. *Dev Neurorehabil*. 2009;12(4):224-238.

107. Munzert J, Lorey B, Zentgraf K. Cognitive motor processes: the role of motor imagery in the study of motor representations. *Brain Res Rev*. 2009;60(2):306-326.

108. Jeannerod M. Neural simulation of action: a unifying mechanism for motor cognition. *NeuroImage*. 2001;14(1 Pt 2):S103.

109. Sharma N, Simmons LH, Jones PS, et al. Motor imagery after subcortical stroke: a functional magnetic resonance imaging study. *Stroke*. 2009;40(4):1315-1324.

110. Page SJ, Levine P, Leonard A. Mental practice in chronic stroke: results of a randomized, placebo-controlled trial. *Stroke*. 2007;38(4):1293-1297.

111. Braun SM, Beurskens AJ, Borm PJ, Schack T, Wade DT. The effects of mental practice in stroke rehabilitation: a systematic review. *Arch Phys Med Rehabil.* 2006;87(6):842-852.

112. Garrison KA, Winstein CJ, Aziz-Zadeh L. The mirror neuron system: a neural substrate for methods in stroke rehabilitation. *Neurorehabil Neural Repair.* 2010;24(5):404-412.

113. Braun S, Kleynen M, Schols J, Schack T, Beurskens A, Wade D. Using mental practice in stroke rehabilitation: a framework. *Clin Rehab.* 2008;22(7):579-591.

114. Molina M, Kudlinski C, Guilbert J, Spruijt S, Steenbergen B, Jouen F. Motor imagery for walking: a comparison between cerebral palsy adolescents with hemiplegia and diplegia. *Res Dev Disabil.* 2015;37:95-101.

115. Spruijt S, van der Kamp J, Steenbergen B. Current insights in the development of children's motor imagery ability. *Front Psychol.* 2015;6:787.

116. Steenbergen B, Craje C, Nilsen DM, Gordon AM. Motor imagery training in hemiplegic cerebral palsy: a potentially useful therapeutic tool for rehabilitation. *Dev Med Child Neurol.* 2009;51(9):690-696.

117. Wilson PH, Adams IL, Caeyenberghs K, Thomas P, Smits-Engelsman B, Steenbergen B. Motor imagery training enhances motor skill in children with DCD: a replication study. *Res Dev Disabil.* 2016;57:54-62.

118. Ezendam D, Bongers RM, Jannink MJ. Systematic review of the effectiveness of mirror therapy in upper extremity function. *Disabil Rehabil.* 2009;31(26):2135-2149.

119. Ramachandran VS, Altschuler EL. The use of visual feedback, in particular mirror visual feedback, in restoring brain function. *Brain.* 2009;132(7):1693-1710.

120. Nojima I, Koganemaru S, Fukuyama H, Kawamata T, Mima T. Effect of mirror visual feedback on human motor plasticity. *Neurosci Res.* 2011;71:e254.

121. Nojima I, Mima T, Koganemaru S, Thabit MN, Fukuyama H, Kawamata T. Human motor plasticity induced by mirror visual feedback. *J Neurosci.* 2012;32(4):1293-1300.

122. Doyle S, Bennett S, Fasoli SE, McKenna KT. Interventions for sensory impairment in the upper limb after stroke. *Cochrane Database Syst Rev.* 2010;6:CD006331.

123. Lisa LP, Jughters A, Kerckhofs E. The effectiveness of different treatment modalities for the rehabilitation of unilateral neglect in stroke patients: a systematic review. *NeuroRehabilitation.* 2013;33(4):611-620.

124. Rothgangel AS, Braun SM, Beurskens AJ, Seitz RJ, Wade DT. The clinical aspects of mirror therapy in rehabilitation: a systematic review of the literature. *Int J Rehab Res.* 2011;34(1):1-13.

125. Auld ML, Russo R, Moseley GL, Johnston LM. Determination of interventions for upper extremity tactile impairment in children with cerebral palsy: a systematic review. *Dev Med Child Neurol.* 2014;56(9):815-832.

126. Laufer Y, Ring H, Sprecher E, Hausdorff JM. Gait in individuals with chronic hemiparesis: one-year follow-up of the effects of a neuroprosthesis that ameliorates foot drop. *J Neurol Phys Ther.* 2009;33(2):104-110.

127. Lannin NA, Ada L. Neurorehabilitation splinting: theory and principles of clinical use. *NeuroRehabilitation.* 2011;28(1):21-28.

128. Kanellopoulos AD, Mavrogenis AF, Mitsiokapa EA, et al. Long lasting benefits following the combination of static night upper extremity splinting with botulinum toxin A injections in cerebral palsy children. *Eur J Phys Rehabil Med.* 2009;45(4):501-506.

129. Jackman M, Novak I, Lannin N. Effectiveness of hand splints in children with cerebral palsy: a systematic review with meta-analysis. *Dev Med Child Neurol.* 2014;56(2):138-147.

130. Copley JKK. *Neurorehabilitation of the Upper Limb Across the Lifespan: Managing Hypertonicity for Optimal Function.* Hoboken, NJ: Wiley-Blackwell; 2014.

SUGGESTED READINGS

College of Occupational Therapists. *Children & Young People with Acquired Brain Injury: Current Practice in Occupational Therapy.* https://www.cot.co.uk/publication/cot-publications/children-and-young-people-acquired-brain-injury-current-practice-occupa. Published August 9, 2015. Accessed March 29, 2017.

Copley J, Kuipers K. *Neurorehabilitation of the Upper Limb Across the Lifespan: Managing Hypertonicity for Optimal Function.* West Sussex, United Kingdom: Wiley Blackwell; 2014.

Hogan L, Uditsky T. *Pediatric Splinting: Selection, Fabrication, and Clinical Application of Upper Extremity Splints.* San Antonio, TX: Therapy Skill Builders; 1998.

Paediatric Stroke Working Group, Royal College of Paediatrics and Child Health London. Stroke in Childhood: Clinical Guidelines for Diagnosis, Management and Rehabilitation. London, United Kingdom: Royal College of Paediatrics and Child Health London; 2017.

8

Communication and Feeding in Children With Stroke

Amy Colin, MA, CCC-SLP and Elizabeth Yeh, MA, CCC-SLP

The goal of this chapter is to provide the reader with a brief overview of symptoms, assessment, and treatment of speech, language, and feeding impairments in infants and children following a stroke. Due to the heterogeneous nature of this population and paucity of research related to treatment of children poststroke in these areas, no single treatment approach has been shown to be comprehensive and reliable. Although various structured speech and language programs have been well researched with adults, further study and validation are needed before the findings can be generalized to the pediatric population. Pediatric speech-language pathologists must employ an eclectic approach pulling from a variety of adult programs and developmental approaches. Involvement of caregivers will be a vital component of treatment to encourage carryover and generalization of skills into natural environments. In general, therapists need to consider the individual strengths and weaknesses of every child and family and develop treatment plans accordingly.

Traditional speech therapy has proven effective in the rehabilitation and recovery of oral feeding, speech, and language functions following a stroke. Progress is most rapid in the first 2 to 3 months post onset[1] and can continue throughout childhood and into adulthood. Initiation of speech therapy services as soon as the child is medically stable is essential to maximize potential for recovery and outcome. Therapy can be provided across the continuum of care, beginning in the acute care setting through outpatient and school-based settings. Providing rehabilitation in the context of functional activities can

optimize the success of generalization of training.[2] The speech-language pathologist should be a core member of the child's rehabilitation team. Even when successful recovery occurs in the young child, it will be important to maintain close monitoring of a child's acquisition of age-expected speech, language, and oral feeding skills over the course of his development.

LANGUAGE

In order to better understand the symptoms of disordered language following a stroke, a general discussion of language is warranted. Language is composed of two modalities: *expressive language* and *receptive language*.

Expressive language is the use of language, spoken, written, or signed, that conveys a meaning or message. It involves use of vocabulary and syntactic rules and morphemes within utterances for communication across many contexts.[3] Expressive language functions that may be vulnerable to impairment poststroke include organization, word retrieval, and fluency.[2]

Receptive language is the comprehension of spoken, signed, or written language. Comprehension of written language can also refer to reading comprehension. Understanding the rules of syntax, morphology, and phonology will aid in comprehension of language across various activities and tasks.[3] This can include following directions, comprehension of basic and complex questions, and following conversations.

Atkinson HL, Nixon-Cave K, Smith SE, eds.
*Pediatric Stroke Rehabilitation: An Interprofessional and
Collaborative Approach* (pp 135-159). © 2018 Taylor & Francis Group.

Within expressive and receptive language, Bloom and Lahey described 3 domains of language: *form, content,* and *use.* They proposed that it is the interaction of these 3 aspects that allows a person to use and understand language[3]:

1. *Form* is the structure and rules for language, primarily consisting of syntax, morphology, and phonology that comprise grammar.

    a. Syntax: The rules of ordering and combining words to create structure within sentences.

    b. Morphology: The rules of structures of words and word forms. Morphemes are the smallest units of meaning in a language (eg, "-ed" for past tense).

    c. Phonology: The sounds of a language and the rules for combining sounds into units of language. A phoneme is the basic unit of sound such as /b/ or /s/.

2. *Content* includes the semantic components of language, including the knowledge of vocabulary, objects, and events.

3. *Use* consists of the functions or rules of language related to pragmatics or social use of language, including what forms to use to achieve those functions (eg, conversation).

APHASIA

The American Speech-Language-Hearing Association defines *aphasia* as a language disorder that results from damage to the parts of the brain responsible for language production and comprehension. When either a partial or complete loss of language functions occurs, speaking, listening, reading, and writing can all be affected.[4]

Acquired childhood aphasia (ACA) refers to the language deficits that may follow a stroke sustained after the age when acquisition of first sentences occurs. The criteria required for a diagnosis of ACA include the stroke occurring after 2 years of age or when first sentences are acquired and the presence of disruption in oral communication.[5]

Congenital aphasia refers to the language deficits that may follow a stroke sustained prior to age 2 disrupting language milestones or developmental language sequence.[5]

There has been conflicting evidence in the literature regarding the influence of age at time of stroke on the reorganization and recovery of language functions. Some literature indicates that early injuries often result in an interhemispheric shift in language functions, whereas later injuries are more likely to result in reorganization of language within the affected hemisphere.[6,7] Based on the principles of neuroplasticity, there is great potential that reorganization of language will occur and shift language function to the contralateral hemisphere to compensate for injured areas. Several studies have shown evidence of language reorganization following early lesions in the left hemisphere through different techniques, including the dichotic listening paradigm and neuroimaging techniques, and most recently, functional magnetic resonance imaging.[7,8] This shifting of language dominance has been shown to enhance recovery and minimize the long-term effects of language-based disorders.

Opposing research indicates that children may grow into their deficits, as developmental expectations are not achieved later in childhood. Chapman and colleagues[9] found poorer outcomes with discourse measures with early age of stroke vs later age of stroke. Kirton and deVeber[10] found that developmental language disorders occur in 20% to 25% of children with history of perinatal stroke, independent of site of lesion. In a study by Avila and colleagues,[11] some aspect of language function was impaired in all of the 32 children and adolescents examined with diagnosis of unilateral ischemic stroke that occurred between the perinatal period and 12 years of age. Whatever the outcome or recovery following neonatal or childhood stroke, ongoing monitoring for the acquisition of age-expected speech and language skills will be critical due to the high potential for disruption of language development at various stages.

The pattern of language problems will vary based on the site and size of lesion in the brain. For the majority of people, the left hemisphere of the cerebral cortex is dominant for speech and language function.[12] The 2 major areas responsible for speech and language skills are located in the frontal lobe and temporal lobe.

Broca's area is located anteriorly in the motor association cortex of the frontal lobe. Lesions located in this area are expected to result in deficits related to speech production and language formulation. Speech will be effortful and nonfluent. Comprehension should be relatively spared; although, comprehension deficits can be present, including understanding complex syntax. Aphasia as a result of lesion to this area is often referred to as *nonfluent aphasia* or *Broca aphasia.* Due to the close proximity to the primary motor strip from Broca's area, lesions in this area may also result in right-sided motor impairments or hemiplegia in addition to weakness of the speech musculature.[13,14]

Wernicke's area is located posteriorly in the left temporal lobe of the brain. Lesions in this area are expected to result in deficits related to comprehension. Speech production is fluent; however, content is often meaningless or illogical. Aphasia as a result of lesion to this area is often referred to as a *fluent aphasia* or *Wernicke aphasia.* Associated motor weakness will most likely not be present with a posterior lesion in this area.[13,14]

The clinical presentation of acquired childhood aphasia can be similar to adults with aphasia based on site of lesion.[15] The dichotomy of fluent vs nonfluent aphasia has not only been observed in the adult population but with children as well. In addition, the proportion of

TABLE 8-1. RECOMMENDED STANDARDIZED MEASURES TO ASSESS LANGUAGE IN CHILDREN WITH STROKE

LANGUAGE AREA	STANDARDIZED MEASURE
Auditory comprehension	■ Clinical Evaluation of Language Fundamentals, Fifth Edition ■ Test of Auditory Processing Skills, Third Edition ■ Test of Narrative Language
Language formulation and organization	■ Clinical Evaluation of Language Fundamentals, Fifth Edition ■ Clinical Evaluation of Language Fundamentals: Metalinguistics ■ Pediatric Test of Brain Injury ■ Test of Narrative Language
Narrative construction	■ Clinical Evaluation of Language Fundamentals, Fifth Edition ■ Test of Written Language, Fourth Edition ■ Test of Narrative Language
Reading comprehension	■ Clinical Evaluation of Language Fundamentals, Fifth Edition ■ Test of Reading Comprehension, Fourth Edition
Word finding	■ Boston Naming Test ■ Expressive One Word Picture Vocabulary Test, Fourth Edition ■ Expressive Vocabulary Test, Second Edition ■ Pediatric Test of Brain Injury ■ Test of Word Finding, Third Edition

nonfluent vs fluent aphasia appears similar in children and adults.[16,17]

ASSESSMENT CONSIDERATIONS

Few, if any, standardized measures have been developed to specifically assess children with acquired aphasia (Table 8-1). Standardized measures designed to assess developmental language disorders in children can provide valuable information and should be used. However, in order to provide a comprehensive assessment of speech and language skills, a combination of standardized and nonstandardized measures must be considered. Comprehensive language batteries for assessment of different aspects of language, including fluency, syntax, auditory comprehension, and repetition, should be used to identify affected language abilities. Naming can be assessed through measures designed for assessment of word retrieval or through single-word vocabulary tests. Divergent word naming tasks can further assess efficiency and accuracy with word retrieval. However, limitations of standardized measures need to be taken into account when making clinical judgments

regarding the child's language abilities and recommendations for treatment.[2,18]

Gathering detailed information regarding the child's communication abilities across settings can give insight into the impact of the child's speech and language deficits on daily functioning. Keeping in mind the child's premorbid language and academic performance compared to current functioning may guide interpretation of results and recommendations even in the setting of average scores. Nonstandardized measures and child and parent report of current functioning will be critical in obtaining a comprehensive picture of the child's language and learning profile. Nonstandardized measures should include a discourse sample, writing sample, and detailed case history following review of health and educational records. Observation of play for a younger child can give information regarding spontaneous speech, organization, and problem-solving skills.

Assessment of reading comprehension should be included using standardized measures or age-equivalent relevant information. General observation of cognitive status (eg, attention, working memory, executive function) and its impact on language performance should occur.[19] Observation of strategy use and testing of higher-level

TABLE 8-2. EXAMPLES OF TYPES OF PARAPHASIAS		
TYPE OF PARAPHASIA	**DEFINITION**	**EXAMPLE**
Semantic	Word related in meaning	"wolf" for "dog"
Phonemic	Sound substitution resulting in nonword	"sog" for "dog"
Mixed	Word related in meaning and sound	"hog" for "dog"
Neologistic	Nonword with many sound substitutions	"pelf" for "dog"

language or cognitive skills during more challenging tasks can provide appreciation into the child's awareness and insight into current deficits. During both assessment and treatment, the child's capacity for new language learning will need to be carefully examined to help guide treatment and academic recommendations.

COMMON SYMPTOMS OF APHASIA

Word Finding

One of the most prevalent symptoms following a stroke is anomia, which is the inability to access and retrieve target words, including nouns and verbs, during conversation or structured tasks.[13,20-22] This is more commonly referred to as *word finding.* Most people have experienced the feeling of a word being "on the tip of their tongue." For people with aphasia, this occurs frequently throughout the day and can be manifested in both spoken and written language.

A child with word finding may require increased time to generate the target word or be unable to access the word at all. During a word-finding episode, the child may demonstrate stalling behaviors to gain extra time to search for the target word. These can include using filler nonwords (eg, I saw a um…um…um…elephant) or repetition of the initial phrase or word of the utterance (eg, the boy, the boy, the boy rode his bike). Common features of word finding include the following:

- *Circumlocution* is the act of talking around a word or describing the key features of the word that the individual cannot access. For example, a child may be trying to say "ball" but instead may say "It's round. It bounces. You can throw it."

- *Paraphasias* are unintended word productions that often interfere with or change the meaning of the child's message (Table 8-2). The child may be aware of these errors and attempt to correct them or appear to be completely unaware that the errors occurred. There are 2 categories of paraphasias. Semantic or verbal paraphasias are word substitutions (eg, *horse* for *cow*), and phonemic paraphasias are sound substitutions within words (eg, *gow* for *cow*).

- *Neologisms* are nonwords composed of multiple sound substitutions. A word is considered neologistic when more than half of the word contains sound substitutions. Neologisms are often produced with jargon seen in fluent aphasia.

- *Perseverations* are repeated productions of a word or phrase in response to different stimuli or questions. For example, a child responded "chicken sandwich" when asked what he ate for lunch. He provided the same response when asked what activities he participated in during physical therapy and during responsive naming tasks. Although aware of the error, he was unable to correct and break the perseveration.

Word-finding difficulties can have a significant impact on communication. A child's ability to make requests, ask or respond to questions, or share information can be affected by word-finding difficulties. It can affect a child's participation in conversation, leading to communication breakdowns that the child is unable to repair independently. This can lead to frustration of the child and listener and abandonment of the communicative interaction.

Word finding can also affect academic performance in the school-aged child. Acquisition of vocabulary can be affected. Test performance, ability to participate in oral debates or group discussions, and formulation of cohesive and coherent written narratives can all be affected. Performance on time-sensitive activities, such as timed tests or pressure situations, including an oral presentation, may lessen as stress may further exacerbate word-finding problems.

Therapy for word finding is often comprised of naming-based tasks and compensatory strategy training. Activities that focus on various naming tasks, including confrontation naming (eg, labeling pictures), generative or divergent naming (eg, naming members in categories), responsive naming, and associative naming (eg, synonyms, analogous statements) may all assist in improving efficiency with access to target vocabulary. The overall goal of naming treatments, despite the approach, is to foster generalization of word-finding abilities beyond the training items within spontaneous speech. Although some studies have shown generalization to untrained words, the majority of studies have reported mostly training-specific effects.[23,24]

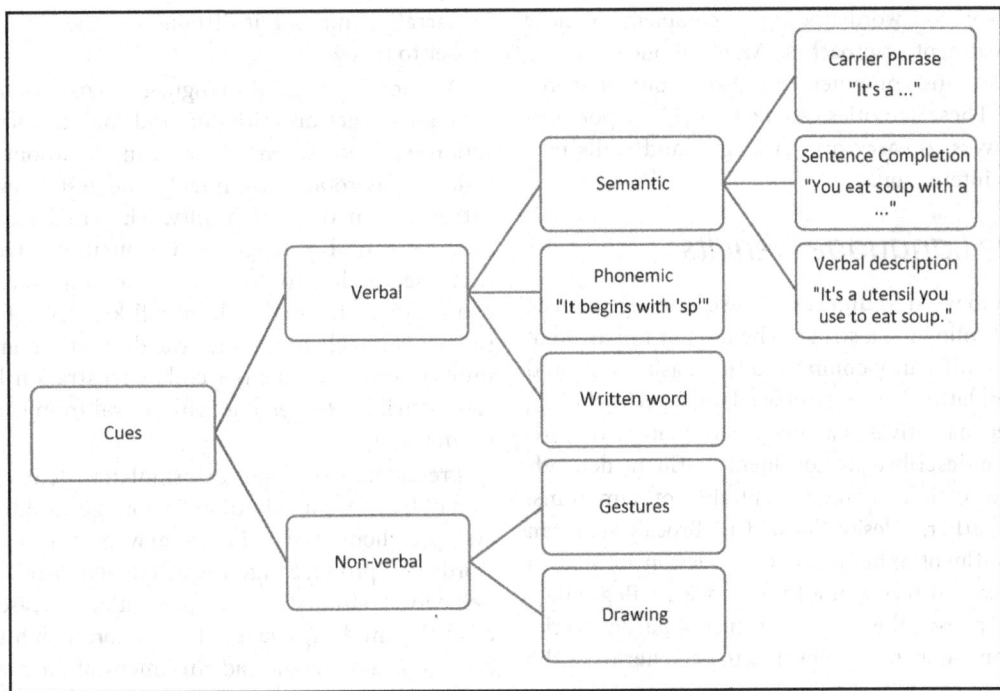

Figure 8-1. Word-finding cues.

Phonological treatments are aimed at incorporating the lexical system to improve naming. This may include training with rhyming words, use of phonemic cues (ie, providing the first sound of the word), and word repetition.[25]

Semantic treatments involve activating the semantic systems to associate concepts with target words. Success has been found in the literature with increasing word retrieval skills in adults with aphasia using Semantic Feature Analysis (SFA).[26-28] SFA is a semantic treatment based on the theory that neural connections between related concepts are strengthened within the semantic system so that access to vocabulary becomes more automatic. Vocabulary is stored within semantic networks consisting of word meanings, creating highly organized associations of words, concepts, and images. When there is a disruption in either the organization of networks or retrieval process, word retrieval becomes inefficient. Generating words or phrases related to target vocabulary should help to recreate or strengthen the connections of networks in an organized fashion. Through SFA, the speech-language pathologist prompts the child to answer a set of description and function questions about the target within feature categories. These responses are recorded in a visual diagram.

Providing word-finding cues to the child during therapy tasks or within conversation can facilitate retrieval of target words (Figure 8-1). Verbal and nonverbal cues can be utilized. Verbal cues include semantic, phonemic, and written cues. Semantic cues, including sentence completion cues, carrier phrases, or verbal description cues, provide additional meaning of the target word. A phonemic cue provides no semantic meaning. Nonverbal cues include gestures and drawing.

Teaching children to use these cues independently can equip them with compensatory strategies leading to more effective and efficient communication.[29] Self-cuing by the child may also provide the listener with sufficient information to assist him or her in generating the desired word if needed. Training the child in the use of strategies and self-cuing early on in the recovery process will not only promote successful communication opportunities. If deficits persist, it will provide the child with the tools and skills to anticipate or correct word-finding episodes so the listener is unaware and the communication interaction is not disrupted.

Compensatory strategy training can be a challenge with younger children, as they have not yet developed the language skills necessary for self-cuing such as defining or describing. A child's vocabulary may not be large enough to access appropriate word substitutions (eg, synonyms) during word-finding episodes. Phonological knowledge may be limited in a preschool-aged child minimizing the success of phonemic cues. Gesturing may be a more effective strategy for younger children. Preschool and young school-age children may need to rely on an adult for cueing to facilitate word retrieval.

Activities and materials within the home and community setting can also facilitate word finding in a natural, engaging manner. Games that focus on vocabulary (eg, Scattergories [Hasbro], Boggle [Hasbro], Hedbanz [Spin Master Games]) can provide natural opportunities for the child to work on word finding to complement more traditional treatment approaches. Many applications on electronic tablets and computers can also encourage word-finding skills. These activities can also provide opportunities for caregivers to carry over strategies and skills in a typical family interaction.

Expressive Language Deficits

In addition to word finding, expressive language deficits can be present following a stroke. The level of impairment can range from difficulty communicating basic wants and needs to formulating more complex language, including oral or written narratives. Language formulation or production can be described as nonfluent or fluent depending on the site of lesion and presentation of symptoms. As described earlier, a lesion located in Broca's area can result in a nonfluent aphasia, whereas a lesion located in Wernicke's area can result in a fluent aphasia. Regardless of the type of aphasia, there will be a shift of burden to the communication partner, who now has to decipher what the child is trying to communicate.

For a child with nonfluent aphasia, formulation of language will be an effortful process. Fluency will be disrupted due to the child's inability to organize language despite a linguistic plan, resulting in a halting speech pattern with unnatural pauses within utterances. Associated word-finding difficulties can be present. Common features include agrammatism; slow, labored production of words and phrases; sparse use of vocabulary; and minimal prosody.[14]

Agrammatism is difficulty organizing words that follow grammatical rules to create sentences. The child is able to convey the meaning of his message with omission or decreased use of grammatical units. Structural errors will exist, including word order and incorrect use or omission of morphological endings (eg, plurals, past tense). Sentence structures will be simplified or incomplete. Mean length of utterance will be reduced. Speech may be referred to as telegraphic speech, similar to a message on a telegram, including only content words such as nouns and verbs. Written language can mirror the same errors in spoken language. For example:

Dog...ball

Mommy...drink...um...juice

Connected speech or discourse can be challenging for the child. Formulating cohesive strings of sentences within conversation or narratives can be extremely difficult for a child with nonfluent aphasia.[9] The child may have difficulty with construction of a cohesive narrative due to decreased use of complex syntax or morphological units to create a cohesive structure. Use of transition vocabulary in order to clearly delineate a beginning, middle, and end within a narrative may be omitted. Decreased organization for structure and content can lead to decreased coherence of narrative, making it difficult for the child's listener or reader to follow.

A school-aged child's language formulation deficits can have an impact on initiation and maintenance of conversation with peers, participation in classroom discussions, written classroom assignments and tests, and communication within the community. The child may have good awareness of his language formulation errors and his decreased ability to effectively communicate. Frustration can occur easily as the child will know what he wants to say but is unable to produce the desired product. It will be important to monitor the child's frustration level, as this can contribute to possible withdrawal from social or classroom activities.

Presentation of language formulation deficits and expression of frustration will differ in younger children. Toddlers and preschool-aged children may be unable to combine words or produce age-expected sentences or phrases. Behavioral outbursts can be present or increase in frequency as the child experiences frustration with his inability to communicate. Further advancement of language development, including the acquisition of age-expected word and sentence structures, may be disrupted.[6,7]

The initial focus of speech therapy should include establishing a functional means for the child to communicate with caregivers. Alternative or augmentative communication systems, including low-tech (eg, picture boards, alphabet boards, writing, drawings) and high-tech (eg, symbol-to-speech and text-to-speech devices) options, may need to be considered with severe nonfluent aphasia. A multimodal approach to communication (speaking, writing, gesturing, augmentative communication systems) should be considered to assist with expression of basic wants and needs.[29] This may only be needed for a brief period as recovery progresses. For a child with chronic severe nonfluent aphasia, a more permanent augmentative communication device may be warranted.

Use of automatic speech tasks (eg, counting, ABCs), familiar nursery rhymes, or songs may facilitate the child's first successful experience with fluent speech poststroke. Incorporating melody or rhythm into spoken language recruits involvement of the unaffected right hemisphere. Melodic Intonation Therapy has been a long-standing treatment program used with adults with chronic severe nonfluent aphasia. Developed in 1973, this treatment uses those musical elements of speech in a systemized manner to improve expressive language. The premise is that recruitment of right hemisphere structures will assist in the facilitation of speech processes.[30,31]

As a child's functional communication abilities progress, focus will shift to recovery of age-expected or premorbid expressive language skills. Sentence formulation with inclusion of age-expected grammatical morphemes and syntax should be targeted starting with simple structures and increasing complexity as able. Organization and flexibility

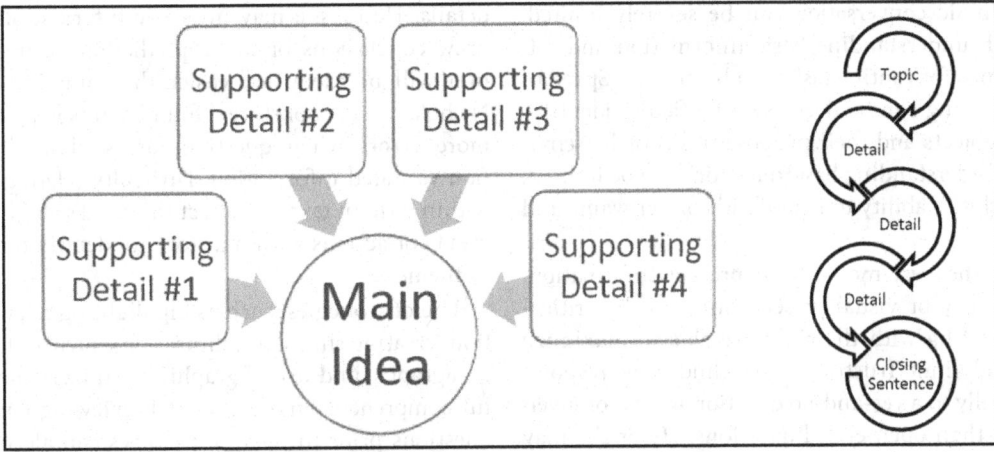

Figure 8-2. Example of graphic organizer for narrative construction.

TABLE 8-3. FLUENT VERSUS NONFLUENT APHASIA	
NONFLUENT APHASIA	FLUENT APHASIA
Halting labored speech	Effortless speech
Sparse vocabulary	Errors in word choice
Agrammatism	Jargon or nonsensical speech
Associated word finding	Frequent paraphasias
Awareness of errors	Poor awareness of errors

of language formulation should always be considered when addressing verbal expression and output. Use of organizational tools (eg, outlines, story maps, or webs) (Figure 8-2) can assist the child in formulating fluent and cohesive narratives. Therapy should not only target improving language behaviors but improving the child's ability to be a better communicator.

For a child with fluent aphasia, formulation of language will be effortless; however, word selection will be impaired. Frequent word-finding errors and paraphasias in the child's utterances can lead to decreased coherence. Content can contain many irrelevant statements, and information gaps may be present. Content of written output will be similar to the child's verbal output. Repetition is poor.[13,14]

Jargon can be another feature of fluent aphasia. When speech makes little sense and is scattered with semantic paraphasias or neologisms, it is referred to as *jargon*.[14] Anosognosia, or poor awareness of errors or difficulties, will further affect the child's communication effectiveness.[14] A child can also present with *press of speech*, which is described as a rapid rate of speech, with frequent interruptions and urgency to speak.

A child with fluent aphasia can have frequent communication breakdowns that he or she is unaware of, leading to confusion for his or her communication partner. His or her verbosity, frequent interruptions, incoherent speech, and poor comprehension will affect his or her communication

abilities across home, community, social, and academic settings. His or her interactions and ability to maintain relationships with peers can be affected (Table 8-3).

Due to the child's impaired comprehension and lack of awareness that is frequently seen with fluent aphasia, remediation can be challenging. Improving comprehension will need to be the first step in improving coherence of speech. Increasing awareness and self-monitoring will also be critical components of therapy in order to decrease jargon and paraphasias. Starting with repetition and naming tasks will allow for increasing awareness in a structured format with less demand on comprehension. Progression to modeling and chaining can then occur as repetition and comprehension increase.[14]

Receptive Language Deficits

Comprehension of spoken and written language can also be impaired following a stroke. It is rarely unaffected poststroke despite the location of the lesion. The severity of comprehension can range from mild to severe and will be dependent on the site and size of lesion. Comprehension can be more affected by larger lesions located within the temporal lobe region. Reading comprehension deficits are often present in addition to auditory comprehension.[32]

For a child with severe comprehension deficits—often seen immediately following a stroke—participation in daily routines and basic conversation can be severely limited. Difficulty with understanding basic information and following directions for routine tasks can be present. Speed of language processing can be decreased. Difficulty identifying common objects and their purpose in his or her environment and understanding basic questions can be limited, affecting the child's ability to identify his or her wants and needs.

Identifying the best modality to present information, including auditory or visual presentation, will be critical so those interacting with the child are able to maximize interaction and limit frustration. A child may respond more successfully to a yes-and-no question format or given choices rather than open-ended questions. He or she may benefit from directions provided in single components or paired with visual support (eg, written text, pictures, gestures) to facilitate understanding. Rate of speech will need to be slowed to account for increased processing time. Use of personally relevant stimuli, such as photos of family members, favorite toys, or highly common objects within therapy sessions may enhance the child's attention, participation, and response. Identifying the child's preferred mode of learning prior to his or her stroke will be valuable information to structuring therapy to optimize the child's learning potential.

As a child recovers and comprehension improves, higher-level deficits can persist. The school-aged child can have difficulty following multiple-step or linguistically complex directions, answering questions requiring critical thinking (eg, why questions), and understanding complex sentence structures (eg, passive voice, subordinate clauses).[32] These deficits can affect comprehension for a variety of activities such as listening to a teacher's lecture, taking tests, reading comprehension for textbooks or novels, or listening to a peer's story.

Therapy tasks should focus on following directions within functional tasks, comprehension of complex syntax in both oral and written presentation, and reading comprehension. Simulating a teacher's lecture and engaging the child in conversation regarding novel topics can work on comprehension in a functional but structured manner. Identification of the most successful mode of presentation (eg, oral vs written) can provide valuable information to professionals working with the child to optimize comprehension and new learning.

Reading comprehension deficits can be present from the word level through written text (eg, textbooks, novels, newspaper articles, and menus). These deficits may further be pronounced based on reading experience, attention, working memory, or visual deficits. For a child who is a new reader, the demand for decoding may be just as great as understanding the information, thus exacerbating reading comprehension difficulties. Paraphasias can be present during oral reading tasks. A child can have difficulty identifying the main idea or gist of the story and supporting

details. He or she may miss key information required to draw conclusions or make predictions. Explicit information will be identified easier than implied information. Nicholas and Brookshire[33] found adults with aphasia made more errors when questions assessed implied information vs stated information. Difficulty relating information within written text will affect the child's ability to integrate events or actions within a story to identify the overall plot or theme.

Use of strategies, such as highlighting relevant information, creating summary phrases or sentences for individual paragraphs, and use of graphic organizers can be successful comprehension aids.[2,34,35] Previewing comprehension questions prior to reading passages can alert the child to key details to look for during reading. Establishing a reading routine, such as the SQ3R learning strategy: survey, question, read, recite, review, may be helpful for some children and adolescents to ensure they are gathering all the key information.[36] Use of graphic organizers will allow for organization of material, providing a clearer picture for the child to better understand the relevance of key information.

Presentation of comprehension deficits in the home and school or daycare setting will differ in younger children. Preschool-aged children may have difficulty participating in classroom activities, such as circle time or completing a table top activity. Play may be altered as the child may be unable to identify how toys work or engage in symbolic play. Caregivers may report that their child has difficulty following directions at home and learning new vocabulary and concepts. Knowledge or acquisition of preacademic concepts, such as identification of colors, shapes, letters, and numbers, may have been lost or be at risk for development as a result of the stroke.

Implementing developmental approaches to learning language in the young child can yield good results for recovery of language.[3] Familiar objects and pictures can be utilized to improve identification of vocabulary across several features (eg, function, attribute, location, associated vocabulary). Use of developmentally appropriate books and play can promote understanding and use of language in natural contexts, leading to generalization of skills within home and school environments. Providing therapy in the child's natural setting will further encourage generalization of language skills and caregiver training and involvement.

Global Aphasia

When a child presents with significant impairment in both expressive and receptive language skills across all modalities, his or her aphasia is considered severe and described as a *global aphasia*.[13] The child will demonstrate little or no ability to write, speak, or gesture paired with very poor language comprehension significantly affecting his or her communication abilities. Reading and writing are severely impaired. Automatized words or phrases or stereotypic utterances may be the only expressive language the child is able to produce. These utterances are produced with any attempt to respond and are perseverative in nature. Caregiver training will be critical in order to facilitate any communication ability the child may have, and the home and school environment will need to be set up for accessible communication opportunities. The child could benefit from an alternative communication evaluation to assess options.

SPEECH MOTOR DISORDERS

Speech motor disorders that impede the planning and execution of speech production may also result from a stroke. These disorders are important to consider in the differential diagnosis of aphasia. They can range from mild to severe.

Dysarthria of Speech

Dysarthria of speech is a speech motor disorder where there is a disruption in the execution of speech production. Dysarthria is most frequently associated with lesions in the primary motor cortex or the descending motor pathways. Difficulty with rate of speech, range of motion, and strength and coordination of articulators comprise the speech production profile. There can be associated effects of poor coordination with the respiratory system affecting phonation, resonance, and articulation. Unilateral weakness of the oral musculature is often present affecting articulatory precision.[37,38]

Weakness will be contralateral to the site of the lesion (eg, left-sided lesion will present as right-sided weakness). This can be evident with facial asymmetry or unilateral facial droop. Drooling may be present due to difficulty containing and managing saliva. Speech characteristics include a slurred, slushy speech quality with articulatory imprecision, sound distortions, altered rate of speech, and reduced intelligibility as utterance length increases. Decreased coordination of all speech subsystems can also affect vocal intensity and quality, length of utterance per breath, and prosody.

The overall goal of therapy for children with dysarthria should be improvement of speech motor control and intelligibility. Therapeutic techniques can include articulation exercises, respiratory exercises, and compensatory training.[37] Not one of these techniques should be completed in isolation but as one integrated approach. Working on articulatory precision should follow a hierarchy of complexity, beginning with single sounds and advancing through connected speech. Drawing awareness to breath support for phonation during these tasks may also increase coordination of these subsystems for increased intelligibility.

Oral reading can be a functional activity that can focus on speech production at the discourse level without the demand for or focus on language formulation.

Ensuring good postural support and position with the child sitting upright with feet flat on the ground or in a supported position will allow for optimal breath support and focus on speech production. Teaching a child compensatory strategies, such as modulating rate of speech, phrasing, or chunking to account for decreased breath support; taking a deep breath prior to phonation; and exaggerating articulation will be instrumental in facilitating functional speech for successful communication opportunities.

Apraxia of Speech

Apraxia of Speech (AOS) is a speech motor disorder that affects speech sound production and prosody due to disruption of motor planning and sequencing. Apraxia is most frequently associated with lesions in Broca's area, insular cortex, and subcortical structures (basal ganglia and thalamus).[37,38] There is no underlying motor weakness associated with AOS. A child with AOS demonstrates articulatory errors characterized by substitutions, omissions, consonant and vowel distortions, and syllable segmentation. Production may deteriorate with multisyllable words or longer utterances. Articulatory groping may occur with speech production attempts. Prosody is affected, with the child often presenting with a monotone voice quality with equal stress across words or syllables. Traditional AOS approaches found to be successful include articulatory-kinematic approaches and rate/rhythm control approaches.[39] Articulatory-kinematic approaches promote improved speech production through articulation practice and feedback. Rate and rhythm control approaches involve modifying the rate of speech or incorporating external rhythm to improve speech production.

It can be difficult to differentiate phonemic paraphasias from sound production errors consistent with apraxia, especially because aphasia and apraxia often co-occur. Phonemic paraphasias are usually produced in a fluent utterance and thus differ from the sound substitutions that arise from a motor speech disorder.[14] Sound substitutions in AOS are thought to be a result of impairment to the motor network, whereas phonemic paraphasias occur due to impairments in the language networks. A hallmark characteristic of AOS is error variability and has been one criteria used to differentiate phonemic paraphasias from motor speech errors. However, recent research has questioned the use of error variability to distinguish between paraphasias and sound errors due to AOS in stroke and traumatic brain injury survivors.[40] Consideration of other factors, including other features of AOS and nonfluent aphasia, present in the child's profile need to be included in the differential diagnosis of aphasia and AOS (Table 8-4).

TABLE 8-4. COMPARISON OF APHASIA, DYSARTHRIA, AND APRAXIA		
DISORDER	RECEPTIVE LANGUAGE	EXPRESSIVE COMMUNICATION
Fluent aphasia	Comprehension impaired	<ul><li>Intact sentence and word structures</li><li>Frequent paraphasias and neologisms</li><li>Jargon</li></ul>
Nonfluent aphasia	Comprehension less impaired compared to fluent aphasia	<ul><li>Agrammatic, halting speech</li><li>Dysfluent</li><li>Sparse vocabulary</li></ul>
Dysarthria	Comprehension intact	<ul><li>Intact sentence and word structures</li><li>Consistent speech production errors</li><li>Articulatory imprecision</li><li>Altered rate of speech</li><li>Impaired respiratory muscle function</li><li>Affected prosody</li></ul>
Apraxia of speech	Comprehension intact	<ul><li>Concomitant with nonfluent aphasia</li><li>Inconsistent speech production errors</li><li>Vowel and consonant distortions</li><li>Affected prosody</li></ul>

RIGHT HEMISPHERE LESIONS

Although right hemisphere lesions do not result in the severity of language deficits seen with left hemisphere lesions, language deficits can still be present. Greater cognitive impairment is often observed. Cognitive skills that can be affected due to right hemisphere lesions include visual spatial skills, attention, memory, executive function, problem solving, reasoning, organization, self-planning, and self-awareness.[41] Basic language processes are typically intact; however, research has shown that 50% to 78% of adults with right hemisphere brain damage exhibit one or more communication impairments.[41]

Communication impairments associated with right hemisphere lesions can have significant impact on performance in social and academic settings. Discourse or connected speech is commonly affected. There is a reduced efficiency and effectiveness in communication due to problems relaying and interpreting intent within messages. There can be significant impact on social use of language or pragmatic language skills. Within discourse, comments or responses can be tangential or off topic, egocentric, and disorganized.[42] A child can present with anosognosia, as seen with fluent aphasia, or have difficulty understanding and using contextual cues and creating links between ideas to understand the gist of the message or story. Comprehension of nonliteral or abstract language, including metaphors, idioms, and sarcasm, can be reduced.

Aprosodia can be a feature of right hemisphere lesions. It is a disorder of prosody that affects both use and interpretation of prosodic features.[43] A child's speech production may sound monotone with poor ability to reflect emotion in his or her speech. He or she can have difficulty identifying the emotional intent in speakers based on the tone of voice.

The communication profile of a child with right hemisphere stroke can lead to impaired social interactions and relationships. The child can have great difficulty contributing appropriately to conversations. He or she may attempt to dominate conversations or miss key information presented either verbally or nonverbally for complete understanding. Interpretation and use of humor and sarcasm can be affected.

Therapy interventions targeting cognitive-communication abilities and pragmatic language deficits will be essential for recovery. Training with social scripts can lead to more successful and appropriate communicative interactions with peers. A social skills group can be an effective approach to targeting appropriate social language behaviors in a structured, controlled environment with age-matched peers. Social skills groups have promoted success with pragmatic language abilities and peer relationships for children with autism and acquired brain injuries.[44-46]

INTERPLAY BETWEEN LANGUAGE AND COGNITION

The relationship between language and cognition is complex and can become even more intricate and entwined in the presence of a brain injury poststroke (Figure 8-3). Processing speed, attention, working memory, and executive function are cognitive processes that are particularly vulnerable to brain injury.[2,47-51] Unfortunately, it can be challenging to understand how an identified deficit in one area affects a child's overall functioning given the interplay between these skills and language. Professionals working with children poststroke need to be mindful of the relationship between cognitive processes and the symptoms of aphasia when assessing a child's response to treatment.[19] In addition, they should consider that language symptoms may be exacerbated by cognitive deficits. Chapter 9 will extensively cover the effects of stroke on cognition, including aphasia's role in the cognitive profile of children with stroke.

THERAPY CONSIDERATIONS

Many speech and language disorders and symptoms were described in this chapter. Despite the type of disorder or severity of impairment, the awareness of the family's needs, developmental sequence of speech and language development, and need for strategy training should help guide the speech-language pathologist in development of treatment plans.

Careful consideration of the family's needs, expectations, and goals should be taken when developing treatment plans. Family-centered care should be in the forefront when developing and providing services to the child. Involving caregivers in the development of goals will ensure that goals are not only child focused but family focused as well. Caregiver training will provide caregivers with the skills to promote communication abilities outside of the therapy room. The child will have opportunities to practice these skills in his or her natural settings and create chances for communication success as a family unit.[52,53]

Incorporating developmental approaches for speech and language disorders into treatment plans will direct the speech-language pathologist to be mindful of the developmental sequence of speech and language skills while identifying the current level of the child. Targeting skills based on the developmental sequence will aid in the organization of treatment focus and ensure the child is working towards reacquisition of premorbid communication skills.[34]

In order to maximize the child's functional outcome, therapy should not only focus on rehabilitation and

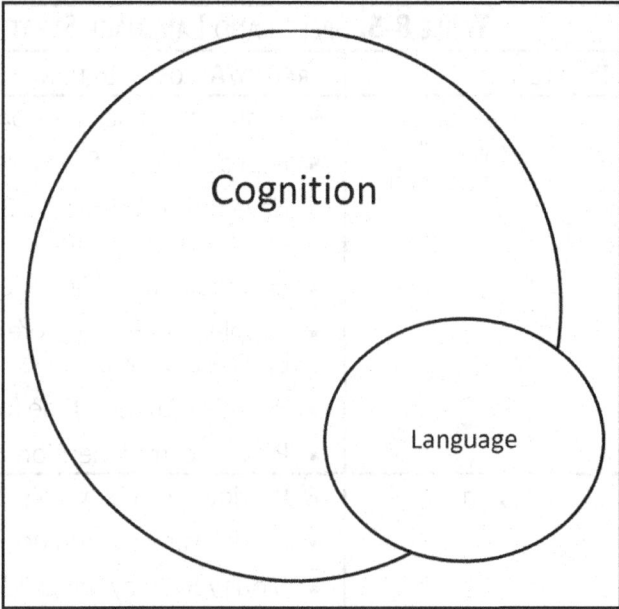

Figure 8-3. Interplay between language and cognition.

recovery but also on compensation. This can be addressed within the therapy session and should be reinforced within home, community, and school environments. It is important to teach children strategies to compensate for speech and language deficits that may not recover. These strategies will prove to be instrumental across settings, especially in the classroom for achievement of academic success. Compensatory strategy training is a vital component of therapy, as children are vulnerable to later language and learning difficulties due to potential disruption of development.[9,10] If effective strategies become a part of a child's daily routine, the impact of later developing language deficits may not be as costly to the child's learning.

TRANSITION RECOMMENDATIONS

When a child is ready to transition back to school, many facets need to be considered in order to create a seamless and successful school re-entry (Table 8-5). Many recommendations, including classroom accommodations, learning support, and communication strategies, can be communicated to the school to facilitate learning and linguistic success. Full discussion on return to school and recommendations will be discussed in Chapter 12. However, recommendations specific to the child's speech, language, and cognitive-communication abilities will be discussed in this chapter.

A school-based speech-language evaluation is usually warranted upon a child's return to school. Most often, a child is still in an emergent period of recovery and will continue to benefit from school-based speech-language intervention. The school-based speech-language pathologist will be an instrumental team member, as he or she will

TABLE 8-5. SPEECH AND LANGUAGE STRATEGIES AND/OR ACCOMMODATIONS FOR SCHOOL	
PROBLEM	STRATEGY/ACCOMMODATION
Comprehension of written or verbally presented information	▪ Reduce the length or complexity of information when teaching novel concepts. ▪ Repeat critical information (topic, main ideas, and directions). ▪ Have the child repeat back directions to ensure he or she has understood the information. ▪ Encourage the child to request repetitions or clarification from the speaker. ▪ Supplement verbally presented information with visual aids (eg, provide an outline of class lectures prior to class). ▪ Provide increased time for taking in information and providing responses. ▪ Provide comprehension questions prior to the reading passage.
Word finding	▪ Provide the child with semantic or phonemic cues to aid with word retrieval. ▪ Focus instruction on use of word-finding strategies for self-cueing. ▪ Modify the way the child provides responses for tests or classwork in order to limit need for word retrieval (eg, true/false, word banks, multiple choice). ▪ Allow the child to be the first or second contributor in class discussions. ▪ Allow extra time for formulation. ▪ Encourage use of augmentative communication if required.
Language organization/ formulation	▪ Encourage use of graphic organizers (eg, story webs, story maps, outlines) prior to narrative construction. ▪ Provide visual aids (eg, checklist, pictures) as a prompt to include all necessary story elements. ▪ Allow the child extra time to formulate written and oral responses.
Speech production	▪ Allow increased time to convey thoughts and ideas. ▪ Encourage use of strategies (eg, slow rate, overarticulation, increased volume) to increase speech intelligibility. ▪ Ensure good posture (eg, feet flat on the floor, trunk well supported, arms on armrest if needed) while speaking. ▪ Encourage use of augmentative communication if child has severe speech production deficits.

be able to provide critical information related to the child's learning and communication needs within the classroom. In-class therapy, in addition to pullout sessions, can be effective in generalization of language skills in the classroom. Enforcement of strategies in the classroom setting will be necessary to further the child's independence and success. As the child is still in an emergent state of recovery, ongoing diagnostic assessment will be crucial, as the child's needs will change and goals and accommodations will need to be adjusted based on his current language and learning status.

It is important to remember that each child is an individual with his or her own learning needs. Identifying the right supports, accommodations, and treatment plan may be a trial-and-error process at the start. Including the child and parents in this process will be necessary in order to create a successful program for the child. If he or she demonstrates awareness and insight into his or her strengths and weaknesses, allowing the child to be an active team member will only empower him or her to be a stronger advocate when problems arise. This will only lead to greater self-assurance, academic success, and achievement of goals.

For children who return to school or begin school with minimal to no speech or language concerns, caregiver knowledge of potential risk for later developing language difficulties secondary to stroke will be paramount. It is the professional's responsibility to provide this education to caregivers at the outset of stroke. Close monitoring for acquisition of age-expected language skills should occur throughout childhood and adolescence. Caregivers should have consistent communication with teachers for any changes in academic performance. Westmacott and colleagues[49] found that children with unilateral neonatal strokes appear to be at risk for cognitive difficulties in the school years, especially with regard to working memory, processing speed, and abstract reasoning. Close attention should be particularly paid during periods of language transitions where the linguistic demands increase and can have a direct impact on academic performance.

The initial transition to school is often a time when children who sustained a stroke in their early years may show language and learning difficulties. Transition from "reading to learn" to "learning to read" around third or fourth grade is a shift in greater reliance on language comprehension to learn academic information. Transitions to middle school and high school are other critical periods where skills related to language organization and comprehension of abstract language may be vulnerable to impairment. Re-evaluations of speech and language skills by a speech-language pathologist at critical periods of language development may be warranted to identify changes in language performance and impact on learning.

FEEDING AND SWALLOWING: INFANTS

Although taken for granted by healthy individuals, swallowing is an extremely complex, precise action that must be performed hundreds of times throughout the day. Safe swallowing requires the dynamic interplay of the central nervous system with the coordinated movement of muscles of the oral cavity, larynx, pharynx, esophagus, and respiratory system. Across the lifespan, stroke is the leading cause of neurogenic dysphagia.[54] Dysphagia is defined as difficulty moving food from the mouth to the stomach and may encompass a variety of oral motor and swallowing issues.[55] It has been reported that 42% to 60% of adults present with dysphagia based on a bedside swallowing evaluation following an acute stroke (Figure 8-4). The percentage increases further to 55% to 72% when a videofluoroscopic swallowing study is completed.[56] Whereas there is an abundance of information concerning adult stroke recovery, little research has been done on swallowing outcomes with neonatal or acquired pediatric stroke. Given the differences between adult and infant anatomy, methods of oral intake, and level of feeding experience prestroke, it is difficult to take results and recommendations from the adult literature and directly apply them to pediatrics. Much more research needs to be conducted in the field of pediatric stroke to better determine the prevalence, severity, and residual effects of dysphagia in this population.

However limited, the existing literature does support the basic assumption that a significant number of infants

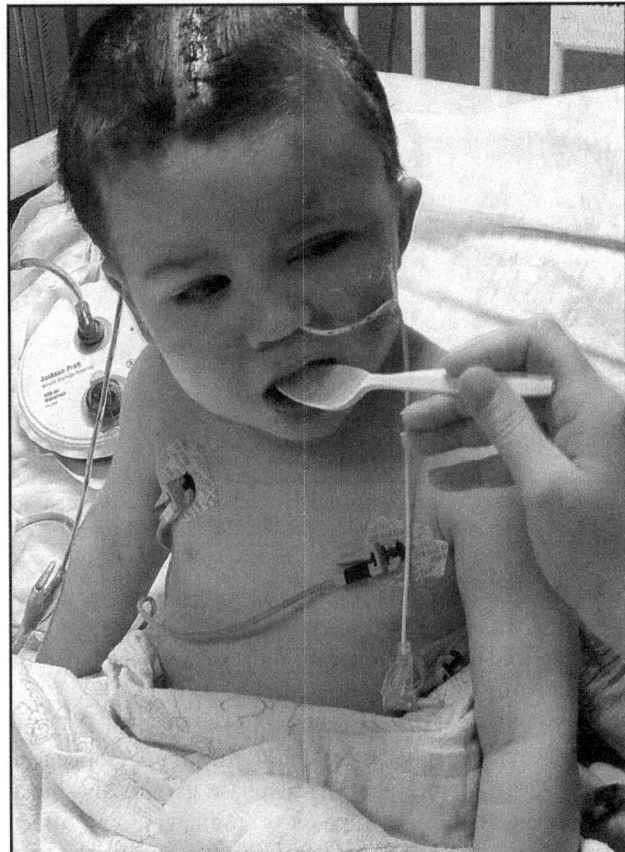

Figure 8.4. Clinical bedside oral feeding assessment in the hospital setting.

will experience oral feeding challenges following a stroke. A retrospective study of 84 children who presented with a neonatal arterial ischemic stroke found that 48% had feeding difficulties. The most common dysfunctions identified in the neonatal period were oral motor disorganization, risk for failure to thrive, and aspiration or risk for aspiration.[57]

When addressing pediatric stroke, the goals of dysphagia therapy are to help establish a safe functional feeding plan that allows the child to consume the least restrictive diet possible while optimizing nutritional intake and minimizing aspiration risk.[58] Throughout the child's recovery, but especially during the initial phase, it is imperative that caregivers and clinicians work together to create the best feeding plan (Figure 8-5). Clinically, one's oral feeding presentation can vary from day to day, or even from meal to meal, so close collaboration, frequent timely discussions, and repeated education with families[59] is necessary to ensure safe intake at all times.

Phases of Swallowing

Before delving into feeding assessments and therapy strategies, a brief overview of swallowing function is warranted. Given the complexity of the swallow mechanism, entire texts have been dedicated to describing the anatomy and physiology required for this seemingly effortless bodily

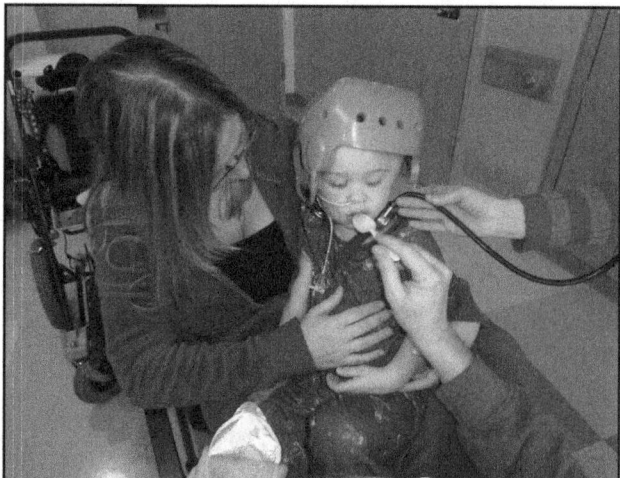

Figure 8-5. Speech-language pathologist collaborating with parent to help support an appropriate seated position during oral feeding.

function. The following is meant as a gross summary, and the reader is encouraged to refer to the suggested reading list at the end of this chapter if a more detailed explanation of swallowing function is desired.

Three phases of the swallow need to be considered. They are the oral phase, pharyngeal phase, and upper esophageal phase. Although the pharyngeal phase garners the most attention, deficits in any phase of swallowing can affect overall function, safety, and the ability to consume the volumes necessary for adequate hydration and nutrition.

1. *Oral phase:* This phase can be further delineated into the oral preparatory stage and the oral stage. The oral preparatory stage includes the acceptance and placement of the bolus into the oral cavity, as well as any manipulation that must be done prior to the bolus being transferred by the tongue. For infants, the oral stage includes rooting and latching to the bottle nipple and extracting liquid by sucking, whereas cup-drinking skills and chewing abilities may be assessed in children and adults. Once the bolus begins to move posteriorly with motion from the tongue, the oral phase of swallowing has been initiated. The midline of the tongue moves with a smooth rolling motion, propelling the bolus backward.[55]

2. *Pharyngeal phase:* The pharyngeal phase is by far the most complex phase of the swallow, requiring multiple actions to occur almost simultaneously and with great coordination. Once a swallow is triggered, the soft palate elevates and retracts to keep the bolus from entering the nasal cavity. The pharyngeal constrictor muscles initiate peristalsis to move the material through the pharynx, and the larynx elevates and closes at 3 points (the glossoepiglottic fold, false vocal folds, and true vocal folds) to prevent the bolus from entering the trachea. The pharyngeal phase of the swallow is completed in approximately one second and relies heavily on intact cranial nerve and muscle functioning.[55]

3. *Esophageal phase:* Once the bolus passes through the pharynx, the upper esophageal sphincter, or cricopharyngeus, relaxes, thus allowing the material to enter the esophagus. Peristalsis then begins.[60]

Oral Feeding Assessment

As we move into assessment and treatment, it should be stated that no feeding strategies or techniques are specifically created for infants who have suffered a stroke. Clinically, an infant poststroke may present similarly to an infant with another neurological condition, such as a hypoxic ischemic injury or a significant seizure disorder. Knowledge of the central nervous system and the impact of neurological injury on feeding and swallowing function are important when working with these babies and their parents. Medical information regarding the extent of an infant's brain injury needs to be given consideration along with clinical performance when making decisions about the safety of oral feeding. Although the frequency of dysphagia with infants poststroke is unknown, the research with adult stroke survivors supports the use of caution and vigilance when initiating oral feeding attempts.

A clinical swallowing assessment is a relatively common practice prior to the initiation or resumption of oral feeding following a stroke.[61-63] In cases of neonatal or infant stroke, it is of vital importance that the professional who performs the swallowing evaluation has specialized education and experience with infant anatomy and physiology. Knowledge of typical feeding skill development in healthy, full-term infants, as well as the feeding challenges encountered by preterm or medically fragile infants, should be a prerequisite to working with those recovering from a neurological insult.

Poststroke, an infant may have difficulty with one or several aspects of oral feeding. During the acute phase of recovery, medication, tenuous medical stability, or the hospital environment may affect a baby's state of control and feeding readiness.[64] It is important to note that when a stroke occurs in the prenatal or perinatal period, those affected do not have a history of oral feeding. Therefore, these infants need to *acquire* adequate feeding and swallowing skills rather than *recover* them. This acquisition can be a challenging and frustrating process for families, as many of these babies physically appear to be healthy. Because infants may not exhibit the same physical manifestations of a stroke that children or adults may, such as a facial paresis[65] or drooling,[66] the presence of the neurological impairment may be less noticeable.

With an infant, the clinical evaluation should begin with a few minutes of observation. Is the baby waking and showing readiness cues, such as mouthing his or her hands or rooting? Is the baby breathing comfortably or with increased effort with retractions or head bobbing? In the hospital setting, having the infant on monitors that record his or her heart rate, respiratory rate, and oxygen saturation levels before, during, and after oral feeding can provide valuable information[67] as significant changes in physiological stability, such as prolonged apnea, may be indicative of swallowing difficulty.[68] An oral motor/feeding assessment should only be initiated if an infant is demonstrating appropriate state control, interest, and stability.

After observation, oral structures and facial muscle tone should be assessed next along with oral and pharyngeal reflexes. These reflexes include the root, gag, suck, and swallow.[64,69] The absence of a gag reflex does not eliminate the possibility of safe oral feeding[70,71]; however, increased caution should be used when feeding anyone who has atypical reflexes. An assessment of non-nutritive skills should be completed prior to offering an oral feed.[72] Although the literature clearly documents the differences between non-nutritive and nutritive sucking,[73,74] important information can be obtained before a feed is ever offered. For instance, is the baby able to maintain a calm awake state with the introduction of oral stimulation? Is the non-nutritive suck strong and coordinated or weak and disorganized? Does secretion management change with stimulation? Is increased work of breathing or significant changes in heart rate or oxygenation levels noted? By gathering information from non-nutritive sucking, the clinician can be better equipped to support the baby with oral feeding and have some indication of what feeding strategies to consider.[75] If an infant demonstrates adequate oral motor reflexes and coordination along with feeding readiness cues, the evaluation should proceed with an oral feeding trial.

When orally feeding an infant who has suffered a stroke, the feeder must closely monitor for adverse reactions and be prepared to immediately adjust the feeding techniques being applied. All phases of the swallow need to be considered, and many questions need to be asked throughout the feed. Is the baby able to successfully root and latch to the breast or bottle? Is the suck strong, rhythmical, organized, and mature? Is the baby efficient, overwhelmed, or inefficient with the nipple offered? Does the swallow appear to be prompt? In addition to answering these questions, the caregiver needs to monitor for signs of aspiration. Aspiration occurs when food or liquid passes through the true vocal folds and enters the trachea and is concerning due to the potentially negative impacts it may have on one's respiratory health or overall medical status.[68,76] Overt signs of aspiration can include coughing, choking, and significant physiological instability, but less notable signs may also be present. Feeding therapists need to be trained to recognize the less obvious markers of swallowing difficulty and utilize information from multiple sources in order to conduct a comprehensive assessment. Cervical auscultation, which involves placing a stethoscope on the infant's neck over the thyroid cartilage, can be a helpful tool to supplement visual observation. This noninvasive technique allows the listener to hear cervical swallowing sounds and obtain some qualitative information on the frequency and promptness of swallowing, as well as the presence of pharyngeal and/or laryngeal congestion that may not be audible to the naked ear.[77] However, due to poor interrater reliability and questionable validity, cervical auscultation should always serve as adjuncts to, and not a substitute for, sound clinical judgment and experience.[78,79]

Compared to adults, infants and young children have a higher incidence of silent aspiration.[80,81] Silent aspiration occurs when food or liquid enters the trachea and no physical response, such as coughing, choking, or a change in breathing pattern, is observed.[80] In 2 studies of infants under 12 months of age who were referred for instrumental swallowing assessments, aspiration was found to be silent in 8 out of 9[82] and 34 out of 42 cases[83], respectively. Silent aspiration is also a more common finding in those with neurological impairment[81] and specifically with stroke.[84,85] Therefore, more subtle indicators of possible aspiration or feeding difficulties, such as increased congestion with feeding, audible gulping, multiple swallows per bolus,[86] drifts in oxygen saturation,[87-89] changes in state control,[90] or wet vocal quality,[84,91,92] need to be attended to throughout the feed. Stress cues, such as finger splays, facial grimacing, or gaze aversion[93,94] in infants may also indicate poor feeding quality. One needs to be able to interpret information from the baby's presentation and caregiver report within the context of the medical findings in order to make the most appropriate feeding recommendations.

Oral Feeding Considerations

Several factors can be manipulated to help improve feeding quality and safety. However, with infants, we are limited to what we can modify to support the baby and foster success, as we cannot "teach" the infant to apply specific swallowing strategies. Factors that can be adjusted include the following:

- *Physical environment:* An infant who appears overwhelmed with feeding may benefit from feeding in a calm, controlled atmosphere with reduced stimuli. Dimming the lights, closing the door, and limiting conversation around the baby can reduce stress cues[64,95,96] and improve the chances of feeding success. To help improve organization, the feeder can provide containment by lightly bundling the baby and bringing her hands to midline.[97]

- *Nipple selection:* When choosing a nipple, one needs to keep in mind the specific oral and pharyngeal concerns. An infant who has difficulty latching may benefit from a firmer nipple, whereas an infant who gulps and dribbles likely needs a slower flow.

Changing the bottle nipple is often the first strategy used to slow liquid flow rate, as it requires no additional caregiver training or education.[98] In general, a nipple with a slower flow rate will allow a smaller bolus to be extracted. Smaller boluses can usually be better controlled and are less likely to overwhelm the baby or lead to oral loss. Use of a slow-flow nipple may be more appropriate than a faster flow when initiating feeds with a medically fragile[99,100] or preterm baby[101,102] who may experience increased work of breathing with the added work of eating.

If the baby is using a disposable hospital nipple, efforts should be made to transition the baby to a commercially available nipple when appropriate. Each nipple brand and type is slightly different, so all nipples marked as the same flow rate are not equal in terms of flow rate, number of holes, and pliability, resulting in variable flow rates.[103] Trialing the particular nipple parents want to use at home is necessary to determine an appropriate, safe plan for home.

- *Pacing:* In a single study of premature infants, use of pacing was found to have clinical and statistical significance, reducing the number of bradycardic events with oral feeds.[104] With pacing, the feeder either removes the nipple from the infant's mouth or tilts the nipple down every few sucks, thus stopping the flow of milk. This allows the baby to take additional swallows to clear pharyngeal residue or additional breaths to help regulate the suck-swallow-breathe pattern and physiological stability.[90,98,99,105]

- *Sidelying:* An infant who has increased respiratory effort with attempts to feed may benefit from being fed while lying on his or her side instead of being held in a more traditional cradled position. The theory behind sidelying is that the lung bases can open more fully, allowing for deeper breaths and reduced respiratory effort, thus allowing for greater physiological stability.[106,107] Reduced respiratory effort can then help to support a more coordinated suck-swallow-breathe pattern.

A feeding plan only works if all caregivers can successfully implement it, from nursing staff in the acute care setting to the grandmother who will babysit once the infant is at home. The hope with all of these strategies is that they can eventually be removed. Over time, with maturation and skill development, many babies demonstrate improved coordination and need less support and modifications to successfully feed.

Oral Feeding Considerations: Breastfeeding

It should be noted that the assessment of oral feeding skills and swallowing safety can be completed with breastfeeding as easily as with bottle feeding. The focus should be the establishment of a safe and functional feeding plan, regardless of modality. Mothers who are interested in breastfeeding should be supported and encouraged to do so, given the substantial literature that details the health and bonding benefits of breastfeeding and breast milk.[108-112] A baby recovering from a stroke may look more or less coordinated with breastfeeding compared to bottle feeding, given the mother's flow rate, milk supply, and the baby's ability to extract liquid. Although oral feeding techniques, such as the use of pacing, are less feasible with breastfeeding, there are still variables that can be manipulated to help increase the chances of success.

For instance, changing the mother and infant's relative positions[113,114] or use of a nipple shield may be considered.[115-117] A mother may try pumping for a few minutes to fully bring milk into the breast prior to feeding attempts for a baby with a weak suck. Conversely, with an infant who gets overwhelmed with milk flow, having the mother put the baby to the breast after pumping through the initial letdown or putting the baby to the breast that produces less milk may be beneficial. Discussion with parents about their interest in breastfeeding and collaboration with lactation consultants can help support the development of breastfeeding skills.

Instrumental Assessment

In cases where pharyngeal dysphagia is suspected, an instrumental assessment may be indicated to further assess swallowing function prior to initiating an oral diet. The primary options consist of a videofluoroscopic swallow study (VFSS) or fiber-optic endoscopic evaluation of swallowing (FEES).

Videofluoroscopic Swallow Study

Often considered to be the gold-standard swallowing assessment,[118,119] the VFSS, which may also be called a *modified barium swallow study*, is a radiographic examination jointly conducted with a feeding specialist and a radiologist. Ideally, the clinician performing the test should have completed a bedside assessment with the baby or child and have tried various feeding techniques and equipment prior to the study. This clinical information can be used to structure the instrumental assessment, thus making it a more streamlined, efficient, and higher-quality test.[120]

During the VFSS, various viscosities of liquid and food that have been mixed with barium sulfate are offered to allow for visualization of the anatomy and physiology of the swallow. All phases of the swallow are captured, typically from a lateral view. If dysphagia is observed, strategies to improve swallowing safety can be applied during the test to determine the effect each change has upon the swallow function,[121] as strategies that work for some may actually worsen dysphagia in others. During the VFSS, all reasonable measures should be taken to minimize radiation exposure and radiation time without compromising the validity and integrity of the test. Collaboration and good communication between the swallowing expert and the radiologist throughout the study can significantly help this effort.

Fiber-Optic Endoscopic Evaluation of Swallowing

An FEES uses an endoscope to evaluate the pharyngeal stage of swallowing. A scope with a lighted camera is passed through the nares to just above the epiglottis. Food coloring is then added to food or liquid and is presented in a typical feeding manner. An FEES has no radiation exposure, no time constraints, and allows for the assessment of swallowing function with an infant's specific formula or mother's expressed breast milk. This assessment also allows for a direct view of the pharynx and upper larynx, including visualization of vocal cord function and structure.[122] The FEES does not provide information about the oral or esophageal phases of the swallow, and whiteout occurs at the moment of the pharyngeal swallow. This whiteout may occur frequently with an infant who engages in a rapid successive swallowing pattern,[123] thus reducing visibility.

Regardless of which test is being performed, with an infant, a variety of nipples with different flow rates and pliability should be available for use. Although most hospitals use disposable nipples that are intended for a single use, trialing commercially available nipples during the instrumental assessment is helpful to mimic real-world options.

Dysphagia Management

When pharyngeal dysphagia is present and requires modifications to the oral feeding plan, our options with infants are somewhat limited. Use of a slower-flow nipple, external pacing, volume or time restrictions, and implementation of specific strategies such as sidelying or thickened liquids may be recommended to help improve swallowing coordination or safety. Thickening feeds in the pediatric population can be a challenge from both a nutritional and gastrointestinal standpoint and should only be considered when other strategies are unsuccessful

in reducing aspiration or aspiration risk.[124] At this time, current practice for thickening oral feeds with infants is to use rice cereal. Concerns have arisen regarding the safety of gum-based thickeners' interactions with the infant gastrointestinal system,[125,126] and commercial cornstarch-based thickeners, such as ThickenUp (Nestlé), are not typically recommended for children under 3 years of age (http://www.nestlenutritionstore.com/product/RESOURCE-THICKENUP.html#.WP-V2ojysdV). Although rice cereal can thicken well with formula, it does not work in the same way with breast milk. Breast milk contains amylase, a polysaccharide-digesting enzyme that breaks down carbohydrates. The issue with thickening breast milk with rice cereal is that the rice cereal will be broken down by the amylase, resulting in a gradually thinner consistency as the feed progresses.[127] Therefore, although a physician may recommend it in cases of reflux, thickening breast milk with rice cereal is not a recommended strategy for dysphagia management. In cases where thickening is deemed appropriate, physician input and approval and the involvement of a dietician are necessary to ensure that hydration and growth will not be adversely affected. It is paramount that all caregivers who will be involved with feeding the baby be educated on the recommended feeding guidelines and the rationale behind them.

FEEDING AND SWALLOWING: CHILDREN

For many families, the resumption of oral feeding is a high-priority goal early on in recovery. Oral feeding is viewed as a normal part of daily life, and any delay in returning to a typical diet can be frustrating for both children and their parents. Unfortunately, children and adolescents may present with oral motor and swallowing issues poststroke that mirror those of adult stroke patients. These deficits may include partial paralysis or paresis of the face or tongue,[65,128,129] which could result in a decreased lip closure on a cup or suction on a straw,[128] oral loss, oral residue, impaired chewing skills and bolus formation, delayed swallowing initiation,[66] and overall decreased swallowing strength and coordination. These deficits not only place the child at increased risk for aspiration, but also can result in insufficient strength and coordination to manipulate many of the foods in his typical diet. Decreased arousal and alertness and reduced energy can affect feeding efficiency and safety,[131] and it may be challenging to remain a full oral feeder, especially in the acute phase of recovery. Supplemental nutrition may be required, at least temporarily,[132,133] to ensure that the child receives adequate nutrition and hydration, which are paramount to recovery.[134] A retrospective study on recovery following arterial stroke found that the vast majority of children initially presented with dysphagia and did require nonoral feeding.[1] Several studies have indicated that the presence of a nasogastric feeding tube does not significantly affect pharyngeal swallow function[135-138] and, therefore, should not be a hindrance to advancing to oral feeding as appropriate throughout recovery.

Whereas significant improvements in feeding are often noted within the first few weeks and months poststroke, adult stroke survivors can suffer from persistent dysphagia. In a review of 112 hospital-referred adult patients with a first acute stroke, clinical evidence of swallowing abnormalities was found in 50% of cases at 6 months after the stroke.[56] Therefore, the potential for longer-term oral or pharyngeal dysphagia should be considered in children poststroke. In the majority of cases, returning to a regular diet poststroke is a process that requires time, patience, and caution. Discussion of this process with the family and the child, as appropriate, is vitally important to help with the development of realistic expectations and therapy goals.[133]

Similarly to an adult, a child who has suffered a stroke may have decreased sensation on the affected side[139] and may not be able to feel if he is having issues with drooling or pocketing food.[140] Self-feeding skills and feeding independence can also be greatly affected by a stroke.[141] For instance, following a stroke, a toddler may no longer be able to lift and hold his sippy cup, and an older child may require help with opening water bottles or cutting meats with a knife. Activities of daily life are discussed in Chapters 6 and 7, but it should be mentioned that the loss of self-feeding skills could further prolong and add stress to meal times, as caregivers need to prepare and assist with feeding. In addition, cognitive and memory deficits following a stroke, including poor insight, impulsivity, agitation, and inattention,[142] play an important role in the selection of appropriate feeding adaptations.[143] One must be able to follow basic motor commands and remember strategies in order for recommended feeding modifications to be useful.

Oral Feeding Assessment

As with infants, we need to address each child's specific feeding challenges when making modifications. A child with decreased sensation or delayed swallowing initiation may benefit from foods with increased sensory input. These include foods or liquids that have more flavor, texture, or temperature input, such as spicy, sour, or crunchy foods or chilled drinks.[144,145] For a child with facial asymmetry or weakness, placement of food on the stronger side during the initial phase of recovery can also be a helpful strategy to increase functionality with solids.[146] Someone who presents with poor tongue movement and reduced control of the bolus may benefit from a liquid or puree wash to clear oral residue, and a dry spoon presentation can facilitate additional swallows in cases of oral or pharyngeal stasis.[146] As appropriate, children and adolescents should be educated on the rationale behind feeding strategies and encouraged to be active participants with feeding recovery.

Dysphagia Management

Compensatory therapy strategies are frequently used with children to improve swallowing safety. These strategies do not change the physiology of the swallow, but instead redirect the flow of the food or liquid[147,148] and may include the use of a chin tuck or chin down, effortful or additional swallows, or a head turn to the affected side.

Chin Tuck or Chin Down

Tilting the chin toward the chest can allow for better bolus control, preventing premature spillage into the pharynx and narrowing the entrance to the trachea.[146] In a study of 30 patients with neurological impairments, the use of a chin-down posture successfully eliminated aspiration for half the subjects.[149] As mentioned previously, it is important to assess the effectiveness of compensatory strategies during objective assessments to validate their impact upon swallowing safety.

Effortful Swallow

Instruct the child to "swallow hard," squeezing all the muscles of the mouth and throat. This increased effort increases posterior tongue base movement and clearance of the bolus from the valleculae.[146]

Head Turn

Rotating one's head to the affected side helps to direct the food or liquid down the stronger side, closing off the pyriform sinus on the weak side.[66,150]

In addition to these strategies, recommendations may be made to restrict or modify one's diet,[77] reduce bite size,[146] limit meal times, or reduce distractions in the environment.[151,152] The performance of specific oral motor exercises to improve muscle strength and coordination may also be used in certain cases. However, given the limited evidence supporting the efficacy of oral motor exercises,[153,154] these exercises should not be used as a blanket approach to treatment and should ideally be applied in the context of speech production or actual feeding. The goal of oral motor exercises should be to improve the functionality of speech, feeding skills, or swallowing ability and should be only one component of the therapy plan.

In cases where there are minimal to no cognitive deficits following a stroke, more complex direct swallowing techniques that have been developed for use in the adult population may be applicable. However, when contemplating use of a more complex swallowing strategy, the motivation and dedication of the child and family need to be considered. Diligence with the application and reinforcement of feeding strategies with all meals and snacks is necessary for the strategies to be successful. Anyone who has experience with teenagers knows that having them adhere to a strict set of rules is challenging. Therefore, when developing a feeding plan for a child, the simpler, the better regardless of the degree of neurological impairment.

An overview of the potential speech, language, and oral feeding impairments following stroke in infants and children has been described throughout this chapter. Various suggestions and techniques have been discussed pertaining to each area of impairment. It is important to ensure that treatment plans are tailored to the specific strengths and weaknesses of each child and family to capitalize one's potential for recovery and growth.

Due to the complexities associated with the ongoing development of an immature brain in the setting of brain injury, working with a child with aphasia or oral feeding difficulties is a dynamic process. These children not only need to recover oral feeding, speech, and language skills acquired prior to their stroke, but they also have a lifetime of learning ahead of them. This process is ever evolving and requires continued surveillance and coordination by the family, medical team, and therapeutic professionals in order to maximize the child's success.

FAMILY FOCUS BOX
FEEDING AND SWALLOWING

Oral feeding difficulties and swallowing dysfunction are very common following a stroke and can encompass anything from decreased interest in eating to poor chewing to coughing and choking during meals. As many infants and children don't show obvious signs of unsafe swallowing, a trained feeding therapist should assess swallowing ability before a diet is initiated. A feeding therapist is typically a speech-language pathologist who has received additional training and education on the anatomy and physiology of the swallowing mechanism. The feeding therapist may recommend that your child only attempt feeding under his or her direct supervision, especially in the first few days or weeks after the stroke. A swallowing test may be needed to ensure that food or liquid isn't entering your child's airway when he or she eats. This is known as aspiration and has the potential to negatively affect your child's overall health.

A feeding tube may be needed after a stroke to help your child get adequate nutrition. Good nutrition is very important to therapeutic progress, as your child needs energy to participate in motor and cognitive therapies. A tube may be placed that goes through the nose and into the stomach. As your child recovers, he or she can start to eat by mouth with the feeding tube still in place.

Your child's feeding therapist should explain why certain strategies and diet recommendations are being made. If you are uncertain how a modification is helping your child to eat and swallow safely, ask for more clarification and education. It's vitally important that you, as your child's best caregiver and advocate, have a solid understanding of the rationale behind all feeding guidelines. The return to a regular diet can be a lengthy process, so on-going collaboration with your child's feeding therapist and nutritionist is extremely important. Your impression of how your child is doing with oral feeding is valuable information and may help shape therapy goals.

FAMILY FOCUS BOX
SPEECH AND LANGUAGE

Stroke can directly affect speech and language abilities, affecting a child's ability to understand and communicate.

Language is composed of *receptive* and *expressive language*.

- *Receptive language* is how one understands language in spoken or written format.

- *Expressive language* is how one uses language to communicate, including speaking, writing, or signing.

Following a stroke, a child can be diagnosed with *aphasia*, a language disorder that results from damage to the parts of the brain responsible for speaking, writing, reading, and understanding. The child can have difficulty understanding conversation, following directions, or listening to and reading stories. He or she can have difficulty forming sentences, finding the words he or she wants to say, and telling stories. School performance can be affected.

A child's speech production can also be affected following a stroke. He or she can have difficulty producing speech sounds clearly, affecting his or her intelligibility when he or she is speaking. The following two types of speech disorders occur with stroke:

- *Dysarthria* is a speech motor disorder that affects the execution of speech production due to underlying weakness of the muscles responsible for speech production. A child's speech may sound slushy or slurred, have low volume, and use a slow or fast rate of speech.

- *Apraxia* is a speech motor disorder that affects speech sound production and prosody due to disruption of motor planning and sequencing. A child with apraxia demonstrates speech production errors that are inconsistent and can include substitutions (ie, "pall" for "ball"), omissions (ie, "og" for "dog"), and consonant and vowel distortions. Speech errors can increase with longer words and sentences. Prosody, which helps to tell the emotion of the message, can be affected, with the child often presenting with a monotone voice quality with no emphasis on syllables within words or words within sentences.

(continued)

FAMILY FOCUS BOX (CONTINUED)
SPEECH AND LANGUAGE

If the child presents with a change in his or her language or speech abilities, a speech-language evaluation is warranted as soon as the child is medically stable. The speech-language pathologist will identify areas of deficit and recommend speech therapy if needed. The earlier the child can initiate speech-language therapy poststroke, the better chance of language success and recovery. Speech therapy can be provided within many settings, including acute care, in- and outpatient rehabilitation, and school. Often, children will require speech therapy services across many of these settings. It will be important for the speech-language pathologist to play a role in preparing the school and family for transition back to school when the child is ready. The school speech-language pathologist will be a vital team member to ensure the child is receiving the appropriate intervention, supports, and accommodations within school to promote academic success.

For the child who does not present with immediate speech and language difficulties following a stroke, close monitoring and surveillance of his speech and language development will be critical, as children with a stroke occurring at birth or in the toddler or preschool years can be vulnerable to future speech and language difficulties.

CASE STUDY

At 2 years of age and with no previous medical history, James* presented to the emergency room with decreased responsiveness after an acute headache and vomiting. He was subsequently diagnosed with a left intracranial hemorrhagic stroke as the result of a ruptured arteriovenous malformation. James had a complex hospital course that included seizure activity, multiple stays in intensive care, and several surgical procedures including a hemicraniectomy, embolization, cranioplasty, ventriculoperitoneal shunt placement, and bone flap removal.

As a result of his stroke, James had significant impairments in his motor skills, language abilities, and swallowing function. Nine days into his first intensive care admission, James received an evaluation by a speech-language pathologist. The initial goals of James's speech therapy were concentrated on maintenance of an awake state, increasing his responsiveness to environmental stimulation, vocalizing with open vowel sounds, smiling, following one-step commands, and accepting small tastes of liquid and puree without physiological instability or overt signs of aspiration. During the first few weeks of his hospitalization, James received nutrition via a nasogastric tube due to the severity of his dysphagia. James participated in daily therapy as appropriate given his tenuous medical status. Once his medical condition improved, James was transferred to an inpatient rehabilitation unit where he could receive more intensive therapy services, including continuation of daily speech therapy services. He remained in the hospital for almost 5 months.

James presented with right-sided facial asymmetry, an open mouth posture, and mild drooling. With therapy, he gradually made progress with oral feeding skills and safety and advanced to a diet of age-appropriate solid foods and thin liquids via a cup or straw. At the time of hospital discharge, James was meeting his nutrition and hydration needs fully by mouth.

When he arrived to the inpatient rehabilitation unit, James was nonverbal and had significant language comprehension deficits. He exhibited irritability, emotional lability, and signs of frustration that decreased over time. Given his diagnoses of expressive aphasia and apraxia of speech, James's speech-language pathologist experimented with several low-tech augmentative communication systems in an attempt to provide James with a functional means to communicate. Increasing James's verbal communication skills was a priority within his speech therapy treatment throughout his admission.

James's parents were actively involved in every step of his rehabilitation, attending and participating in therapy sessions to support James and to learn the therapeutic strategies and interventions that could help facilitate the recovery of his speech and language skills. James's parents consistently reinforced communication strategies outside of speech therapy sessions and were instrumental to James's recovery and success.

Upon discharge, James demonstrated significant progress in his receptive and expressive language skills. He was able to follow 1- and 2-step commands and demonstrated understanding of basic spatial concepts. James was communicating functionally via the use of adapted sign language and gestures. He was beginning to combine 2 signs to request. James was able to vocalize with a variety of vowels and the consonant /m/ and spontaneously produce several single words (apple, ball, bubbles). He could not produce single words on command. James presented with persistent aphasia and apraxia and continued with outpatient speech therapy services following discharge from his inpatient rehabilitation program. Although James did not fully recover speech and language abilities by time of discharge, marked progress was achieved due to the intensity of rehabilitation services provided and his strong parental support and involvement.

*Pseudonym

References

1. Kim C-T, Han J, Kim H. Pediatric stroke recovery: a descriptive analysis. *Arch Phys Med Rehabil.* 2009;90:657-662.

2. Ylivasker M. *Traumatic Brain Injury Rehabilitation: Children and Adolescents,* 2nd ed. Newton, MA: Butterworth-Heinemann; 1998.

3. Bloom L, Lahey M. *Language Development and Disorders.* New York, New York: John Wiley & Sons; 1978.

4. American Speech-Language and Hearing Association. *Clinical Topics: Aphasia.* http://www.asha.org/Practice-Portal/Clinical-Topics/aphasia. Accessed March 29, 2017.

5. Van Hout A. Acquired aphasia in children. *Semin Pediatr Neurol.* 1997;4:102-108.

6. Chilosi AM, Cipriani P, Pecini C, et al. Acquired focal brain lesions in childhood: effects on development and reorganization of language. *Brain Lang.* 2008;106:211-225.

7. Ilves P, Tomberg T, Kepler J, et al. Different plasticity patterns of language function in children with perinatal and childhood stroke. *J Child Neurol.* 2014;29(6):756-764.

8. Tillema JM, Byars AW, Jacola LM, et al. Cortical reorganization of language functioning following perinatal left MCA stroke. *Brain Lang.* 2008;106:184-194.

9. Chapman SB, Max JE, Gamino JF, McGlothlin JH, Cliff SN. Discourse plasticity in children after stroke: age at injury and lesion effects. *Pediatr Neurol.* 2003;29:34-41.

10. Kirton A, deVeber G. Life after perinatal stroke. *Stroke.* 2013;44:3265-3271.

11. Avila L, Riesgo R, Pedroso F, et al. Language and focal brain lesion in childhood. *J Child Neurol.* 2010;25:829-833.

12. Vargha-Khadem F, O'Gorman AM, Watters GV. Aphasia and handedness in relation to hemispheric side, age at injury and severity of cerebral lesion during childhood. *Brain.* 1985;108:677-696.

13. Chapey R. *Language Intervention Strategies in Aphasia and Related Neurogenic Communication Disorders* 5th ed. Baltimore, MD: Lippincott Williams and Wilkins; 2008.

14. Davis GA. *Aphasiology: Disorders and Clinical Practice.* Needham Heights, MA: Allyn & Bacon; 2000.

15. Van Hout A, Evrard PH, Lyon G. Positive semiology of acquired aphasia. *Dev Med Child Neurol.* 1985;27:231-241.

16. Van Dongen HR, Paquier PF, Creten WL, Van Borsel J, Catsman-Berrevoets CE. Clinical evaluation of conversational speech fluency in the acute phase of acquired childhood aphasia: does a fluency/nonfluency dichotomy exist? *J Child Neurol.* 2001;16:345-351.

17. Paquier PF, Van Dongen HR. Review of research on the clinical presentation of acquired childhood aphasia. *Acta Neurologica Scandinavic.* 1996;93:428-436.

18. Cooper JA, Flowers CR. Children with a history of acquired aphasia: residual language and academic impairments. *J Speech Hear Disord.* 1987;52:251-262.

19. Lambon Ralph MA, Snell C, Fillingham JK, Conroy P, Sage K. Predicting the outcome of anomia therapy for people with aphasia post CVA: both language and cognitive status are key predictors. *Neuropsychol Rehabil.* 2010;20(2):289-305.

20. Van Hout A. Acquired aphasia in childhood and developmental dysphasias: are the errors similar? Analysis of errors made in confrontation naming tasks. *Aphasiology.* 1993;7:525-531.

21. Marshall RC. Word retrieval of aphasic adults. *J Speech Hear Disord.* 1976;41:444-451.

22. Hynd GW, Leathem J, Semrud-Clikerman M, Hern KL, Wenner M. Anomic aphasia in Childhood. *J Child Neurol.* 1995;10(4):289-293.

23. Raymer A, Kohen F. Word-retrieval treatment in aphasia: effects of sentence context. *J Rehabil Res Dev.* 2006;43:367-378.

24. Kiran S, Sandberg C, Sebastian R. Treatment of category generation and retrieval in aphasia: effect of typicality of category items. *J Speech Lang Hear Res.* 2011;54:1101-1117.

25. Kendall DL, Pompon RH, Brookshire CE, Minkina I, Bislick L. An analysis of aphasic naming errors as an indicator of improved linguistic processing following phonomotor treatment. *Am J Speech Lang Pathol.* 2013;22:240-249.

26. Boyle M, Coelho C. Application of semantic feature analysis as a treatment for aphasic dysnomia. *Am J Speech Lang Pathol.* 1995;4:94-98.

27. Boyle M. Semantic feature analysis treatment for anomia in two fluent aphasia syndromes. *Am J Speech Lang Pathol.* 2004;13:236-249.

28. Rider JD, Wright HH, Marshal RC, Page JL. Using semantic feature analysis to improve contextual discourse in adults with aphasia. *Am J Speech Lang Pathol.* 2008;17:161-172.

29. Rose M. Releasing the constraints on aphasia therapy: the positive impact of gesture and multimodality treatments. *Am J Speech Lang Pathol.* 2013;22:227-239.

30. Sparks RW, Holland AL. Method: melodic intonation therapy for aphasia. *J Speech Hear Disord.* 1976;61:287-297.

31. Conklyn D, Novak E, Boissy A, Bethoux F, Chemali K. The effects of modified melodic intonation therapy on nonfluent aphasia: a pilot study. *J Speech Lang Hear Res.* 2012;55:1463-1471.

32. DeDe G. Reading and listening in people with aphasia: effects of syntactic complexity. *Am J Speech Lang Pathol.* 2013;22(4):579-590.

33. Nicholas LE, Brookshire RH. Comprehension of spoken narrative discourse by adults with aphasia, right-hemisphere brain damage, or traumatic brain injury. *Am J Speech Lang Pathol.* 1995;4:69-81.

34. Blosser JL, DePompei R. *Pediatric Traumatic Brain Injury: Proactive Intervention,* 2nd ed. Clifton Park, NY: Delmar Learning; 2003.

35. Edmonds MS, Vaughn S, Wexler J, et al. A synthesis of reading interventions and effects on reading comprehension outcomes for older struggling readers. *Rev Educ Res.* 2009;79(1):262-300.

36. Tadlock DF. SQ3R: why it works, based on an information processing theory of learning. *J Read.* 1978;22:110-112.

37. Paul R. *Language Disorders from Infancy through Adolescence: Assessment and Intervention.* St. Louis, MO: Mosby; 2000.

38. Strand EA. Neurologic substrates of motor speech disorders. *Perspect Neurophysiol Neurogenic Speech Lang Disord.* 2013; 23(3):98-104.

39. Dworkin PJ. *Motor Speech Disorders: A Treatment Guide.* St. Louis, MO: Mosby, Inc.; 1991.

40. Wambaugh J, Mauszycki S, Ballard K. Advances in the treatment for acquired apraxia of speech. *Perspect Neurophysiol Neurogenic Speech Lang Disord.* 2013;23(3):95-119.

41. Haley KL, Jacks A, Cunningham T. Error variability and the differentiation between apraxia of speech and aphasia with phonemic paraphasia. *J Speech Lang Hear Res.* 2013;56:891-905.

42. Blake ML, Frymark T, Venedictov R. An evidence-based systemic review on communication treatments for individuals with right hemisphere brain damage. *Am J Speech Lang Pathol.* 2013;22:146-160.

43. Blake ML. Clinical relevance of discourse characteristics after right hemisphere brain damage. *Am J Speech Lang Pathol.* 2006;15:255-267.

44. Rodriguez AD. Aprosodia secondary to right hemisphere damage. *Perspect Neurophysiol Neurogenic Speech Lang Disord.* 2009;19(3):71-76.

45. Laugeson EA, Frankel F, Gantman A, Dillon A, Mogil C. Evidence-based social skills training for adolescents with autism spectrum disorders: the UCLA PEER program. *J Autism Dev Disord.* 2012;42:1025-1036.

46. Hickey EM, Saunders JN. Group intervention for adolescents with chronic acquired brain injury: the future zone. *Perspect Neurophysiol Neurogenic Speech Lang Disord.* 2010;20:111-119.

47. Barakat LP, Hetzke JD, Foley B, et al. Evaluation of a social skills training group intervention with children treated for brain tumors: pilot study. *J Pediatr Psychol.* 2003;28(5):299-307.

48. Murray LL. Attention and other cognitive deficits in aphasia: presence and relation to language and communication measures. *Am J Speech Lang Pathol.* 2012;21:51-64.

49. Lee JB, Sohlberg MM. Evaluation of attention training and metacognitive facilitation to improve reading comprehension in aphasia. *Am J Speech Lang Pathol.* 2013;22:18-33.

50. Westmacott R, MacGregor D, Askalan R, deVeber G. Late emergence of cognitive deficits after unilateral neonatal stroke. *Stroke.* 2009;40:2012-2019.

51. Helm-Estabrooks N. Treating attention to improve auditory comprehension deficits associated with aphasia. *Perspect Neurophysiol Neurogenic Speech Lang Disord.* 2011;21:64-71.

52. Helm-Estabrooks N. Cognition and aphasia: a discussion and a study. *J Commun Disord.* 2002;35:171-186.

53. King G, King S, Rosenbaum P, Goffin R. Family-centered caregiving and well-being of parents of children with disabilities: linking process with outcome. *J Pediatr Psychol.* 1999;24:41-53.

54. Bamm EL, Rosenbaum P. Family-centered theory: origins, development, barriers, and supports to implementation in rehabilitation medicine. *Arch Phys Med Rehabil.* 2008;89:1618-1624.

55. Donovan NJ, Daniels SK, Edmiaston J, Weinhardt J, Summers D, Mitchell PH; American Heart Association Council on Cardiovascular Nursing and Stroke Council. Dysphagia screening: state of the art. *Stroke.* 2013;44:e24-e31.

56. Logemann JA. *Evaluation and Treatment of Swallowing Disorders*, 2nd ed. Austin, TX: Pro-Ed; 1998:1, 27-32.

57. Mann G, Hankey G, Cameron D. Swallowing function after stroke: prognosis and prognostic factors at 6 months. *Stroke.* 1999;30:744-748.

58. Barkat-Masih M, Saha C, Hamby D, Ofner S, Golomb M. Feeding problems in children with neonatal arterial ischemic stroke. *J Child Neurol.* 2009;25(7):867-872.

59. DePippo KL, Holas MA, Reding MJ, Mandel FS, Lesser Ml. Dysphagia therapy following stroke: a controlled trial. *Neurology.* 1994;44:1655-1660.

60. Rogers H, Bond S, Curless R. Inadequacies in the provision of information to stroke patients and their families. *Age Ageing.* 2001;30:129-133.

61. Ertekin C, Aydogdu I. Neurophysiology of swallowing. *Clin Neurophysiol.* 2003;114:2226-2244.

62. Ramsey DJC, Smithard DG, Kaira L. Early assessments of dysphagia and aspiration risk in acute stroke patients. *Stroke.* 2003;34:1252-1257.

63. Luker JA, Wall K, Bernhardt J, Edwards I, Grimmer-Somers K. Measuring the quality of dysphagia management practices following stroke: a systematic review. *Int J Stroke.* 2010;5:466-476.

64. Daniels S, Anderson J, Wilson P. Valid items of screening dysphagia in patients with stroke: a systematic review. *Stroke.* 2012;43:892-897.

65. Vergara ER, Bigsby R. *Developmental and Therapeutic Interventions in the NICU.* Baltimore, MD: Paul H. Brookes Publishing Co., Inc; 2004.

66. Goldstein LB, Simel D. Is this patient having a stroke? *JAMA.* 2005;293(19):2371-2402.

67. Corbin-Lewis K, Liss JM, Sciortino K. Physiological bases of neurogenic dysphagia and treatment strategies. In: *Clinical Anatomy and Physiology of the Swallow Mechanism.* Independence, KY: Thomson Delmar Learning; 2004:151-179.

68. Lau C. Interventions to improve oral feeding performance of preterm infants. *Persepct Swallowing Disord Dysphagia.* 2014;23(1):23-45.

69. Tutor JD, Gosa MM. Dysphagia and aspiration in children. *Pediatr Pulmonol.* 2012;47:321-337.

70. Miller AJ. Oral and pharyngeal reflexes in the mammalian nervous system: their diverse range in complexity and the pivotal role of the tongue. *Crit Rev Oral Biol Med.* 2002;13(5):409-425.

71. Leder SB. Gag reflex and dysphagia. *Head Neck.* 1996;18(2):138-141.

72. Bleach NR. The gag reflex and aspiration: a retrospective analysis of 120 patients assessed by videofluoroscopy. *Clin Otolaryngol Allied Sci.* 1993;18(4):303-307.

73. Sundseth Ross E. Feeding in the NICU and issues that influence success. *Persepct Swallowing Disord Dysphagia.* 2008;17:94-100.

74. Barlow SM. Oral and respiratory control for preterm feeding. *Curr Opin Otolaryngology Head Neck Surg.* 2009;17(3):179-186.

75. Lau C. Oral feeding in the preterm infant. *NeoReviews.* 2006;7(1):e19-e27.

76. Arvedson J. Assessment of pediatric dysphagia and feeding disorders: clinical and instrumental approaches. *Dev Dis Res Rev.* 2008;14:118-127.

77. Seddon PC, Khan Y. Respiratory problems in children with neurological impairment. *Arch Dis Child.* 2003;88:75-78.

78. Logemann J. Screening, diagnosis, and management of neurogenic dysphagia. *Semin Pediatr Neurol.* 1996; 16(4): 319-327.

79. Borr C, Hielscher-Fastabend M, Lucking A. Reliability and validity of cervical auscultation. *Dysphagia.* 2007;22:225-234.

80. Leslie P, Drinnan MJ, Finn P, Ford GA, Wilson JA. Reliability and validity of cervical auscultation: a controlled comparison using videofluoroscopy. *Dysphagia.* 2004;19:231-240.

81. Arvedson J, Rogers B, Buck G, Smart P, Msall M. Silent aspiration prominent in children with dysphagia. *Int J Pediatr Otorhinolaryngol.* 1994;28:173-181.

82. Weir K, McMahon S, Taylor S, Chang A. Oropharyngeal aspiration and silent aspiration in children. *Chest.* 2011;140(3):589-597.

83. Newman LA, Keckley C, Petersen MC, Hamner A. Swallowing function and medical diagnoses in infants suspected of dysphagia. *Pediatrics.* 2001;108(6):e106-106. doi: 10.1542/peds.108.6.e106.

84. Uhm KE, Yi SH, Chang HJ, Cheon HJ, Kwon JY. Videofluoroscopic swallowing study findings in full-term and preterm infants with dysphagia. *Ann Rehabil Med.* 2013;37(2):175-182.

85. Horner J, Massey EW, Riski JE, Lathrop DL, Chase KN. Silent aspiration following stroke: clinical correlates and outcomes. *Neurology.* 1988;38:317-319.

86. Daniels SK, Brailey K, Priestly DH, Herrington LR, Weisberg LA, Foundas AL. Aspiration in patients with acute stroke. *Arch Phys Med Rehabil.* 1998;79:14-19.

87. Wolf LS, Glass RP. Clinical feeding evaluation. In: *Feeding and Swallowing Disorders in Infancy: Assessment and Management.* San Antonio, TX: Therapy Skill Builders; 1992:127-128.

88. Collins MJ, Bakheit AMO. Does pulse oximetry reliably detect aspiration in dysphagia stroke patients? *Stroke.* 1997;28:1773-1775.

89. Sherman B, Nisenboum JM, Jesberger BL, Morrow CA, Jesberger JA. Assessment of dysphagia with the use of pulse oximetry. *Dysphagia.* 1999;14:152-156.

90. Smith H, Lee S, O'Neill P, Connolly M. The combination of bedside swallowing assessment and oxygen saturation monitoring of swallowing in acute stroke: a safe and humane screening tool. *Age Ageing.* 2000;29:495-499.

91. Shaker C. Nipple feeding preterm infants: an individualized, developmentally supportive approach. *Neonatal Network.* 1999;18(3):15-22.

92. Weir K, McMahon S, Barry L, Masters IB, Chang AB. Clinical signs and symptoms of oropharyngeal aspiration and dysphagia in children. *Eur Respir J.* 2009;33(3):604-611.

93. Durvasula VSPB, O'Neill AC, Richter GT. Oropharyngeal dysphagia in children: mechanism, source, and management. *Otolaryngol Clin N Am.* 2014;47:691-720.

94. McGrath JM, Bodea Braescu AV. State of the science: feeding readiness in the preterm infant. *J Perinat Neonatal Nurs.* 2004;18(4):353-368.

95. Als H, Lawhon G. Theoretic perspective for developmentally supportive care. In: Kenner C, McGrath JM, eds. *Developmental Care of Newborns and Infants: A Guide for Health Professionals.* St Louis, MO: Mosby; 2004:52-57.

96. Glass RP, Wolf LS. A global perspective on feeding assessment in the neonatal intensive care unit. *Am J Occup Ther.* 1994;48(6):514-526.

97. Wilson Jones M, Morgan E, Shelton JE. Dysphagia and oral feeding problems in the premature infant. *Neonatal Network.* 2002;21(2):51-57.

98. Altimier L, Phillipa RM. The neonatal integrative developmental care model: seven neuroprotective core measures for family-centered developmental care. *Newborn Infant Nurs Rev.* 2013;13:9-22.

99. Sundseth Ross E, Philbin K. Supporting oral feeding in fragile infants: an evidence-base method for quality bottle-feedings of preterm, ill and fragile infants. *J Perinat Neonatal Nurs.* 2011;25(4):349-357.

100. Sundseth Ross E, Browne JV. Developmental progression of feeding skills: an approach to supporting feeding in preterm infants. *Semin Neonatal.* 2002;7:469-475.

101. Jadcheria SR, Peng J, Moore R, et al. Impact of personalized feeding program in 100 NICU infants: pathophysiology-based approach for better outcomes. *J Gastroenterol Nutr.* 2012;54(1):62-70.

102. Oommen MP. Breathing patterns of preterm infants during bottle feeding: role of milk flow. *J Pediatr.* 1991;119:960-965.

103. Chang YJ, Lin CP, Lin CH. Effects of single-hole and cross-cut nipple units on feeding efficiency and physiological parameters in premature infants. *J Nurs Res.* 2007;15(3):215-223.

104. Jackman KT. Go with the flow: choosing a feeding system for infants in the neonatal intensive care unit and beyond based on flow performance. *Newborn Infant Nurs Rev.* 2013;13:31-34.

105. Law-Morstatt L, Judd DM, Snyder P, Baier RJ, Dhanireddy R. Pacing as a treatment technique for transitional sucking patterns. *J Perinatol.* 2003;23:483-488.

106. Ludwig SM, Waitzman KA. Changing feeding documentation to reflect infant-driven feeding practice. *Newborn Infant Nurs Rev.* 2007;7(3):155-160.

107. Clark L, Kennedy G, Pring T, Hird M. Improving bottle feeding in preterm infants: investigating the elevated side-lying position. *Infant.* 2007;3(4):154-158.

108. Park J, Thoyre S, Knafl G, Hodges E, Nix W. Efficacy of semielevated side-lying positioning during bottle-feeding of very preterm infants. *J Perinat Neonatal Nurs.* 2014;28(1):69-79.

109. Scariati PD, Grummer-Strawn LM, Fein SB. A longitudinal analysis of infant morbidity and the extent of breastfeeding in the United States. *Pediatrics.* 1997;99(6):e5.

110. Leung AKC, Sauve RS. Breast is best for babies. *JAMA.* 2005;97(7):1010-1019.

111. Meier PP, Engstrom JL, Patel A, Jegier BL, Bruns NE. Improving the use of human milk during and after NICU stay. *Clin Perinatol.* 2010;37:217-245

112. Hauck FR, Thompson JM, Tanabe KO, Moon RY, Vennemann MM. Breastfeeding and reduced risk of sudden infant death syndrome: a meta-analysis. *Pediatrics.* 2011;128(1):103-110.

113. Eidelman AI, Schanler RJ, Johnston M, et al. Breastfeeding and the use of human milk. *Pediatrics.* 2012;129(3):e827-e841. doi:10.1542/peds.2011-3552.

114. Colson S. Maternal breastfeeding positions: have we got it right? *Pract Midwife.* 2005;8(11):29-32.

115. Colson SD, Meek JH, Hawdon JM. Optimal positions for the release of primitive neonatal reflexes stimulating breastfeeding. *Early Hum Dev.* 2008;84:441-449.

116. Chertok IR, Schneider J, Blackburn S. A pilot study of maternal and term infant outcomes associated with ultrathin nipple shield use. *J Obstet Gynecol Neonatal Nurs.* 2006;35(2):265-272.

117. McKechnie AC, Eglash A. Nipple shields: a review of the literature. *Breastfeed Med.* 2010;5(6):309-314.

118. Meier PP, Furman LM, Degenherdt M. Increased lactation risk for late preterm infants and mothers: evidence and management strategies to protect breastfeeding. *J Midwifery Womens Health.* 2007;52(6):579-587.

119. Martino R, Foley N, Bhogal S, Diamant N, Speechley M, Teasell R. Dysphagia after stroke: incidence, diagnosis, and pulmonary complications. *Stroke.* 2005;36:2756-2763.

120. Martin-Harris B, Brodsky MB, Michel Y, et al. MBS Measurement Tool for Swallow Impairment (MBSImp): establishing a standard. *Dysphagia.* 2008;23(4):392-405.

121. Linden-Castelli P. Treatment strategies for adult neurogenic dysphagia. *Semin Speech Lang.* 1991;12(3):255-261.

122. East L, Nettles K, Vassant A, Daniels SK. Evaluation of oropharyngeal dysphagia with the videofluoroscopic swallowing study. *J Radiol Nurs.* 2014;33(1):9-13.

123. Langmore SE, Schatz K, Olsen N. Fiberoptic endoscopic examination of swallowing safety: a new procedure. *Dysphagia.* 1988;2:216-219.

124. Willging JP, Miller CK, Link DT, Rudolph CD. Use of FEES to assess and manage pediatric patients. In: Langmore SE, ed. *Endoscopic Evaluation and Treatment of Swallowing Disorders.* New York, NY: Thieme; 2001:213-232.

125. Gosa M, Schooling T, Coleman J. Thickened liquids as a treatment for children with dysphagia and associated effects: a systematic review. *ICAN.* 2011;3(6):344-350.

126. Woods CW, Oliver T, Lewis K, Yang Q. Development of necrotizing enterocolitis in premature infants receiving thickened feeds using Simply Thick. *J Perinatol.* 2012;32:150-152.

127. Beal J, Silverman B, Bellant J, Young T, Klontz K. Late onset necrotizing enterocolitis in infants following use of a xanthan gum-containing thickening agent. *J Pediatr.* 2012;161(20):354-356.

128. Almeida MB, Almeida JA, Moreira ME, Novak FR. Adequacy of human milk viscosity to respond to infants with dysphagia: experimental study. *J Appl Oral Sci.* 2011;19(6):554-559.

129. Han TR, Paik NJ, Park JW. Quantifying swallowing function after stroke: a functional dysphagia scale based on videofluoroscopic studies. *Arch Phys Med Rehabil.* 2001;82:677-682.

130. Hallett M. Plasticity of the human motor cortex and recovery from stroke. *Brain Res Rev.* 2001;36:169-174.

131. McLaren SMG, Dickerson JWT. Measurement of eating disability in an acute stroke population. *Clin Eff Nurs.* 2000;4(3):109-120.

132. Westergren A, Ohlsson O, Hallberg IR. Eating difficulties, complications and nursing interventions during a period of three months after a stroke. *J Adv Nurs.* 2001;35(3):416-426.

133. Bouziana SD, Tziomalo K. Malnutrition in patients with acute stroke. *Nutr Metab.* 2011; doi:10.1155/2011/167898.

134. Crary MA, Groher ME. Reinstituting oral feeding in tube-fed adult patients with dysphagia. *Nutr Clin Pract.* 2006;21:576-586.

135. James R, Gines D, Menlove A, et al. Nutrition support (tube feeding) as a rehabilitation intervention. *Arch Phys Med Rehabil.* 2005;86(2):82-92.

136. Huggins PS, Tuomi, SK, Young, C. Effects of nasogastric tubes on the young, normal swallowing mechanism. *Dysphagia.* 1999;14:157-161.

137. Dziewas R, Warnecke T, Hamacher C, et al. Do nasogastric tubes worsen dysphagia in patients with acute stroke? *BMC Neurol.* 2008;8(28): doi: 10.1186/1471-2377-8-28.

138. Leder SB, Suiter D. Effect of nasogatric tubes on incidence of aspiration. *Arch Phys Med Rehabil.* 2008;89:648-651.

139. Wang TG, Wu MC, Chang YC, Hsiao TY, Lien IN. The effect of nasogastric tubes on swallowing function in persons with dysphagia following stroke. *Arch Phys Med Rehabil.* 2006;87:1270-1273.

140. Kirshner H. Causes of neurogenic dysphagia. *Dysphagia.* 1989;3:184-188.

141. Gariballa SE, Sinclair AJ. Assessment and treatment of nutritional status in stroke patients. *Postgrad Med J.* 1998;74:395-399.

142. Westergren A, Karlsson S, Andersson P, Ohlsson O, Hallberg IR. Eating difficulties, need for assisted eating, nutritional status and pressure ulcers in patients admitted for stroke rehabilitation. *J Clin Nurs.* 2001;10:257-269.

143. Avery-Smith W, Dellarosa DM. Approaches to treating dysphagia in patients with brain injury. *Am J Occup Ther.* 1994;48(3): 235-239.

144. O'Neil KH, Purdy M, Falk J, Gallo L. The Dysphagia Outcome Severity Scale. *Dysphagia.* 1999;14:139-145.

145. Hamdy S, Jilani S, Price V, et al. Modulation of human swallowing behavior by thermal and chemical stimulation in health and after brain injury. *Neurogastroenterol Motil.* 2003;15(1):69-77.

146. Logemann JA, Pauloski BR, Colangelo L, et al. Effects of a sour bolus on oropharyngeal swallowing measures in patients with neurogenic dysphagia. *J Speech Hear Res.* 1995;38:556-563.

147. Huckabee ML, Pelletier CA. *Management of Adult Neurogenic Dysphagia.* San Diego, CA: Singular Publishing Group; 1999:93-145.

148. Daniels S. Neurological disorders affecting oral, pharyngeal swallowing: Part 1 Oral cavity, pharynx, and esophagus. *GI Motility online.* 2006; doi:10.1038/gimo34.

149. Carnaby-Mann G, Lenius K, Crary MA. Update on assessment and management of dysphagia post stroke. *Northeast Florida Med.* 2007;58(2):31-34.

150. Shanahan TK, Logemann JA, Rademaker AW, Pauloski BR, Kahrilas PJ. Chin-down posture effect on aspiration in dysphagic patients. *Arch Phys Med Rehabil.* 1993;74:736-739.

151. Ney D, Weiss J, Kind A, Robbins J. Senescent swallowing: impact, strategies, and interventions. *Nutr Clin Pract.* 2009;24(3):395-413.

152. Sura L, Madhavan A, Carnabt G, Crary MA. Dysphagia in the elderly: management and nutritional considerations. *Clin Interv Aging.* 2012;7:287-298.

153. Galvan TJ. Dysphagia: going down and staying down. *Am J Nurs.* 2001;101(1):37-43.

154. Arvedson J, Clark H, Lazarus C, Schooling T, Frymark T. The effects of oral-motor exercises on swallowing function on children: an evidence-based systematic review. *Dev Med Child Neurol.* 2010;52(11):1000-1013.

155. Lazarus C, Clark H, Arvedson J, Schooling T, Frymark T. Evidence-based systematic review: effects of oral sensory-motor treatment on swallowing in adults. In: *ASHA's National Center for Evidence-Based Practice in Communication Disorders.* Rockville, MD: 2011: 1-42.

SUGGESTED READINGS

Anatomy and Physiology and Dysphagia Treatment Techniques

Corbin-Lewis K, Liss JM, Sciortino K. *Clinical Anatomy and Physiology of the Swallow Mechanism.* Boston, MA: Thomson Delmar Learning; 2004.

Huckabee ML, Pelletier CA. *Management of Adult Neurogenic Dysphagia.* San Diego, CA: Singular Publishing Group; 1999.

Works by Jeri Logemann, Joan Arvedson

Stroke Incidence, Presentation, and Treatments

American Heart Association/American Stroke Association: http://stroke.ahajournals.org/

Infant Developmental Care in the Preterm or Hospitalized Infant

Sundseth-Ross E, Browne JV Feeding outcomes in preterm infants after discharge from the neonatal intensive care unit (NICU): a systematic review. *Newborn Infant Nurs Rev.* 2013;13:87-89

Shaker C. Improving feeding outcomes in the NICU: moving from volume-driven to infant-driven feeding. *SIG 13.* 2010;19:68-74

Als H, Lawhon G, Duffy F, McAnulty G, Gibbs-Grossman R, Blickman J. Individualized developmental care for the very low birth weight pre-term infant: medical and neurofunctional effects. *JAMA.* 1994;272(11):853-858.

Aphasia and Cognition

Blosser JL, DePompei R. *Pediatric Traumatic Brain Injury: Proactive Intervention,* 2nd ed. Clifton Park, NY: Delmar Learning; 2003.

Ylivasker M. Traumatic *Brain Injury Rehabilitation: Children and Adolescents,* 2nd ed. Newton, MA: Butterworth-Heinemann; 1998.

9

Cognitive Changes and Potential in Children With Stroke

Amanda Fuentes, PhD, C Psych and Robyn Westmacott, PhD, C Psych, ABPP

Stroke is an important cause of acquired brain injury in the pediatric population. Strokes are diagnosed in approximately 1 in every 4000 live births/year and have an annual incidence of 0.6 to 13/100,000 children/year with a recurrence rate of 6% to 40%.[1] Despite growing awareness of the prevalence of pediatric stroke and its negative impact on neurodevelopment, cognitive outcomes following pediatric stroke remain poorly understood. The assessment of long-term cognitive outcomes in the pediatric stroke population is important for several reasons. First, this population offers a unique opportunity to examine the impact of early focal injury on development, thus increasing our knowledge of brain–behavior relationships and plasticity of the immature brain. Second, a better understanding of the predictors of long-term outcomes assists with prognosis and allows for the identification of high-risk subgroups. To this end, this information is critical for directing interventions and assisting with academic planning. Finally, this research serves an important role in providing informed guidance and support to families, teachers, and clinicians. In this chapter, we review the outcomes of both perinatal and childhood stroke in a variety of cognitive domains, including overall cognitive ability/intellectual functioning, visual-spatial processing, memory and learning, attention, executive functioning, working memory, and social cognition. Furthermore, the influence of possible determinants of cognitive outcomes, such as age at stroke, time since stroke/age at assessment, sex, lesion location, lesion laterality, lesion volume, neurological impairment, and seizures, is discussed. Finally, implications and recommendations for

neuropsychological assessment and cognitive rehabilitation are reviewed. In particular, the importance of understanding the neuropsychological sequelae commonly associated with pediatric stroke and variables influencing cognitive outcomes, advocating for the child and family, and conducting sequential assessments is highlighted.

EFFECT OF PEDIATRIC STROKE ON COGNITIVE OUTCOMES

Intellectual Functioning/Overall Cognitive Ability

Intelligence can be broadly defined as the "ability to understand complex ideas, to adapt effectively to the environment, to learn from experience, to engage in various forms of reasoning, [and] to overcome obstacles by taking thought."[2] There remains a lack of consensus regarding the nature of the construct of intelligence (for review, see Neisser et al,[2] Nettelbeck and Wilson[3]). Briefly, variations in approaches to defining and measuring intelligence stem from the heterogeneity that exists across cultures, developmental theories (eg, Piaget,[4] Vygotsky[5]), and perceptions of intelligence as a general ability (eg, Spearman's *g*) or as multiple forms (eg, theories proposed by Gardner[6] and Sternberg[7]).[2,3] The intelligence quotient (IQ) describes overall performance on intelligence tests

Atkinson HL, Nixon-Cave K, Smith SE, eds.
Pediatric Stroke Rehabilitation: An Interprofessional and Collaborative Approach (pp 161-183). © 2018 Taylor & Francis Group.

and is converted to a standard score in order to allow for comparisons between a child's performance and his or her same-age peers. Nettelbeck and Wilson[3] caution, however, that intelligence and IQ should be viewed as distinct constructs on the basis that IQ does not capture the multiple domains within intelligence and evidence of the steady increase in IQ scores over the past century (ie, *Flynn effect*). IQ scores have been shown to remain fairly stable throughout development and to correlate with a number of characteristics, including school achievement, years of education, and job performance.[2] Moreover, research indicates that individual differences in intelligence are attributable to contributions from both genes and the environment, as IQ has been shown to have high heritability and to also be influenced by a range of environmental factors, particularly duration of schooling.[2,3]

Studies on global intellectual outcomes after pediatric stroke consistently indicate that overall intelligence is generally within the broad range of average, although compromised compared to normative samples.[8-14] For example, a large cross-sectional study of cognitive outcomes (as assessed by the age-appropriate Wechsler scales) in children with unilateral arterial ischemic stroke (AIS; $n = 145$) sustained between the perinatal period and 16 years revealed that overall intelligence (ie, Full Scale Intelligence Quotient; FSIQ), Verbal Comprehension/Verbal IQ, Working Memory, and Processing Speed Indices were significantly lower in children with AIS than the normative sample means (all $P < 0.01$).[8] Importantly, mean group averages fell within the average range (range of mean composite scores = 92.1 to 95.9).[8] These findings were recently replicated by Studer et al,[9] who found that children with AIS ($n = 99$) sustained between 1 month and 16 years performed in the average range across all 5 Wechsler index measures (range of mean composite scores = 93.4 to 103.1), despite scoring significantly lower than the normative sample mean on the Processing Speed Index ($P = 0.004$) and trending toward lower performance on the Verbal Comprehension ($P = 0.12$), Perceptual Reasoning ($P = 0.07$), and Working Memory ($P = 0.07$) Indices. Similar findings were reported by Ballantyne et al,[10] who found that children with perinatal AIS ($n = 29$) scored significantly lower than healthy controls ($n = 24$) on Verbal IQ ($P < 0.0001$), Performance IQ ($P = .002$), and FSIQ ($P < 0.0001$) when tested at preschool and school age, despite all 3 index measures falling within the average range (range at Time 1 = 92.8 to 96.6, range at Time 2 = 93.5 to 98.7). In keeping with these findings, a recent cross-sectional study found that children with perinatal AIS ($n = 29$) exhibited significantly lower performance compared to the normative sample on FSIQ ($P = 0.001$), Performance IQ ($P = 0.001$), and Verbal IQ ($P = 0.003$) measures, although still within the low end of the average range (range = 86.2 to 90.2).[11] Moreover, findings were generally similar in children with periventricular

hemorrhagic infarction ($n = 21$), with children scoring lower than the normative sample on FSIQ (mean = 86.1; $P = 0.001$) and Performance IQ (mean = 79.8; $P < 0.001$), but not Verbal (mean = 94.0; $P = 0.158$).[11] A recent cross-sectional study of cognitive outcomes following perinatal or childhood AIS ($n = 36$) also found nonsignificant trends toward poorer performance in children with AIS compared to controls with asthma ($n = 15$) on measures of expressive vocabulary, ($P = 0.34$), visual abstract reasoning, ($P = 0.29$) and transcriptions ($P = 0.05$), although statistical power to detect effects was likely underpowered due to the small sample size.[12] In one of the few studies to assess cognitive outcomes following cerebral sinovenous thrombosis (CSVT), Hetherington et al[13] reported overall intellectual functioning in the average range (mean FSIQ = 97.8). Finally, Everts et al[14] similarly reported that overall cognitive ability fell within the average (mean FSIQ = 96.5) for children with stroke sustained between birth and 18 years ($n = 21$); although more deficits were detected in specific cognitive domains than expected in typically developing children. More specifically, children with stroke scored significantly lower than the normative sample on Performance IQ ($P < 0.001$) and Digit Span ($P < 001$), Arithmetic ($P = 0.007$), Divided Attention ($P = 0.028$), and Alertness ($P = 0.002$) subtests.[14] Moreover, Verbal IQ was found to be significantly better than Performance IQ in 13/17 patients, independent of the hemispheric side of the lesion, prompting Everts et al[14] to propose that verbal abilities may be more resilient to brain injury. That is, Everts et al[14] proposed that nonverbal abilities develop later than verbal abilities, which renders this domain less capable of reorganization.

Taken together, these studies indicate that children with stroke are at risk for compromised intellectual functioning relative to typically developing children, although difficulties are subtle and do not represent genuine deficits. With the exception of the findings reported by Everts et al,[14] studies also document similar verbal and nonverbal intellectual outcomes, with composite scores falling within the low end of the average range. The fact that only subtle difficulties are evident relative to normative samples could be interpreted as evidence that the developing brain is generally able to compensate for early injury, but perhaps not to the point that a complete recovery is achieved. Of note, given that the majority of studies have focused on children with AIS, caution is warranted in extending these findings to children with CSVT or hemorrhagic stroke. Further, recent evidence indicates that intellectual outcomes following pediatric stroke vary according to demographic (ie, age at stroke, time since stroke, sex), lesion (ie, size, laterality, location), neurological, and stroke characteristics (ie, stroke type, vascular classification, etiology—discussed in the following section), suggesting that more accurate predictions of overall cognitive functioning are achieved by taking these factors into account.

TABLE 9-1. DIFFICULTIES ASSOCIATED WITH VISUOSPATIAL DEFICITS

VISUOSPATIAL DEFICIT	ASSOCIATED DIFFICULTIES
Visual acuity	Differentiating visual details, loss of sharpness in vision, blurred vision
Visual fields	Perceiving portions of visual space
Depth perception	Perceiving distances of objects in space
Visual attention	Visual scanning, attending to objects or body parts in space
Visual figure-ground discrimination	Differentiating visual details from background
Visual-motor integration	Copying, drawing, building, coordination
Visual memory	Memory for faces, designs, etc; reading
Spatial orientation	Confusion of left/right, navigating environment, getting lost

Visuospatial Processing

Visuospatial processing encapsulates a wide range of cognitive abilities required for understanding spatial information that vary from "the basic ability to analyze how parts or features of an object combine to form an organized whole, to the dynamic and interactive spatial processes required to track moving objects, to visualize displacement, and to localize, attend, or reach for objects or visual targets in a spatial array."[15] Visuospatial processing abilities are governed by the ventral and dorsal processing pathways, which process patterns and objects (ie, "what") and movement and location (ie, "where"), respectively (for review, see Stiles et al[15]). The 3 main functions of the ventral processing pathway are global-local processing (ie, analyzing the holistic features or details of a visual stimulus, respectively), face processing, and spatial construction (eg, drawing, block assembly).[15] Conversely, dorsal stream processing includes functions such as spatial localization (ie, analyzing the perceptual locations of visual stimuli), spatial attention (ie, orienting, attending, and shifting attention to different visual stimuli), and mental rotation (ie, the ability to move mental representations of objects).[15] Both the ventral and dorsal pathways begin at the retina and project from the lateral geniculate nucleus to the primary visual cortex.[15] The ventral pathway projects to the posterior and anterior areas of the inferior temporal lobe, and the dorsal pathway projects to the medial areas of the temporal lobe and the inferior parietal lobe.[15] Both pathways project to regions of the prefrontal cortex.[15] Visuospatial processes governed by the dorsal pathway have been shown to be particularly vulnerable to brain injury, which is hypothesized to be due to later maturation of the dorsal pathway.[15] Table 9-1 provides examples of difficulties that children with deficits in visuospatial processing may present with.

Children with histories of stroke demonstrate subtle, persistent deficits in visuospatial processing.[16-21] A longitudinal analysis of the copying task of the Rey-Osterrieth Complex Figure among children with perinatal stroke documented impaired performance at ages 6 to 7, with children with right hemisphere damage ($n = 9$) omitting significantly ($P < 0.01$) more configural elements than children with left hemisphere damage ($n = 10$).[16] Conversely, children with left hemisphere damage were found to produce more errors on detail placement ($P < 0.05$).[16] Notable improvements were observed by age 12, and discrepancies between the profiles of children with right vs left hemisphere damage were no longer evident.[16] However, children with perinatal stroke continued to evince a nonstrategic, piecemeal approach, indicating the persistence of subtle deficits.[16] Stiles et al[17] conducted a longitudinal analysis of the performance of children with early stroke (ie, prenatal to 6 months) on a free-drawing task of possible and impossible houses and similarly found a gradual improvement with development. Interestingly, children with right hemisphere damage demonstrated more limited use of strategies during the impossible house task.[17] These results were interpreted as reflecting persistent difficulty in the capacity of the right hemisphere group to reorganize spatial patterns.[17]

Evidence has been found for lateralized deficits (ie, hemispheric specialization of cognitive functions) in children with histories of stroke on spatial reconstruction tasks and memory for visual-spatial patterns.[18,19] After studying both the processes and final products of block reconstructions in 4- to 5-year-old children with prenatal or perinatal stroke, Stiles et al[18] discovered that children with right hemisphere injuries were more delayed than children with left hemisphere injuries. Interestingly, both groups exemplified a less strategic approach relative to controls.[18] Schatz et al[19] analyzed the specific types of errors produced by children aged 6 to 12 years with histories of perinatal stroke on block reconstruction tasks and found evidence for lateralized differences in hierarchical processing patterns, with children with damage to the right hemisphere ($n = 12$) producing more global errors (44.4%) compared to children with left hemisphere ($n = 10$) damage (13.3%), and children with damage to the left hemisphere producing more local errors (74.9%) than children with right hemisphere damage (23.6%). Of note, both groups obtained similar scores ($P = 0.41$) that generally fell within the average to low-average range.[19] These findings were interpreted as support for the proposal that the left hemisphere is specialized for processing visual details, whereas the right hemisphere is specialized for global visual processing.[19] In keeping with these findings, Stiles et al[20] documented a double dissociation in global-local processing (ie, processing the overall gestalt or whole vs focusing on specific details) after comparing children with right ($n=19$) vs left ($n=19$) perinatal brain lesions on memory reproduction for hierarchical forms. That is, children with right hemisphere damage were impaired on global accuracy, whereas children with left hemisphere damage were impaired on local accuracy.[20] Similarly, in a cross-sectional study comparing visual search, global-local processing, and spatial judgments (ie, estimating the locations of objects in space) in children with unilateral right ($n=7$), left ($n=14$), and bilateral ($n=12$) stroke secondary to sickle cell disease (SCD), SCD without infarction ($n=25$), and healthy siblings ($n=18$), the right and bilateral injury groups were found to demonstrate impaired global processing and coordinate spatial judgments, whereas the left injury group was found to show intact processing and spatial judgments and a general impairment of response time.[21] Both the left and right injury groups displayed impaired visual search for the field contralateral to their injury, whereas the bilateral injury group showed impaired visual search across visual fields.[21]

In summary, it appears that the hemispheric side of the lesion and age at assessment are important variables in visuospatial processing profiles in children with stroke. Of note, given that the majority of studies consist of samples of children with perinatal stroke, caution is warranted in extending these findings to children with stroke occurring in later childhood. This limitation points to the importance of conducting future studies on visual-spatial processing in children with stroke occurring later in development, as profiles may be dependent on the time of injury.

Memory and Learning

Research indicates that there are multiple memory systems (for review, see Gathercole[22] and Siegel[23]). A key distinction is made between short-term memory and long-term memory. *Short-term memory* has a limited capacity and refers to memory for events in the immediate past (ie, occurring seconds or minutes ago).[22] The immediate or short-term memory system consists of sensory memory (ie, retention of stimuli lasting less than a second) and working memory (ie, temporary storage and manipulation of information; discussed in more detail later).[23] *Long-term memory* has a potentially unlimited capacity and refers to memory for events that occurred hours, days, or years ago.[22] Long-term memory is distinguished according to 2 types: declarative or explicit memory (ie, consciously accessible) and nondeclarative or implicit memory (ie, cannot be consciously accessed).[23] Nondeclarative memory includes

implicit learning processes such as perceptual priming (ie, enhancing accessibility of stimuli through previous experience), classical conditioning (ie, association between an environmental stimuli and a naturally occurring stimuli), and procedural memory (ie, memory for skills).[23] Nondeclarative memory is present at birth and mediated by the limbic regions, basal ganglia, and perceptual cortices.[23] Declarative memory is further divided into episodic memory (ie, memory for events) and semantic memory (ie, factual knowledge about the world). Declarative memory emerges during the first 1 to 2 years of life in conjunction with the maturation of the medical temporal lobe (including the hippocampus) and prefrontal cortex.[23] The hippocampus is crucial for memory encoding (ie, processing and organizing information for later recall) and consolidation (ie, process by which information becomes a permanent part of long-term memory).[23] Moreover, the hippocampus is responsible for functions such as sequencing and the development of an "internal map," thereby providing one with a sense of time and space.[23] The prefrontal cortex plays an important role in the organizing or executive processes of memory. Specifically, the ventrolateral prefrontal region is implicated during incidental learning (ie, informal learning that takes places in situations in which there is not a direct intention to learn), and the dorsolateral prefrontal region is implicated during evaluation or monitoring retrieval (ie, recalling previously learned information) processes.[23] Table 9-2 presents examples of difficulties associated with specific memory impairments.

Previous studies indicate that stroke renders children vulnerable to subtle deficits in memory and learning.[25-28] For example, Block et al[25] reported subtle, nonlateralized verbal learning and functional memory deficits in children with unilateral ischemic stroke sustained between 6 months and 16 years ($n=11$) relative to controls ($n=11$) matched on age, sex, and socioeconomic status (SES) after examining performance on the California Verbal Learning Test, Children's Version (CVLT-C) and the Rivermead Behavioral Memory Test. Similarly, Lansing et al[26] found evidence for subtle, nonlateralized verbal memory deficits after comparing CVLT-C performance among children with ischemic or hemorrhagic stroke sustained between the perinatal period and 13 years ($n=26$) and age-, gender-, and SES-matched orthopedic controls ($n=26$). Specifically, children with stroke recalled fewer words on initial learning, long-delay free recall, and cued recall trials and were more susceptible to proactive interference (all $P<0.05$).[26] However, no differences were found with respect to consistency of word recall, forgetting rates, and discriminability (ie, recognizing previously presented information through cued recall).[26] A recent cross-sectional study comparing children with neonatal ($n=21$) or childhood ($n=10$) ischemic or hemorrhagic stroke and age- and sex-matched healthy controls ($n=31$) also revealed significantly lower performance in both stroke groups on Sentence Repetition

TABLE 9-2. DIFFICULTIES ASSOCIATED WITH SPECIFIC MEMORY IMPAIRMENTS[24]	
MEMORY IMPAIRMENTS	**ASSOCIATED DIFFICULTIES**
Process	
Encoding	Processing and organizing new information for later recall
Consolidation	Poor long-term memory storage of facts, events, etc; overreliance on rote memorization
Retrieval	Recalling previously learned information, monitoring accuracy of recall
Modality	
Auditory	Recalling orally presented information (eg, phone numbers, lists, instructions, facts)
Visual	Recalling visuospatial information (eg, locations, figures, designs, faces)
Motor (procedural)	Remembering information that involves physical skills (eg, riding a bicycle, driving a car)

and Memory for Faces measures, with large effect sizes (Cohen's *d* =1.46 and -.88, respectively).[27] In a recent study, McCauley and Pedroza[28] used a computerized measure of event-based prospective memory (EB-PM) (ie, memory for planned actions when the circumstances present themselves) to examine whether performance differed between children with SCD and no stroke (*n* = 23), SCD and silent infarct (*n* = 9), SCD and overt stroke (*n* = 9), and controls (*n* = 27). All 3 SCD groups demonstrated compromised performance compared to controls, with children with overt stroke (*P* < 0.001) and silent stroke (*P* = 0.01) showing the most pronounced deficits.[28] Interestingly, EB-PM performance was found to improve in all groups after the presentation of a distinctive cue, with one exception, the overt stroke group.[28] McCauley and Pedroza[28] suggested that damage to anterior brain regions may reduce one's capacity to benefit from PM cues. It is important to note that, given that the sample consisting of children with SCD, these findings may not be representative of the general pediatric stroke population. Together, the data suggest that memory and learning are compromised following pediatric stroke. More research is needed to explore a broad range of memory functioning (eg, visual, autobiographical, implicit), as well as to examine the relation between memory performance and other domains of functioning (eg, social, academic).

Attention

According to the seminal multicomponent model of attention put forward by Mirsky et al,[29] attention is a complex set of processes consisting of 4 elements: focus-execute, sustain, shift, and encode. Moreover, each of these processes has its own unique neural correlates.[29] The *focus-execute*

element refers to the ability to selectively attend to target information and execute a response.[29] These functions are governed by the inferior parietal, superior temporal, and striatal regions.[29] The *sustain* element is responsible for maintaining focus over time and is supported by rostral midbrain structures.[29] The *shift* component refers to the capacity to adaptively change focus and is governed by the prefrontal cortex.[29] Finally, the hippocampus and amygdala are responsible for *encoding* of stimuli.[29] The model proposed by Mirksy et al[29] has been validated in both children and adults. Table 9-3 provides examples of difficulties associated with the focus-execute, sustain, and shift components of attention (see Table 9-2 for difficulties associated with the encode component).

Although there are few studies exploring attentional processes following pediatric stroke, emerging evidence indicates that attention problems are a common consequence.[30-33] For example, Max et al[30] documented an incidence of 46% (13/28) of attention deficit hyperactivity disorder (ADHD) in children with ischemic or hemorrhagic stroke sustained prenatally or in childhood, compared to only 17% (5/29) of orthopedic controls. Further, children with stroke with ADHD traits were found to have reduced Verbal IQ (*P* < 0.04), arithmetic achievement (*P* < 0.04), executive function (*P* < 0.005), and motivation (*P* < 0.005) compared to children without ADHD traits.[30] In a separate series of analyses using the same sample, Max et al[31] documented alerting and sensory-orienting attention deficits in children with stroke relative to orthopedic controls. Similarly, Elias and Moura-Ribeiro[32] reported auditory selective attention deficits in children with ischemic unilateral stroke (*n* = 13) compared to healthy controls (*n* = 13). Finally, a recent study examining attention and social outcomes in children with malformations of cortical

TABLE 9-3. DIFFICULTIES ASSOCIATED WITH DEFICITS IN THE COMPONENTS OF ATTENTION PROPOSED BY MIRSKY ET AL[29]	
ATTENTION COMPONENTS	ASSOCIATED DIFFICULTIES
Focus-execute	Attending to target stimuli while ignoring other stimuli, distractibility (eg, paying attention in class while others are talking, completing work in a noisy environment, etc.)
Sustain	Attending to stimuli over an extended period, increasing vulnerability to distractions over time, fatigue, need for frequent breaks
Shift	Paying attention to more than one stimulus, alternating between tasks, multitasking (eg, taking notes while listening to a lecture)

development (MCD) ($n = 14$) or stroke ($n = 14$) reported higher levels of impairment for the group overall in both domains than normative samples.[33] However, children with stroke exhibited more favorable social and attention outcomes than children with MCD, as indicated by their higher scores in shifting attention ($P = 0.027$, $\eta^2 = 0.19$), divided attention ($P = 0.024$, $\eta^2 = 0.18$) and teacher ratings of peer problems ($P = 0.025$, $\eta^2 = 0.19$), peer relations ($P = 0.008$, $\eta^2 = 0.25$), school adjustment ($P = 0.021$, $\eta^2 = 0.20$), and prosocial ($P = 0.039$, $\eta^2 = 0.16$) scales.[33] Further, lower performance on attention shifting was moderately correlated with greater peer problems ($r = -0.54$, $P < 0.01$).[33] Overall, these studies emphasize the vulnerability of attentional problems in children with stroke and highlight the reciprocal nature between attention and academic and social outcomes.

Executive Function

Executive function (EF) is an umbrella term referring to a collection of higher-level cognitive processes required for goal-directed behavior.[34,35] In one of the most influential developmental models of EF to date, Anderson[34] conceptualized EF as comprising 4 independent, interrelated components: 1) attentional control, 2) cognitive flexibility, 3) goal setting, and 4) information processing. Attentional control encompasses the ability to selectively attend to environmental stimuli while filtering out distracting stimuli, as well as to monitor and regulate behavior.[34] Cognitive flexibility includes the ability to divide attention, effectively respond to feedback in the environment, shift between different ways of responding, and hold multiple pieces of information in the mind simultaneously and manipulate that information in order to solve a problem (ie, working memory, discussed later).[34] Goal setting includes the capacity to reason abstractly, plan strategically, and initiate a response.[34] Finally, information processing refers to the ability to take in new information and produce a response in a timely manner.[34] Given the wide range of abilities that fall under the umbrella of EF, it is not surprising that dysfunction in this domain can manifest in many forms.

For example, a child with EF dysfunction may evince difficulties with impulsivity, self-regulation, problem solving, planning, perseveration, organization, self-monitoring, inhibition, initiation, and mental rigidity.[34] EF processes emerge as early as infancy and develop rapidly throughout childhood and well into adulthood.[35] Moreover, different developmental trajectories are associated with Anderson's[34] 4 EF components, which correspond roughly with maturational processes in the area of the brain proposed to regulate EF, the frontal lobes. Although the prefrontal cortex is posited to have a key role in EF, it is important to note that it has many connections with cortical and subcortical brain regions, thereby rendering it a "necessary, but not sufficient condition for intact EF."[34] Consequently, EF dysfunction can result from network disconnections or damage to other nonfrontal brain regions.[34,35] Table 9-4 provides examples of difficulties associated with the many skills falling under the umbrella of EF.

Although research is limited, new lines of evidence indicate that children with stroke are vulnerable to EF impairments.[36-40] For example, Long et al[36] reported deficits in 3 of the 4 EF components outlined in Anderson's[35] model in children with ischemic or hemorrhagic stroke ($n = 28$). Specifically, children with stroke performed significantly worse ($P < 0.05$) than the normative population on attentional control, cognitive flexibility, and information processing.[36] However, it is important to note that, despite these significant group differences, the mean scores of children with stroke generally fell within the low end of the average range.[36] Moreover, elevated levels of everyday EF dysfunction were common, with 25% of parent ratings on the Behavioral Regulation, Metacognition, and Global Executive Composite Indices on the Behavior Rating of Executive Function (BRIEF) falling in the clinical range (ie, T score ≥ 65) and 25% to 61% of teacher ratings reaching the clinical range on these composite measures.[36] A separate analysis conducted by Long et al[37] in the same sample of children revealed that these EF difficulties were present irrespective of lesion location (ie, frontal vs extrafrontal, cortical vs subcortical), thereby highlighting

TABLE 9-4. DIFFICULTIES ASSOCIATED WITH SPECIFIC EXECUTIVE FUNCTION DEFICITS	
EXECUTIVE FUNCTIONS	**ASSOCIATED DIFFICULTIES**
Planning	Goal setting, breaking large tasks into individual chunks, formulating a step-by-step plan, tendency to become overwhelmed by large tasks
Organization	Messiness (eg, desk, room, closet), tendency to misplace belongings
Time management	Following a timeline, estimating how long it will take to complete tasks, prioritizing importance of tasks and devoting time accordingly
Metacognition	Error monitoring, knowing when to seek help, insight into personal strengths/weaknesses, evaluating own performance
Inhibition	Interrupting others, inappropriate comments during social interactions
Self-regulation	Low frustration tolerance, easily upset
Initiation	Getting started on tasks
Flexibility	Getting stuck on one approach, adapting to change, thinking creatively when problem solving, reliance on routines

the wide network of brain regions implicated in EF (noted earlier). After comparing a sample of Mexican youth with hemophilia with ($n=10$) and without ($n=6$) intracranial hemorrhage and healthy controls ($n=10$), Morales et al[38] documented impaired performance in the children with intracranial hemorrhage on measures of cognitive flexibility and planning, with 40% to 70% achieving scores below average on these measures compared to 16.7% to 50% of children with hemophilia alone and 10% to 40% of controls. Of note, caution is warranted in interpreting these findings, as it is unclear as to whether or not they extend to children with stroke without hemophilia. Finally, impairments in inhibitory control[12] and phonemic fluency[39] have also been documented in children with stroke. In contrast, others have failed to find evidence for EF dysfunction in this population.[11,27] Overall, evidence points to the presence of diffuse EF dysfunction in children with stroke relative to normative samples, regardless of lesion location.

Working Memory

Working memory is the mental system that allows us to keep information active for a brief amount of time while performing a task. The multicomponent model proposed by Baddeley and Hitch[40] and later extended by Baddeley[41] has been one of the most influential models of working memory to date. The original model put forward by Baddeley and Hitch[40] consists of 3 components. The phonological loop refers to the storage and rehearsal mechanisms of verbal material, whereas the visuospatial sketchpad represents a similar system that is specialized for the storage and processing of visual information.[40] Collectively, the visuospatial sketchpad and the phonological loop are conceived of as *slave systems* that subserve the central executive.[40] The central executive component is responsible for the activation

of long-term memory and the coordination between the phonological loop and the visuospatial sketchpad.[40] In the latest revision of the model, Baddeley[41] proposed that the working memory system consists of a fourth component—the episodic buffer. This component is responsible for integrating the separate components of working memory and long-term memory into a single representation.[41]

Several studies in adults indicate that working memory is compromised following stroke.[42-44] Moreover, hemispheric side and lesion location are associated with different working memory deficits. Left cortical damage has been shown to result in impairment in the phonological loop.[43,44] Conversely, right cortical damage results in deficits in both the phonological loop and visuospatial sketchpad, thus indicating the critical role of the right cortex for multimodal working memory processes.[43]

In contrast, much less is known about the consequences of pediatric stroke on working memory performance. Emerging evidence indicates that children with stroke demonstrate subtle working memory difficulties, with performance typically falling within the low-average range.[8,26,45,46] These subtle deficits are associated with younger age at stroke[8,26] and are reported to emerge during the school years.[45] Different lesion locations may result in different patterns of working memory performance in children. For example, White et al[47] found differential patterns of working memory among children with anterior ($n=4$), posterior ($n=4$), and diffuse ($n=12$) infarcts secondary to SCD after examining performance on a word span task. Specifically, children with anterior infarcts demonstrated a reduced word length effect (ie, performance did not improve with shorter words), despite the fact that their overall memory span was not significantly different from controls.[47] Children with diffuse infarcts recalled fewer words but showed an intact word length effect.[47] In contrast, the performance of children with posterior infarcts was comparable to controls.[47] White et al[47] hypothesized that anterior infarcts caused dysfunction in the phonological loop and diffuse infarcts impaired the central executive. Of note, these findings are difficult to interpret because the sample of participants with stroke was small and composed only of children with stroke secondary to SCD, a condition characterized by multiple and silent infarcts. Finally, in the first study to date to systematically asses the 3 components of the working memory model proposed by Baddeley and Hitch[40] in children with stroke, Fuentes[46] reported significantly lower performance in children with AIS ($n = 32$) relative to healthy controls ($n = 32$) on the phonological loop ($P = 0.001$), visuospatial sketchpad ($P = 0.005$), and the verbal ($P = 0.017$) and visual ($P = 0.023$) aspects of the central executive (as assessed by the Working Memory Test Battery for Children [WMTB-C]). Further, these results were corroborated by parent reports indicating significantly more working memory dysfunction in everyday life (as assessed by the BRIEF) in children with AIS compared to controls ($P < 0.001$).[46] Of note, despite these significant group differences, children with stroke consistently performed within the average range (range of mean composite scores on the WMTB-C = 90.3 to 98.5 and mean T score on the BRIEF = 61.6).[46] These results indicate that children with stroke are at risk for developing subtle challenges in all 3 components of working memory, but not to the extent that they would be considered impaired. In everyday life, these subtle working memory difficulties may be evinced by struggles with following multistep directions, multitasking, mental arithmetic, incomplete or inaccurate recall of information, etc.

Social Cognition

Although social cognition is a broad construct encompassing many abilities, there is a general consensus that it refers to the "ability to construct representations of the relation between oneself and others and to use those representations flexibly to guide social behaviour."[48] The sociocognitive integration of abilities (SOCIAL) model proposed by Beauchamp and Anderson[49] provides a useful developmental framework for understanding social cognition by highlighting its biological, psychological, and environmental underpinnings. The model identifies 3 core types of cognitive abilities underlying social behavior: 1) attention-executive (ie, higher-order thinking abilities such as attentional control, working memory, goal setting, problem solving, planning); 2) communication (ie, abilities that allow individuals to understand and express messages in social interactions); and, 3) socioemotional (ie, affective processes such as face/emotion perception, intent attribution, theory of mind, moral reasoning).[49] The emergence of these core cognitive abilities is mediated by internal and external factors (eg, personality and temperament, physical attributes, family function, SES, culture) and brain development.[49] Many brain regions are implicated in social cognition, with the amygdala, basal ganglia, insula, and superior temporal sulcus being particularly of note for their roles in encoding social information and the prefrontal cortex being crucial for its role in the higher-order thinking skills involved (for review, see Yeates et al[50]). Essentially, it follows from the SOCIAL model[49] that the emergence of the cognitive functions required for successful social outcomes relies on normal brain development within an optimal environment. Table 9-5 presents examples of difficulties associated with specific social impairments in the SOCIAL model.[49]

Although there is a paucity of research examining social outcomes following pediatric stroke, previous studies indicate subtle deficits in this domain.[46,51-55] In particular, evidence points to difficulties in social information processing (SIP) following pediatric stroke.[46,51,52] Crick and Dodge[56] conceive of SIP as a form of "on-line brain performance" consisting of 6 problem-solving steps: encoding, interpretation, clarification of goals, response construction, response decision, and enactment. Previous studies suggest that children's SIP following stroke is marked by subtle difficulties in the first 2 steps of Crick and Dodge's[56] model: encoding and interpretation. For example, Ballantyne and Trauner[51] observed subtle deficits in facial recognition in children and adolescents with prenatal or perinatal stroke ($n = 40$) relative to controls ($n = 40$), regardless of hemispheric side of the lesion ($P = 0.003$). Right and left parietal lobe involvement was found to correlate with worse facial recognition performance, thus highlighting the pivotal role of this region for facial discrimination early in development.[51] Boni et al[52] similarly found that children with stroke secondary to SCD ($n = 21$) performed worse on measures of facial and vocal social cue encoding compared to children with SCD without stroke ($n = 31$). Closer examination of the patterns of performance revealed that the stroke group performed worse when social cues were ambiguous.[52] Conversely, children with stroke achieved greater success when the social situations were straightforward and well-learned.[52] In the first study to date to systematically examine all 6 steps of SIP in children with unilateral AIS ($n = 32$), Fuentes[46] discovered isolated difficulties in social cue encoding and decoding relative to healthy controls ($n = 32$). Specifically, children with AIS exhibited significantly lower ($P = 0.007$) encoding scores on an experimental structured interview measure of SIP involving 4 video vignettes of children in ambiguous social situations.[46] Further, children with AIS demonstrated significantly lower performance than controls on an experimental facial decoding measure ($P = 0.029$).[46] In contrast, children with AIS performed similarly to controls across the remaining steps of the Crick and Dodge[56] model, and no significant differences were found on parent ratings of social skills.[46]

TABLE 9-5. DIFFICULTIES ASSOCIATED WITH DEFICITS IN COMPONENTS OF THE SOCIAL MODEL[50]	
SOCIAL COMPONENT	ASSOCIATED DIFFICULTIES
Attention-executive	Attending to social cues, impulsivity, generating and carrying out strategies to solve social dilemmas, responding to feedback, regulating affect, monitoring own responses in social responses, inhibiting inappropriate responses
Communication	Joint attention, expressive language, receptive language, interpreting nonverbal forms of communications (eg, body language)
Socioemotional	Interpreting facial expressions, recognizing faces, identifying attributions and perspectives of others (ie, theory of mind), moral reasoning, empathy

Studies utilizing questionnaire measures to assess social outcomes following pediatric stroke also indicate subtle difficulties. For example, Trauner et al[53] documented that children with perinatal stroke were rated by parents as having more social impairments compared to controls on the Personality Inventory for Children. Similarly, studies examining quality of life in children with stroke have documented lower socialization scores compared to normative samples.[57,58] A recent prospective study of quality of life in children with ischemic stroke (AIS or CSVT) sustained in the neonatal period ($n = 34$) or after 1 year of age ($n = 78$) revealed poor quality of life in 17.8% of children with histories of stroke, particularly in relation to school and play; however, mean scores fell within the adequate range.[54] Deficits in cognitive/behavioral functioning and low verbal IQ predicted poorer quality of life and socialization.[54] In contrast, Lo et al[59] failed to detect significant differences in children with neonatal or childhood AIS ($n = 36$) and controls with asthma ($n = 15$) on parent reports of social participation, social adjustment, and social problems; however, higher IQ correlated with fewer social adjustment problems. The study conducted by Everts et al[14] also showed that self-reported ratings of autonomy and social acceptance were more frequently below the normal range compared to the normative sample. Unlike adults, the hemispheric side of the lesion may not correlate with social functioning following pediatric stroke. In a study pairing adults and children with similar unilateral stroke lesions ($n = 29$ adult–child pairs), Mosch et al[55] found laterality effects in caregiver ratings of social functioning of adults but not children. Adults with right hemisphere lesions showed significantly worse social functioning compared to adults with left hemisphere lesions.[55] In contrast, children showed mild to moderate deficits in social functioning, regardless of lesion location.[55] Taken together, these findings suggest that children with histories of stroke are at increased risk for developing social difficulties. It will be crucial for future studies to conduct more detailed analyses of the precise nature of these social impairments and to examine this in relation to lesion characteristics and age at injury.

FACTORS INFLUENCING COGNITIVE OUTCOMES

Demographic Variables

Age at Stroke

Contrary to the previous proposal that the immature brain is more resilient to damage due to increased plasticity allowing for the redistribution of cognitive functions to undamaged regions (ie, plasticity hypothesis), evidence suggests that the immature brain is in fact more vulnerable to damage to the resulting disruption of cerebral development (ie, early vulnerability hypothesis). Studies show that children with histories of stroke sustained before 1 year of age exhibit worse cognitive outcomes compared to children with histories of stroke sustained later in childhood.[8,9,26,39,60] For example, Westmacott et al[8] showed that children with unilateral AIS sustained during the perinatal period ($n = 46$) exhibited significantly lower verbal reasoning than children who suffered stroke during early childhood (ie, between 1 month and 5 years; $n = 57$) or late childhood (ie, between 6 and 16 years; $n = 42$). Moreover, working memory and overall intellectual functioning indices were also significantly lower (all $P < 0.05$) in the perinatal group than the late childhood group.[8] Similarly, Studer et al[9] found that children with early AIS (ie, sustained between 1 month and 2 years, 11 months; $n = 24$) performed significantly worse across all intelligence measures compared to the preschool (ie, AIS sustained between 3 years and 5 years, 11 months; $n = 22$), middle childhood (ie, AIS sustained between 6 years and 9 years, 11 months; $n = 22$), and late childhood (ie, AIS sustained after age 10; $n = 31$) groups. In addition, a retrospective analysis of the neuropsychological sequelae of children with unilateral AIS revealed that children who suffered a stroke between 1 month and 1 year ($n = 12$) were significantly ($P < 0.05$) more impaired on nonverbal reasoning indices on the age-appropriate Wechsler scales than children who suffered a stroke between 1 and 6 years ($n=11$) or 6 to 16 years ($n=21$).[39] In the study of verbal learning and memory conducted by Lansing et al,[26] children who experienced a stroke before one year of age ($n=16$) performed worse on the long-delay free recall ($P<0.05$, Cohen's $d=-1.01$) and discriminability ($P=0.05$, Cohen's $d=-0.69$) indices of the CVLT-C than children who experienced stroke after 1 year of age ($n=10$). After examining group differences among controls and children with early stroke (ie, stroke before 1 year of age, $n=17$),"late stroke (ie, stroke after 1 year of age, $n=12$), and orthopedic controls ($n=29$), Max et al[60] reported larger group differences (in favor of controls) for the early stroke group compared to the late stroke group, with large effect sizes (Cohen's $d\geq0.80$) for written expression, visual-spatial processing, and memory; medium effect sizes (Cohen's $d=0.50$ to 0.79) for reading, spelling, and language; and small effect sizes (Cohen's $d=0.20$ to 0.49) for intellectual functioning, arithmetic, and working memory. Of concern, the early stroke group also had a higher number of psychiatric diagnoses than the late stroke group (Cohen's $d=0.37$).[60] This collection of findings indicates that children with early stroke represent a high-risk subgroup for cognitive deficits.

Emerging evidence indicates that the *early vulnerability hypothesis* may not relate linearly to all cognitive outcomes, such that there is a protective effect for strokes occurring during midchildhood.[14,39,46] For example, Allman and Scott[39] found that children who experienced stroke during midchildhood (ie, between 1 and 6 years) exhibited higher verbal reasoning than children who experienced stroke during infancy (ie, before 1 year of age) or late childhood (ie, between 6 and 16 years) (both $P<0.01$). Moreover, unlike the infancy and late childhood groups, the verbal, nonverbal, working memory, and processing speed indices of the age-appropriate Wechsler scales were not significantly lower in the midchildhood stroke group compared to the normative sample.[39] Similar findings were found in the memory domain, with only the infancy and late childhood groups demonstrating significantly lower performance across a number of indices on the Children's Memory Scale (CMS) and the CVLT-C compared to the normative sample.[39] Everts et al[14] also reported a trend toward better visual-spatial reasoning in children who experienced a stroke between 5 and 10 years compared to children who experienced a stroke before age 5 or between 10 and 18 years. After conducting a retrospective analysis of parent ratings of social skills (as assessed by the Behavior Assessment System for Children, second edition [BASC-2]) of a large sample of children with unilateral AIS ($n=129$), Fuentes[46] also found partial support for a protective effect of midchildhood stroke, as children with a stroke sustained between 1 month and 5 years ($n=53$) were rated more favorably than children with a stroke sustained between 6 and 14 years ($n=20$, $P=0.040$); however, significant differences were not found between children with perinatal

stroke ($n=56$) and the other 2 groups. Researchers suggest that the capacity for reorganization in the immature brain is not realized very early in development due to the rapid changes in brain development occurring during this time.[8,14] Moreover, early injury is thought to disrupt the course of myelination, particularly in the frontal lobes, thereby rendering the developing brain less capable of supporting higher-level cognitive skills.[31] Conversely, although brain networks may be less vulnerable in the older brain, the potential for plasticity is also lower.[39] Of note, it remains unclear as to the precise age range associated with the most optimal cognitive outcomes, as the findings reported by Allman and Scott[39] indicate that the best outcomes are found in children with a stroke occurring between 1 and 5 years, whereas those reported by Everts et al[14] report that the best outcomes are associated with a stroke occurring between 5 and 10 years. Further, new data point to an interaction between age at stroke and lesion location.[8] More specifically, Westmacott et al[8] discovered that cortical and subcortical lesions were associated with different periods of peak vulnerability, with children with subcortical lesions sustained during the perinatal period showing worse intellectual outcomes compared to children with subcortical lesions sustained between 1 month and 5 years and 6 to 14 years, and children with cortical strokes sustained between 1 month and 5 years showing worse intellectual outcomes than children with cortical strokes sustained during the perinatal period and between 6 and 16 years. Taken together, these findings suggest that although the early vulnerability hypothesis holds true when comparing children with early stroke (ie, before age 1) to children with stroke sustained later in childhood (ie, after age 1), it does not apply when comparing children with stroke sustained in midchildhood and children with stroke sustained in later childhood. That is, evidence points to a nonlinear relationship between age at stroke and cognitive outcomes that is moderated by lesion location.

Time Since Stroke

The influences of time since stroke remain unclear, as some studies report the emergence of deficits in school age,[45,61] whereas others report stability[10,62] or improvements[14] in cognitive outcomes over time. Westmacott et al's[45] longitudinal analysis of cognitive outcomes in children with unilateral neonatal AIS ($n=26$) revealed the emergence of deficits between preschool and school age. More specifically, 69% of children exhibited a decline in one or more indices between preschool and school age and, unlike the preschool period, demonstrated significantly lower performance than the normative sample on overall intelligence ($P<0.01$), working memory ($P<0.01$), processing speed ($P<0.01$), and perceptual reasoning ($P<0.05$) indices at school age.[45] Similarly, Levine et al's[61] longitudinal analysis of children with early (ie, before 1 year of age) unilateral stroke ($n=15$) found a decrease in intelligence scores over time, regardless of lesion laterality or seizure status. It is important to note that these data reflect the emergence of difficulties in higher-order cognitive functions over time, as opposed to a worsening or plateauing in cognitive functioning over time. In contrast, neither Ballantyne et al[10] or Aram and Eisele[62] detected discrepancies between test–retest intervals in children with stroke on a range of intelligence, academic, and language measures. Complicating matters further, Everts et al[14] detected a trend toward better cognitive functioning with stroke occurrence more than 5 years before the assessment. It is possible that differences in sample characteristics may have led to the conflicting findings. For example, several of the studies included children with histories of seizure disorders,[10,61] whereas others excluded children with neurological comorbidities.[45,62] The test–retest intervals also varied between studies, with the minimum time between assessments ranging from 6 months[62] to 18 months[8,45,61] and the maximum time ranging from about 8 years[10,45,62] to 15 years.[61] Clearly, the conflicting findings pertaining to the influence of time since stroke limit the clinician's ability to prognosticate about cognitive outcomes following pediatric stroke and warrant further investigation. It is likely that the influence of time since stroke depends on a host of other factors, such as the cognitive domain being assessed, stroke subtype, lesion characteristics, and neurological characteristics.

Sex

Previous studies indicate that pediatric stroke is sex dimorphic in terms of prevalence, with males showing a predominance.[63-65] However, the possibility of sex dimorphism with respect to cognitive outcomes following pediatric stroke remains unknown, as few studies examining sex differences in this population have been conducted, and those that have yielded conflicting results. For example, the longitudinal analysis conducted by Westmacott et al[45] indicated that males with neonatal AIS displayed a greater decline than females in nonverbal ability between preschool and school age ($P = 0.01$) and were trending toward a greater decline in overall intellectual functioning ($P = 0.19$). In contrast, sex differences were not found in the large sample ($n = 635$) of children and adults with focal lesions analyzed by Braun et al[66] However, males were found to be more likely than females to suffer epilepsy as a complication following brain injury.[66] Interestingly, an interaction between lesion laterality and sex was found for verbal ability, with left hemisphere damage being associated with higher verbal ability in females and right hemisphere damage being associated with higher verbal ability in males.[66] Although more work is needed to elucidate the influence of sex on cognitive outcomes, the data thus far indicate that this factor represents yet another variable in which the specific impact depends on the cognitive domain in question and the lesion location.

Lesion Characteristics

Lesion Location

Combined cortical-subcortical lesions have been shown to be more detrimental to cognitive outcomes compared to cortical or subcortical lesions alone.[8,9,12,59] For example, Hajek et al[12] found that, unlike children with cortical or subcortical lesions, children with combined lesions exhibited worse inhibitory control than children with asthma (Cohen's $d = 0.68$). Regression analyses also showed that combined lesions accounted for a significant proportion of variance in processing speed outcomes, but only once neurological impairment was included in the analysis.[12] Further, both Westmacott et al[8] and Studer et al[9] found that children with combined lesions performed more poorly than children with cortical or subcortical lesions across all intelligence indices. In contrast, the correlational analyses conducted by Lo et al[59] revealed an association between combined lesions and poorer adaptive, but not intellectual, functioning.

Anterior and posterior lesions have been linked with differential social outcomes in children with stroke. For example, Trauner et al[53] found that children with non-frontal lesions ($n = 7$) were rated less favorably by parents on social competence compared to controls ($n = 23$) and children with frontal lesions ($n = 10$, $P = 0.0002$). On the other hand, children with frontal lesions were rated as having the highest amount of cognitive dysfunction ($P < 0.0001$).[53] Children with perinatal stroke involving the parietal lobe have also been found to demonstrate significantly ($P = 0.046$) poorer facial recognition skills compared to children with lesions involving the frontal, temporal, or occipital lobes.[51] Taken together, these findings indicate that combined cortical-subcortical lesions represent a risk factor for compromised intellectual outcomes following pediatric stroke, whereas posterior lesions render children vulnerable to social impairments.

Lesion Laterality

As previously discussed, laterality effects have been well-documented in visuospatial processing following pediatric stroke.[16-21] Conversely, research indicates that these laterality effects do not extend to other cognitive domains, including intellectual functioning,[8,10,14,61] facial recognition skills,[51] verbal learning and memory,[25,26] and social functioning.[53,55] The 2 exceptions appear to be the studies conducted by Allman and Scott[39] and Aram and Eisele.[62] More specifically, Allman and Scott[39] found that children with left hemisphere lesions ($n = 21$) exhibited poorer working memory ($P < 0.05$), delayed verbal memory ($P < 0.01$), and receptive language ($P < 0.05$) performance compared to children with right hemisphere lesions ($n = 18$). However, further analysis examining these effects according to age at stroke (ie, before age 1, 1 to 6 years, 6 to 16 years) revealed that laterality effects were present only in children with stroke occurring before age 1, with children with left hemisphere damage performing more poorly than children with right hemisphere damage on measures of perceptual reasoning and processing speed (both $P < 0.05$).[39] In contrast, Aram and Eisele[62] found that children with right hemisphere lesions ($n = 8$) exhibited worse intellectual outcomes than children with left hemisphere lesions ($n = 18$). These discrepancies highlight the need for further investigation of laterality effects following pediatric stroke, with a focus on examining the possible interaction between hemispheric side of the lesion and age at injury.

Lesion Volume

Not surprisingly, findings generally point to a deleterious effect of large lesion volume on cognitive outcomes following pediatric stroke.[12,14,36,59,61,67] More specifically, associations have been reported between larger lesion volume and poorer processing speed,[14] intellectual functioning,[12,59,61] executive functioning,[36] and quality of life.[36,37] However, the effect of lesion volume does not appear to be straightforward, as evidence indicates that it is mediated by neurological impairment[12] and time since stroke.[61] Moreover, new findings suggest the presence of a threshold effect (ie, cognitive impairment occurs after reaching or surpassing a specific lesion volume).[67] Evidence regarding the mediating effects of neurological impairment on the relationship between lesion volume and cognitive outcomes stems from findings reported by Hajek et al,[12] in which lesion volume was found to account for a significant proportion of variance ($R^2 = 0.35$) on processing speed measures only after neurological impairment was included in the hierarchical regression model. Findings reported by Levine et al[61] point to similar mediating effects for time since stroke on the relationship between lesion volume and cognitive outcomes, with larger lesions being associated with more impairing, immediate, and stable cognitive deficits and smaller lesions being associated with milder cognitive deficits that emerge over time. Finally, Lo et al[67] found that hemorrhages greater than 4% of cerebral volume predicted poorer outcomes, indicating the presence of a threshold effect. Of note, it is unclear as to whether or not a threshold effect may be present for pediatric ischemic stroke. Overall, these findings indicate that larger lesion volume is a risk factor for worse cognitive outcomes following pediatric stroke.

Neurological and Cognitive Impairment

Previous studies indicate that persisting neurological deficits are correlated with worse cognitive, social, and adaptive outcomes following pediatric stroke.[9,12,39,59] For example, Allman and Scott's[39] retrospective analysis of children with unilateral AIS showed that children with neurological deficits such as hemiplegia and visual field deficits ($n = 19$) performed worse than children without neurological deficits ($n = 25$) on all 5 indices of the age-appropriate Wechsler scales, as well as immediate and delayed verbal memory, delayed visual memory, and visual-spatial recall. Similar findings were reported by Studer et al[9] after comparing intellectual outcomes among children with ($n = 31$) and without neurological impairment ($n = 39$). In addition, inverse correlations have been found between scores on the Pediatric Stroke Outcome Measure and expressive vocabulary and psychomotor expression in children with perinatal or childhood AIS.[12] Moreover, children with neurological impairment have been found to fare worse than children with low-severity stroke on social and adaptive measures.[59]

Not surprisingly, cognitive impairment itself is a risk factor for poor social adjustment and quality of life.[54,59] For example, Lo et al[59] reported a significant negative correlation between the Social Problems subscale of the Child Behavior Checklist (CBCL) and FSIQ ($r = -0.377$, $P = 0.030$) in children with AIS. Similarly, cognitive impairment was identified as an important predictor of quality of life (assessed using the Center for Health Promotion's Quality of Life Profile) in a large ($n = 112$) prospective study of children with ischemic stroke, accounting for more than 50% of the variance in this domain.[54] Further, cognitive impairment was found to be most detrimental to quality of life for older children and females.[54] These findings suggest that neurological and cognitive impairment represent reliable markers of risk for negative cognitive and social outcomes following pediatric stroke.

Seizure Disorders

The negative consequences of seizure disorders on cognitive outcomes have been well documented in the pediatric stroke literature.[1,9-12,68] For example, children who evince epilepsy as a consequence of stroke have consistently been shown to demonstrate worse overall intellectual functioning[9-11] and show less cognitive improvements over time[10] compared to children without seizure disorders. Epilepsy appears to be particularly common in children with presumed perinatal stroke (ie, diagnosis is made retrospectively after the child displays neurological symptoms and imaging reveals remote infarct).[68] For example, a retrospective analysis of children with presumed perinatal stroke ($n = 45$) documented epilepsy in 38% of the sample, which was significantly correlated with cognitive disability ($P = 0.05$).[68] These data suggest that children who suffer epilepsy as a complication of stroke represent another high-risk subgroup for cognitive sequelae and that children with presumed perinatal stroke are particularly vulnerable to this complication.

ROLE OF NEUROPSYCHOLOGICAL ASSESSMENT IN PEDIATRIC STROKE

Clinical neuropsychology is defined as the "applied science that examines the impact of both normal and abnormal brain functioning on a broad range of cognitive, emotional, and behavioral functions."[69] A pediatric neuropsychologist is a licensed psychologist with training in the neurological bases of behavior.[69] A key role of the pediatric neuropsychologist is to conduct a neuropsychological assessment, interpret the results, and communicate the findings to the child (when appropriate) and those involved in the child's care. A neuropsychological assessment consists of formal testing designed to measure a broad range of functioning, including intelligence, language, visual-spatial abilities, memory and learning, attention, executive functioning, academic performance, and social-emotional functioning. In addition, the neuropsychologist gathers information about the child's history through the review of available reports (eg, report cards, previous evaluations); medical records; and interviews with the child, caregivers, and teachers (when possible). The primary aims of the neuropsychological assessment include 1) describing cognitive functioning, 2) assisting in diagnosis, 3) documenting and monitoring neurocognitive development, and 4) assisting with treatment and academic planning.[70] The results arising from the neuropsychological assessment are documented in a written report and communicated to the child, family, interdisciplinary team members, and school personnel. The neuropsychological assessment acts as a foundation for understanding the child's brain-related patterns of cognitive strengths and weaknesses.[70] This information is used to determine whether or not the child meets the criteria for specific learning, neurodevelopmental, or behavioral disorders (eg, intellectual disabilities, ADHD, learning disorders, depressive disorders, anxiety disorders, disruptive/conduct disorders). In addition, this information acts as a basis for designing interventions, developing individualized education programs (IEPs), and monitoring treatment efficacy. To this end, the results arising out of the neuropsychological assessment are crucial for determining a baseline of cognitive functioning and documenting development over time. The selection of test measures depends on the referral question, child's age, time since stroke, whether or not the assessment is intended as a baseline or follow-up, and presence or absence of persisting neurological impairment (eg, vision problems, motor difficulties). Table 9-6 provides a list of domains that should be assessed and recommended test measures (language and academic domains are excluded, as they are reviewed in Chapters 8 and 13, respectively).

Several key considerations are unique to the assessment of children with histories of stroke. First, it is paramount that the pediatric neuropsychologist has a solid understanding of the neuropsychological sequelae commonly associated with pediatric stroke. As previously discussed, pediatric stroke is associated with subtle deficits in a broad range of domains, including intellectual functioning, visual-spatial processing, memory and learning, attention, executive functioning, working memory, and social cognition. Second, the pediatric neuropsychologist must have a strong understanding of the multiple factors influencing cognitive outcomes following pediatric stroke. More specifically, the effects of age at stroke, time since stroke/age at assessment, lesion characteristics (location, laterality, volume), sex, presence of seizures, and presence of persisting neurological deficits on cognitive outcomes must be taken into account. To this end, reflection must be given to the interactive effects that exist among these factors. In addition, consideration must be given to any comorbid medical conditions. In this way, assessment is guided by a broad working knowledge of the neuropsychological profile associated with pediatric stroke and the unique demographic and neurological characteristics of the child. Third, the pediatric neuropsychologist must be equipped to translate this information within the context of assessment findings in a way that is easily accessible to families, school personnel, and interdisciplinary team members. In particular, special emphasis should be placed on the ways in which the area of the brain damaged by the stroke relates to learning and behavior and the impact on development. Fourth, given the limited awareness concerning stroke in childhood, the pediatric neuropsychologist must be prepared to act as an advocate on behalf of the child by educating others involved in his or her care about stroke and the unique needs of the child. Finally, it is imperative that the pediatric neuropsychologist have an appreciation of the evolving nature of the neurocognitive profiles evinced by children with stroke throughout development. In practice, this entails following the child over time and acting as a consultant when needed, carrying out sequential assessments, and updating treatment plans and recommendations. Of note, the intervals between assessments often vary depending on the clinical setting; however, it is recommended that follow-up assessments be completed during key transition periods (eg, 6 months poststroke, 1 to 2 years poststroke, entry to high school, entry to postsecondary school).

REHABILITATION STRATEGIES TO IMPROVE COGNITIVE FUNCTION

A useful Pediatric Neurocognitive Interventions (PNI) model was recently developed by Limond et al[71] to guide clinicians in the planning and implementation of cognitive rehabilitation strategies for children with acquired brain injury (ABI). The model emphasizes the role of cognitive development in intervention planning.[71] Accordingly, a

DOMAIN	RECOMMENDED MEASURES
	TABLE 9-6. RECOMMENDED MEASURES IN THE NEUROPSYCHOLOGICAL ASSESSMENT OF CHILDREN WITH STROKE
Intellectual functioning	• Wechsler Intelligence Scale for Children, Fourth Edition • Wechsler Preschool and Primary Scale of Intelligence, Fourth Edition • Wechsler Adult Intelligence Scale, Fourth Edition • Stanford Binet Intelligence Scales, Fifth Edition
Visual-spatial processing	• Beery-Buktenica Developmental Test of Visual-Motor Integration, Sixth Edition • Rey-Osterrieth Complex Figure Test • Test of Visual Perceptual Skills, Third Edition • Judgment of Line Orientation
Memory and learning	• CVLT-C • CMS • Wide Range Assessment of Memory and Learning, Second Edition
Attention	• The Test of Everyday Attention for Children • Conners' Continuous Performance Test, Second Edition • Conners' Rating Scales, Third Edition
Executive functioning	• Delis-Kaplan Executive Function System • A Developmental NEuroPSYcological Assessment, Second Edition • Wisconsin Card Sorting Test • Children's Category Test • BRIEF
Working memory	• Working Memory Test Battery for Children
Social-emotional functioning	• CBCL • Teacher Report Form • Youth Self-Report • BASC-2
Adaptive functioning	• Adaptive Behavior Assessment System, Second Edition • Vineland Adaptive Behavior Scale, Second Edition

sequential bottom-up approach to intervention that aligns with cognitive development is proposed.[71] Psychosocial factors that take into account the child's social and family environment form the foundation of the model and are deemed to be a prerequisite for successful PNI.[71] That is, Limond et al[71] emphasize the need to continually monitor and manage issues such as family stability, parenting skills, mental health needs of the child and family, sensory impairments, and health needs. The model then outlines 4 sequential levels of interventions: A) compensatory strategies to develop semantic knowledge and adaptive functioning, B) remediation of core cognitive skills, C) developing and supporting evaluation skills, and D) independent strategies for specific cognitive impairments.[71] At the lowest level, caregivers are encouraged to assist children through prompting/cued support with utilizing compensatory strategies such as precision teaching, errorless learning, elaborative encoding, and rehearsal.[71] Level B entails targeting core cognitive skills (eg, working memory, processing speed, inhibitory control, sequencing) through intensive practice.[71] In practice, this may entail engaging children in computerized remediation training programs.[71] Level C involves assisting children with developing evaluation skills (eg, metacognition, supervisory processes, reasoning) through training in goal management skills, prospective reminding, and

TABLE 9-7. COGNITIVE REHABILITATION STRATEGIES[71-76]

DOMAIN	INTERVENTION STRATEGIES/ACTIVITIES
Visuospatial processing	Puzzles, object flashcards, building blocks/Lego (The Lego Group), visual memory games, visual perceptual games
Memory and learning	External aids to prompt memory, mnemonic strategies (eg, visual imagery, chunking, elaborative rehearsal), metacognitive strategies, individualized memory notebook
Attention	Attention process training, cognitive behavioral strategies to reduce distractibility
Executive functioning	Organizational aids, creation of step-by-step plans, pictorial cues, graphic organizers, breaking tasks into smaller components, external cues to monitor progress, teaching problem-solving steps (eg, identify problem, goal, relevant information, identify possible solutions, evaluate solutions, make a decision, create a plan, monitor and evaluate), structured routine
Working memory	Computerized working memory training
Social cognition	Web-based cognitive-behavioral therapy, Building Friendships process, art therapy, functional communication training, online Family Problem Solving, Pediatric Acquired Brain Injury Community Outreach Program, socialization/community group, self-advocacy group

self-regulation.[71] At the highest level, persisting cognitive deficits (eg, episodic memory, visual-spatial processing) are targeted through specific strategies.[71] Overall, the PNI model proposed by Limond et al[71] provides a means for developing and organizing cognitive intervention goals that effectively address the developmental needs of the child and family.

No studies have specifically examined the efficacy of cognitive intervention programs in children with histories of stroke. Moreover, the literature on cognitive rehabilitation programs in the pediatric brain injury population at large is also minimal. However, reviews of the literature have highlighted a number of cognitive rehabilitation strategies that may be applicable to the treatment of children with stroke.[72-77] Of note, studies consistently highlight the importance of educating and involving the family in cognitive interventions. Although a full discussion of the cognitive rehabilitation literature in the pediatric ABI population is beyond the scope of this chapter, a list of recommended cognitive intervention strategies stemming from these reviews is provided in Table 9-7 in an effort to guide clinicians and families.

SUMMARY

Data on cognitive and behavioral outcomes in children with histories of stroke show that this population experiences subtle deficits in overall intellectual functioning, visual-spatial processing, memory and learning, attention, executive functioning, working memory, and social cognition. Studies of intellectual functioning suggest that children with stroke generally perform in the low end of the average range, although compromised compared to normative samples.[8-14,39,45,60] Children with histories of stroke demonstrate subtle, lateralized deficits in visual-spatial processing.[16-21] Specifically, evidence has been found for a double-dissociation in global-local processing in perinatal stroke, with right hemisphere damage resulting in global processing deficits and left hemisphere damage resulting in local processing deficits.[19-21] In contrast, verbal memory and learning profiles in children with stroke are marked by subtle, nonlateralized deficits.[25-28] A high incidence of attentional difficulties has also been documented in children with stroke, and reports indicate that these difficulties often go hand in hand with academic and social impairments.[27,30-33] Similarly, emerging evidence points to compromised EF following pediatric stroke.[12,36-39] Working memory represents an EF domain of particular concern, as subtle difficulties have been documented in all 3 components (ie, phonological loop, visuospatial sketchpad, central executive) of Baddeley and Hitch's[40] theoretical model.[8,26,45,46] Finally, a growing body of evidence indicates that subtle difficulties in social cognition are a common consequence of pediatric stroke.[46,51-55]

FAMILY FOCUS BOX

1. The cognitive difficulties exhibited by children following stroke are subtle and influenced by a range of demographic and stroke factors.

2. Cognitive outcomes following pediatric stroke depend on the following: 1) age of the child at the time of the stroke; 2) amount of time that has passed since the stroke; 3) age of the child at the time of the assessment; 4) sex of the child; 5) the size, side, and specific location of the brain region damaged by the stroke; 6) presence of persisting neurological impairment; and 7) presence of seizures

3. Neuropsychological assessments are an important tool for better understanding the child's cognitive strengths and weaknesses, academic planning, and cognitive rehabilitation.

4. Cognitive interventions for children with histories of stroke must involve the family and take into account developmental factors.

CASE STUDIES

Case #1: Difficulties With Visual-Motor Development, Attention, and Working Memory Following Perinatal Stroke

Reason for Referral

- Four-year-old girl (M) with history of left hemisphere perinatal stroke associated with right-side hemiparesis
- Referred for neuropsychological assessment to evaluate cognitive abilities and assist with academic planning

Background

- M and twin sister born at 35 weeks' gestation by emergency C-section due to concerns about blood flow in umbilical artery for twin B (M)
- Birth weight = 3 lbs, 5 oz
- Early left hand preference observed at 6 months
- Brain magnetic resonance imaging (MRI) at age 1 revealed remote infarct involving left middle cerebral artery (MCA) (area of damage = left frontal, parietal, and temporal cortex; parts of left basal ganglia and thalamus)
- Moderate right hemiparesis
- Some visual field loss in upper right quadrant
- No other medical concerns
- Milestones: Walked late (22 months), language and motor milestones achieved a few months later than twin sister
- Rehabilitation: Early intervention services, physical therapy, occupational therapy
- Speech-language assessment indicated age-appropriate development

Behavioral Observations

- Cooperative and sociable
- Difficulties focusing and sustaining attention
- Fidgety, but no significant signs of hyperactivity or impulsivity
- Speech and language age appropriate
- Minimal fine motor ability with right hand
- Fisted pencil grip with left hand

(continued)

CASE STUDIES (CONTINUED)

Test Results

- Intellectual functioning: Average overall (FSIQ = 42nd percentile), with discrepancy between verbal and nonverbal intellectual abilities (68th and 16th percentiles, respectively)

- Language: Average core language skills (ie, expressive and receptive vocabulary, grammatical expression, verbal concepts)

- School-readiness: Age-appropriate knowledge of colors, shapes, numbers, letters, size comparisons, classification

- Visual-motor skills: Visual-motor integration average, but difficulties with motor coordination and visual perception (tasks discontinued)

- Difficulties with attention and working memory reported by parents and teacher and indicated during formal testing

Recommendations

- Activities to promote fine-motor and visual-motor development (eg, ongoing occupational therapy, practice through arts and crafts, puzzles)

- Extra in-class support

- Strategies to facilitate attention and learning (eg, structured environment, minimize distractions, reward system)

- Follow-up assessment in 2 years

Case #2: Learning Difficulties Following Childhood Stroke

Reason for Referral

- Six-year-old girl (P) who experienced left basal ganglia stroke at age 5 secondary to focal vasculitis

- Referred for neuropsychological assessment to evaluate cognitive abilities and assist with academic planning

Background

- Born following healthy pregnancy and delivery

- Developmental milestones age appropriate

- Medical history unremarkable prior to stroke

- Stroke event at age 5:

    □ Signs: Right facial droop, slurred speech, clumsiness, speech difficulties, right-sided weakness

    □ Brain MRI: Acute stroke involving left basal ganglia (caudate, putamen, globus pallidus)

    □ Treatment: Steroids, anticoagulation, enoxaparin

    □ Follow-up: Resolution of MCA stenosis

- Secondary stroke prevention: Aspirin (40 mg daily)

- Neurological examination revealed subtle difficulties with right hand fine motor control and subtle signs of residual articulation difficulties

- Six-week stay at inpatient rehabilitation setting

- Academic/behavioral concerns following stroke: Reading and spelling, distractibility, working memory, word finding, anxiety, fatigue

(continued)

CASE STUDIES (CONTINUED)

Behavioral Observations

- Cooperative and sociable
- Difficulties focusing and sustaining attention
- Restless and fidgety
- Speech and language skills marked by mild articulation and word-finding difficulties

Test Results

- Intellectual functioning: Average overall (General Ability Index [GAI]=37th percentile), with equally well-developed verbal and nonverbal intellectual abilities (both 37th percentile), solid processing speed (42nd percentile), and a specific weakness in working memory (9th percentile)
- Language: Solid expressive language and verbal reasoning, but difficulties with word retrieval
- Memory and learning: Average memory skills with relative weakness in rote verbal learning
- Attention: Difficulties with sustained auditory attention, attention to visual detail, divided attention, inhibitory control
- Academic functioning: Difficulties with reading (word recognition, fluency, comprehension, phonological processing), spelling, printing, mathematics (borderline to low-average range performance)
- Visual-motor skills: Visual-motor integration average, but slow right-hand fine-motor speed

Summary and Recommendations

- Diagnosis: Learning disorder
- Identification, Placement, and Review Committee (formal meeting process in which decisions are made concerning the identification of the student, areas of exceptionality, and appropriate placement), designation of learning disability, and development of IEP
- Assistive technology (eg, word processing, text-to-speech software, word prediction, mind mapping, etc.)
- Strategies to maximize attention and learning (eg, structured environment, reduce multitasking, opportunities for preteaching, repetition)
- Occupational therapy focusing on letter formation and printing
- Strategies for facilitating writing skills (eg, extra time, outlines, templates)
- Follow-up assessment in 2 to 3 years

Case #3: Follow-Up Neuropsychological Assessment of Adolescent With Moyamoya Disease

Reason for Referral

- Seventeen-year-old girl (J) who was diagnosed with moyamoya disease at age 12 and underwent 3 revascularization surgeries, with postoperative strokes each time
- Initial neuropsychological assessment at age 13 indicated strong overall cognitive abilities
- Referred for follow-up assessment to obtain updated cognitive profile and assist with academic planning

Background

- Born following healthy pregnancy and delivery
- Developmental milestones age appropriate
- Immigrated to Canada from Bangladesh at age 5

(continued)

CASE STUDIES (CONTINUED)

- Family history: Moyamoya disease, depression
- Medical history: Seizures at ages 1 and 3 (treatment deemed unnecessary), otherwise unremarkable until age 12 when diagnosed with moyamoya
- Moyamoya diagnosis:
  - Signs/symptoms: Recurrent episodes of hemiparesis over course of 1 week, headaches for approximately 1 year
  - MRI: Multiple small strokes in left frontoparietal white matter and cortex
  - Angiogram: Significant narrowing of main arteries on both sides of brain (anterior cerebral artery, MCA, posterior cerebral artery), more pronounced on left
- Initial neuropsychological assessment at age 13:
  - Strong cognitive profile overall
  - Strengths: Nonverbal reasoning, abstract thinking, flexible problem solving, working memory
  - Weaknesses: Sustained attention, vocabulary
- Revascularization surgeries:
  - Age 13: Left hemisphere pial synangiosis, small postoperative stroke in left caudate, no focal deficits following stroke, continuation of headaches and transient ischemic attacks
  - Age 14: Right hemisphere pial synangiosis, postoperative multifocal stroke involving mesial right frontal, right parietal, and right temporal cortex; residual weakness of left leg
  - Age 16: Bilateral pial synangiosis and cerebrovascular bypass undergone after brain imaging revealed progression of moyamoya and new lesions involving bilateral caudate and corona radiata, postoperative right MCA stroke affecting right prefrontal cortex and temporoparietal cortex; left hemiparesis
- Seven-week stay at inpatient rehabilitation setting after second surgery and participation in day rehabilitation program after third surgery
- Current concerns: Difficulties with concentration, energy level, memory, information processing, academics, sleep disturbance, low mood

Behavioral Observations

- Cooperative and polite
- Quiet and withdrawn
- Difficulties with oral expression (eg, elaboration, expressing complex thoughts)
- Difficulty with visual scanning
- Slow to complete tasks
- Minimal use of left arm and hand

Test Results

- Intellectual functioning: low average overall (GAI=10th percentile), with a relative strength in verbal intellectual abilities (19th percentile) and notable declines in visual-spatial (10th percentile), processing speed (8th percentile), and working memory (13th percentile) abilities
- Memory and learning: Verbal memory unchanged since initial assessment (average), but visual memory weaker (borderline to low average)

(continued)

CASE STUDIES (CONTINUED)

- Academic functioning: Average word recognition and reading comprehension, significant weaknesses in math (calculations, applied problem solving)
- Fine motor skills: Left-hand weakness, but average right-hand fine motor speed, dexterity, and grip strength
- Social-emotional functioning: Concerns about low mood and withdrawal raised by teacher and mother

Summary and Recommendations

- Diagnosis: Math learning disability
- Updates to IEP with focus on learning disability designation and acknowledgement of neurological history
- Academic accommodations (eg, extended time and reduced workload, assistive technology, access to a resource teacher, individualized math curriculum)
- Strategies to manage weaknesses in working memory and information processing (eg, frequent review of new material, present information in manageable chunks, teach strategies for organizing new information, use of an agenda)
- Intervention for depression (ie, counseling referral)

Given the heterogeneity of the pediatric stroke population, it is crucial to consider the influences of variables such as age at stroke, time since stroke/age at assessment, sex, lesion characteristics, neurological impairment, and seizures, as well as their interactions with one another, on cognitive outcomes. With respect to the influence of age at stroke, early stroke (ie, before 1 year of age) has been identified as a risk factor for less favorable cognitive outcomes.[8,9,26,39,60] However, the relationship between age at stroke and cognitive outcomes is nonlinear and moderated by lesion location.[8,14,39,46] Inconsistencies in the literature on time since stroke/age at assessment make it difficult to arrive at any conclusions concerning the influence of these variables[10,14,45,61,62] and point to the likely interactions that this variable has with other factors (eg, cognitive domain in question, age at stroke, sex, stroke subtype, etiology), which are yet to be explored. The possible sex dimorphism of cognitive outcomes following pediatric stroke also remains unclear, and evidence indicates that this variable may be moderated by lesion laterality.[66] Regarding the influence of lesion location, combined cortical-subcortical lesions have been consistently identified as an overall risk factor for negative cognitive outcomes,[8,9,12,59] whereas the impact of anterior vs posterior lesions or damage to specific brain lobes appears to be contingent on the cognitive ability being assessed.[47,51,53] Findings generally indicate that larger lesion volume is a risk factor for negative cognitive outcomes[12,14,59,61,67]; however, new evidence indicates that the influence of this variable is moderated by neurological impairment and time since stroke.[12] The effect of lesion laterality is contingent on the cognitive domain in question—although effects of the hemispheric side of the lesion on visual-spatial processing outcomes have been well documented, studies have generally failed to find laterality effects on intellectual functioning,[8,10,14,61] facial recognition skills,[51] verbal learning and memory,[25,26] and social functioning.[53,55] Lastly, both seizures[1,9-11,14,68] and neurological impairment[9,12,39,59] have been identified as risk factors for negative cognitive outcomes following pediatric stroke.

The information provided in this chapter has important implications for the neuropsychological assessment and cognitive rehabilitation of children with histories of stroke. Neuropsychological assessments should be guided by a strong working knowledge of the overall cognitive profiles of children with histories of stroke and an understanding of the multiple factors influencing outcomes. In practice, this requires that the neuropsychologist be aware of the subtle nature of the cognitive difficulties exhibited by children with histories of stroke in intellectual, visual-spatial processing, memory and learning, attention, EF, and social domains, and take into account the effects of age at stroke, time since stroke, lesion characteristics (location, laterality, volume), sex, presence of seizures, and presence of persisting neurological deficits. Furthermore, it is critical to consider the interactions among these variables. Interactions particularly of note include the following: 1) age at stroke × lesion location[8]; 2) lesion characteristics (ie, volume, location) × neurological impairment[12]; 3) lesion volume × time since stroke[61]; 4) sex × lesion laterality[66]; and 5) presence of seizures × time since stroke.[10] Moreover, the cognitive ability in question consistently emerges as a key factor affecting these complex relationships. Cognitive rehabilitation efforts should be guided by models that take into account cognitive developmental mechanisms and the importance of the role of the family. The PNI model recently put forward by Limond et al[71] and specific intervention strategies stemming from the ABI cognitive rehabilitation literature (see Table 9-7) are particularly useful in this regard.

In conclusion, the cognitive difficulties exhibited by children with histories of stroke may be subtle and moderated by a host of variables such as age at stroke, time since stroke, sex, lesion characteristics, neurological impairment, and seizures. Future research is now required to follow children with histories of stroke into adulthood in order to further clarify enduring neuropsychological consequences. Moreover, longitudinal analysis will be helpful with differentiating between permanent patterns of cognitive deficits vs delays in development. To this end, future studies should examine how specific cognitive domains are differentially affected by lesion characteristics and age at stroke. This research will be critical for designing interventions to promote better cognitive and social outcomes in children with histories of stroke, improving our understanding of prognosis in this population, and enhancing our knowledge of brain–behavior relationships.

REFERENCES

1. Hartel C, Schilling S, Sperner J, Thyen U. The clinical outcomes of neonatal and childhood stroke: review of the literature and implications for future research. *Eur J Neurol.* 2004;11:431-438.
2. Neisser U, Boodoo G, Bouchard TJ. Intelligence: knowns and unknowns. *Am Psychol.* 1996;51:77-101.
3. Nettelbeck T, Wilson C. Intelligence and IQ: what teachers should know. *Educ Psychol.* 2005;25:609-630.
4. Piaget J. *The Psychology of Intelligence.* Totowa, NJ: Littlefield Adams; 1972.
5. Vygotsky L. *Mind in Society: The Development of Higher Psychological Processes.* Cambridge, MA: Harvard University Press; 1978.
6. Gardner H. *Frames of Mind: The Theory of Multiple Intelligence.* New York, NY: Basic Books; 1983.
7. Sternberg RJ. *Beyond IQ: A Triarchic Theory of Human Intelligence.* New York, NY: Cambridge University Press; 1985.
8. Westmacott R, Askalan R, MacGregor D, Anderson P, deVeber G. Cognitive outcome following unilateral arterial ischaemic stroke in childhood: effects of age at stroke and lesion location. *Dev Med Child Neurol.* 2010;52:386-393.
9. Studer M, Boltshauser E, Capone A, et al. Factors affecting cognitive outcome in early pediatric stroke. *Neurology.* 2014;82: 784-792.
10. Ballantyne AO, Spilkin AM, Hesselink J, Trauner DA. Plasticity in the developing brain: intellectual, language and academic functions in children with ischaemic perinatal stroke. *Brain.* 2008;131:2975-2985.
11. van Buuren LM, van der Aa NE, Dekker HC, et al. Cognitive outcome in childhood after unilateral perinatal brain injury. *Dev Med Child Neurol.* 2013;55:934-940.
12. Hajek CA, Yeates KO, Anderson V, et al. Cognitive outcomes following arterial ischemic stroke in infants and children. *J Child Neurol.* 2014;29(7):887-994.
13. Hetherington R, Tuff L, Anderson P, Miles B, deVeber G. Short-term intellectual outcome after arterial ischemic stroke and sinovenous thrombosis in childhood and infancy. *J Child Neurol.* 2005;20:553-559.
14. Everts R, Pavlovic J, Kaufmann F, et al. Cognitive functioning, behavior, and quality of life after stroke in childhood. *Child Neuropsychol.* 2008;14:323-338.
15. Stiles J, Akshoomoff N, Haist F. The development of visuospatial processing. In: Rubenstein JLR, Rakic P, eds. *Comprehensive Developmental Neuroscience: Neural Circuit Development and Function in the Brain.* Amsterdam, Netherlands: Elsevier; 2013: 271-296.
16. Akshoomoff NA, Feroleto CC, Doyle RE, Stiles J. The impact of early unilateral brain injury on perceptual organization and visual memory. *Neuropsychologia.* 2002;40:539-561.
17. Stiles J, Trauner D, Engel N, Nass R. The development of drawing in children with congenital focal brain injury: evidence for limited functional recovery. *Neuropsychologia.* 1997;35:299-312.
18. Stiles J, Stern C, Trauner D, Nass R. Developmental change in spatial grouping activity among children with early focal brain injury: evidence from a modeling task. *Brain Cogn.* 1996;31:46-62.
19. Schatz AM, Ballantyne AO, Trauner DA. A hierarchical analysis of block design errors in children with early focal brain damage. *Dev Neuropsychol.* 2000;17:75-83
20. Stiles J, Stern C, Appelbaum M, Nass R, Trauner D, Hesselink J. Effects of early focal brain injury on memory for visuospatial patterns: selective deficits of global-local processing. *Neuropsychology.* 2008;22:61-73.
21. Schatz J, Craft S, Koby M, DeBaun MR. Asymmetries in visual-spatial processing following childhood stroke. *Neuropsychology.* 2004;18:340-352.
22. Gathercole SE. The development of memory. *J Child Psychol Psychiatry.* 1998;39:3-27.
23. Siegel DJ. Memory: an overview with emphasis on the developmental, interpersonal, and neurobiological aspects. *J Am Acad Child Adolesc Psychiatry.* 2001;40:997-1011.
24. Skeel RL, Edwards S. The assessment and rehabilitation of memory disorders. In: Johnstone B, Stonnington HH, eds. *Rehabilitation of Neuropsychological Disorders: A Practical Guide for Rehabilitation Professionals,* 2nd ed. New York, NY: Psychology Press; 2009: 47-73.
25. Block GW, Nanson JL, Lowry NJ. Attention, memory, and language after pediatric ischemic stroke. *Child Neuropsychol.* 1999;5:81-91.
26. Lansing AE, Max JE, Delis DC, et al. Verbal learning and memory after childhood stroke. *J Int Neuropsychol Soc.* 2004;10:742-752.
27. Kolk A, Ennok M, Laugesaar R, Kaldoja M, Talvik T. Long-term cognitive outcomes after pediatric stroke. *Pediatr Neurol.* 2011;44:101-109
28. McCauley SR, Pedroza C. Event-based prospective memory in children with sickle cell disease: effect of cue distinctiveness. *Child Neuropsychol.* 2010;16:293-312.
29. Mirsky AF, Anthony BF, Duncan CC, Ahearn MB, Kellam SG. Analysis of the elements of attention: A neuropsychological approach. *Neuropsychol Rev.* 1991;2:109-145.
30. Max JE, Matthews K, Manes FF, et al. Attention deficit hyperactivity disorder and neurocognitive correlates after childhood stroke. *J Int Neuropsychol Soc.* 2003;9:815-829.
31. Max JE. Effects of side of lesion on neuropsychological performance on childhood stroke. *J Int Neuropsychol Soc.* 2004;10:698-708.
32. Elias KMI, Moura-Ribeiro MVL. Stroke caused auditory attention deficits in children. *Arch Neuropsychiatry.* 2013;71:11-17.
33. Gomes AM, Spencer-Smith MM, Jacobs RK, Coleman L, Anderson VA. Attention and social functioning in children with malformations of cortical development and stroke. *Child Neuropsychol.* 2012;18:392-403.

34. Anderson P. Assessment and development of executive function (EF) during childhood. *Child Neuropsychol.* 2002;8:71-82.

35. Alvarez JA, Emory E. Executive function and the frontal lobes: A meta-analytic review. *Neuropsychol Rev.* 2006;16:17-42.

36. Long B, Anderson V, Jacobs R, et al. Executive function following child stroke: the impact of lesion size. *Dev Neuropsychol.* 2011;36:971-987

37. Long B, Spencer-Smith MM, Jacobs R, et al. Executive function following child stroke: the impact of lesion location. *J Child Neurol.* 2011;26:279-287.

38. Morales G, Matute E, Murray J, Hardy DJ, O'Callaghan ETO, Tlacuilo-Parra A. Is executive function intact after pediatric intracranial hemorrhage? A sample of Mexican children with hemophilia. *Clin Pediatr.* 2013;52:950-959.

39. Allman C, Scott R. Neuropsychological sequelae following pediatric stroke: a nonlinear model of age at lesion effects. *Child Neuropsychol.* 2011;19:97-107.

40. Baddeley AD, Hitch GJ. Working memory. In: Bower G, ed. *The Psychology of Learning and Motivation.* New York, NY: Academic Press; 1974:47-89.

41. Baddeley A. The episodic buffer: a new component of working memory? *Trends Cogn Sci.* 2000;4:417-423.

42. Hommel M, Miguel ST, Naegele B, Gonnet N, Jaillard A. Cognitive determinants of social functioning after a first ever mild to moderate stroke at vocational age. *J Neurol Neurosurg Psychiatry.* 2009;80:876-880.

43. Philipose LE, Alphs H, Prabhakaran V, Hillis AE. Testing conclusions from functional imaging of working memory with data from acute stroke. *Behav Neurol.* 2007;18:37-43.

44. van Geldorp B, Kessels RPC, Hendriks MPH. Single-item and associative working memory in stroke patients. *Behav Neurol.* 2013;26:199-201.

45. Westmacott R, MacGregor D, Askalan R, deVeber G. Late emergence of cognitive deficits after unilateral neonatal stroke. *Stroke.* 2009;40:2012-2019.

46. Fuentes A. Social information processing and working memory following pediatric stroke (unpublished doctoral dissertation). Toronto, ON: York University; 2014.

47. White DA, Salorio CF, Schatz J, DeBaun M. Preliminary study of working memory in children with stroke related to sickle cell disease. *J Clin Exp Neuropsychol.* 2000;22:257-264.

48. Adolphs R. The neurobiology of social cognition. *Curr Opin Neurobiol.* 2001;11:231-239.

49. Beauchamp MH, Anderson V. SOCIAL: An integrative framework for the development of social skills. *Psychol Bull.* 2010;136:39-64.

50. Yeates KO, Bigler ED, Dennis M, et al. Social outcomes in childhood brain disorder: a heuristic integration of social neuroscience and developmental psychology. *Psychol Bull.* 2007;133:535-556.

51. Ballantyne AO, Trauner DA. Facial recognition in children after perinatal stroke. *Neuropsychiatry Neuropsychol Behav Neurol.* 1999;12:82-87.

52. Boni LC, Brown RT, Davis PC, Hsu L, Hopkins K. Social information processing and magnetic resonance imaging in children with sickle cell disease. *J Pediatr Psychol.* 2001;26:309-319.

53. Trauner DA, Panyard-Davis JL, Ballantyne AO. Behavioral differences in school age children after perinatal stroke. *Assessment.* 1996;3:265-276.

54. Friefeld SJ, Westmacott R, MacGregor D, deVeber G. Predictors of quality of life in pediatric survivors of arterial ischemic stroke and cerebral sinovenous thrombosis. *J Child Neurol.* 2011;26:1186-1192.

55. Mosch SC, Max J, Tranel D. A matched lesion analysis of childhood versus adult-onset brain injury due to unilateral stroke. *Cogn Behav Neurol.* 2005;18:5-17.

56. Crick NR, Dodge KA. A review and reformulation of social-information processing mechanisms in children's social adjustment. *Psychol Bull.* 1994;115:74-101.

57. Hurvitz E, Warschausky S, Berg M, Tsai S. Long-term functional outcomes of pediatric stroke survivors. *Top Stroke Rehabil.* 2004;11:51-59.

58. O'Keeffe F, Ganesan V, King J, Murphy T. Quality-of-life and psychosocial outcome following childhood arterial ischaemic stroke. *Brain Injury.* 2012;26:1072-1083.

59. Lo W, Gordon A, Hajek C, et al. Social competence following neonatal and childhood stroke. *Int J Stroke.* 2013;9(8). doi: 10.1111/ijs.12222

60. Max JE, Bruce M, Keatley E, Delis D. Pediatric stroke: plasticity, vulnerability, and age of lesion onset. *J Neuropsychiatry Clin Neurosci.* 2010;22:30-39.

61. Levine SC, Kraus R, Alexander E, Suriyakaham LW, Huttenlocher PR. IQ decline following early unilateral brain injury: a longitudinal study. *Brain Cogn.* 2005;59:114-123.

62. Aram D, Eisele JA. Intellectual stability in children with unilateral brain lesions. *Neuropsychologia.* 1994;32:85–95.

63. Fullerton HJ, Wu YW, Zhao S, Johnston SC. Risk of stroke in children: ethnic and gender disparities. *Neurology.* 2003;61:189-194.

64. Golomb MR, Dick PT, MacGregor DL, Curtis R, Sofronas M, deVeber G. Neonatal arterial ischemic stroke and cerebral sinovenous thrombosis are more commonly diagnosed in boys. *J Child Neurol.* 2004;19:493-497.

65. Golomb MR, Fullerton HJ, Nowak-Gottl U, deVeber G. Male predominance in childhood ischemic stroke: findings from the International Pediatric Stroke Study. *Stroke.* 2009;40:52-57.

66. Braun CMJ, Montour-Proulx I, Daigneault S, Rouleau I, Kuehn S, Piskopos M. Prevalence, and intellectual outcome of unilateral focal cortical brain damage as a function of age, sex, and aetiology. *Behav Neurol.* 2002;13:105-116.

67. Lo WD, Hajek C, Pappa C, Wang W, Zumberge N. Outcomes in children with hemorrhagic stroke. *JAMA Neurol.* 2013;70:66-71.

68. Fitzgerald KC, Williams LS, Garg BP, Golomb MR. Epilepsy in children with delayed presentation of perinatal stroke. *J Child Neurol.* 2007;22:1274-1280.

69. American Academy of Clinical Neuropsychology. American Academy of Clinical Neuropsychology (AACN) practice guidelines for neuropsychological assessment and consultation. *Clin Neuropsychol.* 2007;21:209-231.

70. Silver CH, Blackburn LB, Arffa S, et al. The importance of neuropsychological assessment for the evaluation of childhood learning disorders. *Arch Clin Neuropsychol.* 2006;21:741-744.

71. Limond J, Adlam A-LR, Cormack M. A model for pediatric neurocognitive interventions: considering the role of development and maturation in rehabilitation planning. *Clin Neuropsychol.* 2014;28:181-198.

72. Agnihotri A, Keightley ML, Colantonio A, Cameron D, Polatajko H. Community integration interventions for youth with acquired brain injuries: a review. *Deve Neurorehab.* 2010;13:369-382.

73. Catroppa C, Anderson V. Planning, problem-solving and organizational abilities in children following traumatic brain injury: intervention techniques. *Pediatr Rehabil.* 2006;9:89-97.

74. Hulse P, Dudley L. Visual perceptual deficiencies in the brain injury population: management from start to finish. *NeuroRehabilitation.* 2010;27:269-274.

75. Laatsch L, Harrington D, Hotz G, et al. An evidence-based review of cognitive and behavioural rehabilitation treatment studies in children with acquired brain injuries. *J Head Trauma Rehabil.* 2007;22:248-256.

76. Limond J, Leeke R. Practitioner review: cognitive rehabilitation for children with acquired brain injury. *J Child Psychol Psychiatry.* 2005;46:339-352.

77. Slomine B, Locascio G. Cognitive rehabilitation for children with acquired brain injury. *Dev Disabil.* 2009;15:133-143.

78. Shaw J. The assessment and rehabilitation of visual-spatial disorders. In: Johnstone B, Stonnington HH, eds. *Rehabilitation of Neuropsychological Disorders: A Practical Guide for Rehabilitation Professionals,* 2nd ed. New York, NY: Psychology Press; 2009: 107-135.

SUGGESTED READINGS

Allman C, Scott R. Neuropsychological sequelae following pediatric stroke: a nonlinear model of age at lesion effects. *Child Neuropsychol.* 2011;19:97-107.

Ballantyne AO, Spilkin AM, Hesselink J, Trauner DA. Plasticity in the developing brain: intellectual, language and academic functions in children with ischaemic perinatal stroke. *Brain.* 2008;131:2975-2985.

Everts R, Pavlovic J, Kaufmann F, et al. Cognitive functioning, behavior, and quality of life after stroke in childhood. *Child Neuropsychol.* 2008;14:323-338.

Lansing AE, Max JE, Delis DC, et al. Verbal learning and memory after childhood stroke. *J Int Neuropsychol Soc.* 2004;10:742-752.

Limond J, Adlam A-LR, Cormack M. A model for pediatric neurocognitive interventions: considering the role of development and maturation in rehabilitation planning. *Clin Neuropsychol.* 2014;28:181-198.

Max JE, Bruce M, Keatley E, Delis D. Pediatric stroke: plasticity, vulnerability, and age of lesion onset. *J Neuropsychiatry Clin Neurosci.* 2010;22:30-39.

Westmacott R, Askalan R, MacGregor D, Anderson P, Deveber G. Cognitive outcome following unilateral arterial ischaemic stroke in childhood: effects of age at stroke and lesion location. *Dev Med Child Neurol.* 2010;52:386-393.

Westmacott R, MacGregor D, Askalan R, deVeber G. Late emergence of cognitive deficits after unilateral neonatal stroke. *Stroke.* 2009;40:2012-2019.

10

Behavioral and Emotional Functioning in Children With Stroke

Lauren Krivitzky, PhD, ABPP-CN and Danielle Bosenbark, PhD

Derek was 17 years old when he had a stroke as a result of a hemorrhage from a cerebral cavernoma in the right pons. He spent several months in the hospital and many more months completing the arduous process of rehabilitation. Derek wrote this blog entry about coping with his stroke when he was 20.

Giving Up

June 4, 2014 by Derek Marshall

"There is no passion to be found in playing it small—in settling for a life that is less than the one you are capable of living."

—Nelson Mandela

When I was a junior in high school I was a varsity wrestler. At first I wasn't on par with my opponents. But I worked hard to become a better competitor. There is one match in particular that still stands out to me. I was fighting off of my back for the entire bout and spent most of the third period in a bridge and lost by "tech fall." Frustrated, I stormed off the mat and threw my headgear!

In the locker room my coach Vince taught me one of the most important lessons of my life: You won't always win, even when you train hard. Vince taught me to take pride in the work I do on myself and that hard work always pays off, even when you don't get exactly what you were striving for, because you end up better than you started!

I have always been a big dreamer. Some might call me fearless, but that is not entirely true. For three long years I have been in recovery. And I'm ashamed to admit that at some point in this match I have gotten discouraged and threw my headgear aside. Two years into my recovery I started to seriously doubt myself. It was at this time that I chose to leave college and join a vocational program. I gave up my dream of becoming a doctor because I felt incapable. During my time in vocational training I was more unhappy and disappointed in myself than I have ever been, because I knew I was capable of far greater things.

Feeling weak was the hardest thing to cope with after my stroke. Often, depression is associated with brain injury. But I don't think this is entirely true in my case. My spirits were high until I made the choice to give up on my dreams because I was afraid to fail. Somehow during my recovery I lost sight of what's most important: Dedication and commitment to working toward a dream and ultimately becoming a better person.

In the end my desire to succeed overcame my fear of failure. I decided to return to college in order to be what I feel I was born to be! I am not saying that I will not fail, I am, however, sure I will not give up.

If ever you consider quitting on anything in life remember this:

"Pain is temporary. It may last a minute, or an hour, or a day, or a year, but eventually it will subside and something else will take its place. If I quit, however, it lasts forever."

—Lance Armstrong

Atkinson HL, Nixon-Cave K, Smith SE, eds.
Pediatric Stroke Rehabilitation: An Interprofessional and Collaborative Approach (pp 185-203).© 2018 Taylor & Francis Group.

INTRODUCTION

In a 2013 review of perinatal stroke syndromes, Kirton and deVeber[1] postulated that emotional and behavioral difficulties following perinatal stroke are common, yet widely understudied. When reviewing prior research on children with a history of neonatal arterial ischemic stroke (AIS), the authors note that "developmental psychology research specific to perinatal stroke is surprisingly lacking despite abundant child psychology issues including physical disability, bullying, and suspected but unproven increases in anxiety and depression."[1] The authors also point out that their early research suggests that parent psychological outcomes are frequently abnormal when their child has a perinatal stroke (more detail on this topic in Chapter 11). This has many implications for the well-being of these stroke survivors in the future, as parenting stress and parental psychological functioning has a very robust relationship to the child's future functioning.

It is even more challenging to study the emotional and behavioral outcomes in older children with a history of stroke, as these groups are often mixed in terms of the etiology of the stroke and the child's age (age both at the time of the stroke and the time of the assessment). Nonetheless, professionals in the field recognize that mental health outcomes often present the most challenges for the patient and have the longest-term impact on the child's and family's functioning. This chapter is a review of what is known regarding these outcomes to date and interventions that may be helpful for children and families coping with the emotional/behavioral sequelae of pediatric stroke.

SCOPE OF THE PROBLEM

Studies Using Nonspecific Measurement Tools of Emotional and Behavioral Outcomes

Although several studies include descriptions of behavioral and emotional outcomes following pediatric stroke, the majority of these studies are nonspecific in their measurement or descriptions of the types of concerns and/or diagnoses that are present. This has resulted in highly variable estimates of poststroke behavioral disturbances ranging from very small numbers (eg, one study finding <5%) to much higher estimates (eg, ~75% of children poststroke having a diagnosable emotional or behavioral

disorder). Part of the difficulty in understanding the prevalence of these disorders is that varying tools have been used to discern the scope of the problem. Such tools have included chart review, physician-completed tools of stroke outcome (typically the Pediatric Stroke Outcome Measure or PSOM), parent-reported behavior rating scales, quality of life (QOL) questionnaires, and structured psychiatric interview measures.

In general, studies using tools like the PSOM have tended to find lower rates of behavioral problems. One study found that 2.9% of children with neonatal stroke and 16.6% of children with childhood stroke had nonspecific behavioral problems.[2] In contrast, another study examined 59 cases of presumed perinatal ischemic stroke using the PSOM and found that cognitive or behavioral deficits were found in 29% of the group; however, more specific information in terms of the types of problems was not described (mean age at follow up = 5.3 years ±2.1, median = 4.1).[3] These authors noted another important limitation in many studies, in that children are often studied at young ages and thus the full extent of their future emotional and behavioral concerns may not yet be apparent.

Another limitation of many studies is that different stroke types with different etiologies are often mixed together. One study presented on a small group of only acute childhood AIS ($n=20$)[4]. At the time of follow up (mean = 7 years), 16 individuals were studied. About half (7/16) reported "increased sensitivity to daily routines," which generally manifested as behavioral problems such as emotional lability, temper tantrums, and aggressive outbursts. In a larger group of subjects with childhood ischemic stroke (various causes $n=90$), 37% of parents reported that they had a concern about their child's behavior based on a parent questionnaire (single question on behavior).[5] These authors noted that in a small follow-up study of children with stroke vs sibling controls, the patient's scores were significantly higher than sibling controls on the withdrawn, social, and attention domains from a parent checklist measure, the Achenbach Child Behavior Checklist.

Similar types of behavioral concerns have been noted in studies of children with perinatal stroke. Thirty-six young children with perinatal stroke were studied retrospectively (mean age at follow-up = 41 months).[6] Study procedures included a comprehensive chart review, which included reviewing for behavioral abnormalities defined as a physician diagnosis of attention problems, hyperactivity, or behavior problems. This study found that 22% of the children studied had a behavioral diagnosis in the chart review, although precise *Diagnostic and Statistical Manual* (DSM) classifications were not obtained.

FAMILY FOCUS BOX

Key concept: The DSM is the *Diagnostic and Statistical Manual of Mental Disorders.* This manual is used by professionals to diagnose and classify mental disorders. The most recent edition, DSM-5, was released in 2013; thus the research studies described in this chapter generally utilized criteria from the DSM-IV.

Studies Utilizing Diagnostic and Statistical Manual of Mental Disorders-IV Criteria for Mental Health Disorders

Despite the limitations of these studies, it is clear from the results that emotional and behavioral difficulties are common following pediatric stroke. One study in particular has gone into greater detail examining the specific types and prevalence of different psychiatric symptoms in a group of children with pediatric stroke.[7] These researchers examined a group of children with a history of stroke (defined as a stroke resulting in focal, nonrecurrent, supratentorial brain parenchymal lesion), including those with early lesions (defined as stroke occurring prior to 12 months, $n = 17$) and late lesions (stroke occurred at ages 12 months or later, $n = 12$). The group included a mix of etiologies: 21 with occlusive ischemic stroke and 8 with hemorrhagic stroke. These children were compared to a control group of children with a history of clubfoot (matched to the early lesion group) and orthopedic injuries (for the late lesion group). Measures in this study included the Schedule for Affective Disorders and Schizophrenia for School-Age children, Present and Lifetime Version, a semistructured interview designed to identify individuals with current or prior psychiatric diagnoses, and the Neuropsychiatric Rating Schedule, a semistructured interview designed to identify personality changes secondary to a general medical condition.

Results of this study found that among the lifetime postmedical condition psychiatric diagnoses (PD), attention deficit hyperactivity disorder (ADHD) was the most common disorder (46% poststroke or 13/28 subjects without prestroke ADHD, 17% postorthopedic).[7] Anxiety disorders were the next most common PD (31% poststroke, 7% postorthopedic). Mood disorders were the third most common PD (21% poststroke, 7% postorthopedic). Comorbidity (having more than one psychiatric diagnosis) did not occur in orthopedic subjects, but was common among those stroke subjects with current psychiatric symptoms (poststroke PD diagnoses mean = 2.2, SD = 1.2). Children in this study with poststroke PD tended to have additional problems, including more cognitive deficits (eg, lower full-scale IQ scores and adaptive functioning) and a history of family psychiatric problems. Children with ongoing seizures also tended to have greater psychiatric issues. The groups were not significantly different regarding age, socioeconomic status (SES), gender (9/18 males vs 8/11 females), early vs late lesion (10/17 vs 7/12), stroke hemisphere (9/13 left; 8/16 right), size of stroke, academic functioning, and family functioning.

FAMILY FOCUS BOX

Key concept: Three most common psychiatric disorders in pediatric stroke survivors

1. ADHD
2. Anxiety disorders
3. Mood disorders

Studies Utilizing Quality of Life Measures

Studies utilizing QOL measures also provide some insight into real-world behavioral and emotional concerns of children with pediatric stroke. Measurement of health-related quality of life (HRQOL) captures essential information that is not captured by traditional outcome indicators,[8] and over the last decade, HRQOL has been increasingly included in outcome research on patients with cerebrovascular disease.[9-12] HRQOL instruments used with children and adolescents evaluate the physical, emotional, social, and behavioral dimensions of well-being[13] and typically include 3 features that distinguish them from other types of health outcome indicators: 1) use multidimensional factors, 2) measure children's and adolescents' health in terms that are important to the child/adolescent and his or her family, and 3) measure the child/adolescent and parent/proxy perspective. Because most children are young at stroke event, parents provide an important proxy for QOL determination.

Studies of HRQOL in pediatric stroke survivors are limited but have shown that it is reduced in a variety of domains including physical, emotional, social, school, and cognitive functioning.[14-18] Studies of HRQOL in pediatric stroke survivors are limited but have shown that it is reduced in a variety of domains including physical, emotional, social, school, and cognitive functioning.[14-18] However, some discrepancy still exists. While some studies have found physical health to be the most affected area of HRQOL,[16,19] others have found it to be least problematic, reporting school and play domains to be most affected.[20] In a prospective study of 76 children with pediatric arterial ischemic stroke (diagnosed at birth through age 17) with a mix of underlying etiologies, parents indicated significantly lower motor functioning, more anxiety, a less positive mood, and more stomach and lung problems.[14] Children (ages 8 to 15) who were able to complete the measure indicated more social problems. The authors of this study noted that impaired QoL was notable both in children with mild disabilities and in those with more severe disabilities, suggesting that QoL may be independent of neurological severity. A further aim was to describe the health of the parents of these children. Seventeen children and adolescents with cerebral infarction in the territory of the middle cerebral artery were enrolled in the study. A new activity limitation measure with a 4-point Likert scale (the Paediatric Stroke Activity Limitation Measure) others have found it to be least problematic, reporting school and play domains to be most affected.[20] In a prospective study of 76 children with PAIS (diagnosed at birth through age 17) with a mix of underlying etiologies, parents indicated significantly lower motor functioning, more anxiety, a less positive mood, and more stomach and lung problems.[14] Children (ages 8 to 15) who were able to complete the measure indicated more social problems. The authors of this study noted that impaired QOL was notable both in children with mild disabilities and in those with more severe disabilities, suggesting that QOL may be independent of neurological severity.

Various predictors have been shown to have an impact on HRQOL in pediatric stroke. Notably, cognitive and behavior deficits have been shown to be related to QOL after pediatric stroke.[15,18] Similar findings have been supported in other areas of pediatric research as well, particularly that deficits in executive function and attention appear to be significantly correlated with poorer parent ratings of QOL in the acquired brain injury population.[21,22]

POSTSTROKE EMOTIONAL AND BEHAVIORAL DISORDERS

Attention Deficit Hyperactivity Disorder

Among poststroke psychiatric disorders, ADHD is the most common to occur in the pediatric population.[8,23] ADHD is a behavioral disorder characterized by age-inappropriate symptoms of inattention, hyperactivity, and impulsivity.[24] Research has shown that those diagnosed with the disorder also experience deficits in multiple domains of cognitive function, with the most prominent impairments consistently occurring in speed of complex information processing, attention, and executive functions (eg, tasks of verbal fluency, inhibition, and set shifting), and working memory.[25]

Identification of Attention Deficit Hyperactivity Disorder

For children, the DSM-5 requires 6/9 symptoms from the Inattention domain to be present for a diagnosis of ADHD—Predominately Inattentive Presentation, 6/9 symptoms from the Hyperactive-Impulsive domain to be present for a diagnosis of ADHD—Predominantly Hyperactive-Impulsive Presentation, and symptoms from both domains to be present for a diagnosis of ADHD—Combined Presentation.[24] Assessment of ADHD may include several techniques including parent interview, child interview, behavioral rating scales, medical exam, and psychological/neuropsychological tests. The specific assessment methods chosen to evaluate a particular child should be driven by the issues involved in the particular case. For children with a history of stroke, the treating neurologist will often work with the child's pediatrician and a pediatric psychologist/neuropsychologist when making this diagnosis. Several free assessment tools are available for screening symptoms of ADHD, although such methods should never be used in isolation to make the diagnosis.

Attention Deficit Hyperactivity Disorder Symptoms in Children With Neurological Disorders

The concept of increased prevalence of ADHD after a pediatric neurological event or injury (eg, traumatic brain injury, pediatric brain tumor treatments) is not uncommon and is often referred to as secondary ADHD (SADHD).[26–30] Although the presentation of the disorder is acquired from a nondevelopmental etiology, the symptomology and neuropsychological difficulties experienced are similar in nature. What remains uncertain is whether the changes in phenotype and symptoms (eg, fewer problems related to hyperactivity) that can occur throughout development in the traditional developmental view of ADHD—occurring as a result of delayed maturation of cortical areas involved in attention and executive functioning—also occur in clinical populations with SADHD, particularly because the etiology is a traumatic insult to their brain rather than a complex interaction of genetics and environmental influences.[31]

An increased rate of ADHD symptoms is also present in children with a history of pediatric stroke. Research has found that symptoms of ADHD occurred more often in children after perinatal stroke than in the normal population (50% vs 3% to 17%).[32] As mentioned earlier, researchers have found that ADHD was the most common disorder in this population.[7] Because symptoms of ADHD occur on a continuum, these examiners further investigated diagnoses of both ADHD (according to DSM-IV) and ADHD traits, a designation given to those with subthreshold symptoms.[23] Results of this study found high rates of ADHD and

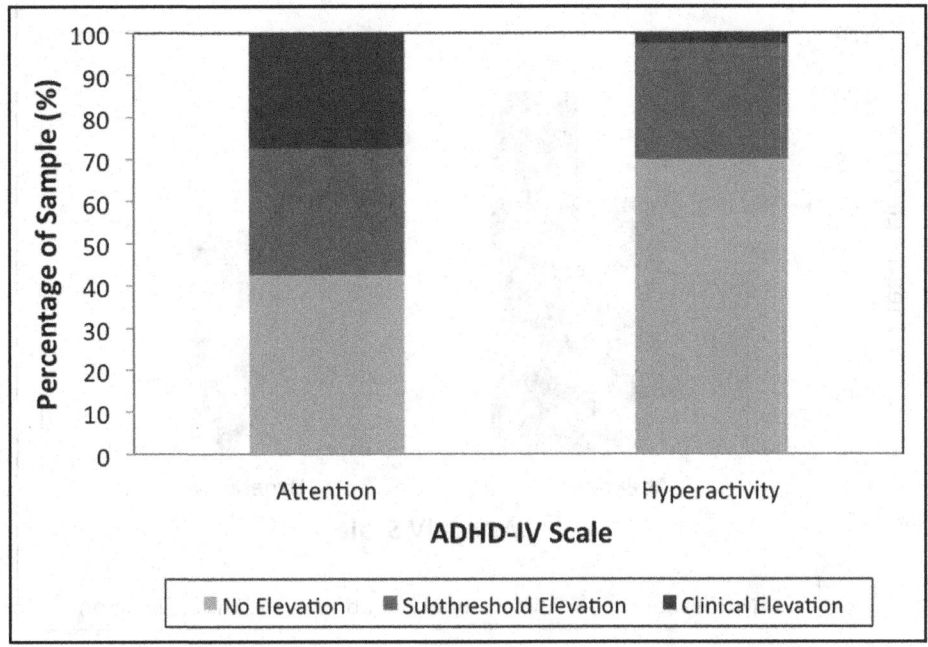

Figure 10-1. Percentage of children with no elevation (< 80th percentile), subthreshold elevation (80th to 90th percentile), and clinical elevation (≥ 93rd percentile) on the Attention and Hyperactivity scales of the ADHD-IV.

FAMILY FOCUS BOX

Key concept: All children with a history of stroke (perinatal or childhood) should be screened for the symptoms of ADHD.

Tools: Several screening tools are available that professionals can use, such as the following:

- ADHD-IV Rating Scales: Home and School
- VADPRS/VADTRS: Vanderbilt ADHD Diagnostic Parent Rating Scale and Teacher Rating Scale

Please see the CHADD* website for more information on screening tools for ADHD: http://www.chadd.org/Understanding-ADHD/Parents-Caregivers-of-Children-with-ADHD/Evaluation-and-Treatment/Rating-Scales-and-Checklists.aspx

Next steps: If red flags emerge about a possible diagnosis, a referral to a mental health provider may be warranted for further assessment and creation of a treatment plan.

*CHADD: Children and Adults with ADHD

ADHD traits in the stroke group. A total of 16 (out of 28, or 57%) children had a history of symptoms (either ADHD or ADHD traits), including 12 diagnosed with ongoing ADHD, 3 with ADHD traits, and 1 with resolved ADHD. This was in contrast to the orthopedic controls, which had a rate of 24% (7/29) with current or resolved symptoms.

One of the most notable findings in this study was the high rate of comorbidity. Specifically, 9 of the 16 children with ADHD/traits also met criteria for other DSM-IV psychiatric disorders, including oppositional defiant disorder, personality change disorder, anxiety disorders, tic/movement disorders, and depressive disorder. In addition, the children from the stroke group with ADHD/traits were significantly more impaired in their verbal IQ scores,

arithmetic scores, and certain executive functioning measures. Also of interest, these increased rates in the stroke group were not related to gender, age, SES, race, family functioning or family history of ADHD, or the presence of a chronic medical condition requiring medical attention.

In a study examining attention and executive functioning outcomes in 40 children with perinatal AIS, nearly one-third of the study cohort (11/40 subjects) were identified as meeting criteria for a diagnosis of ADHD.[33] Moreover, children identified as having ADHD were more likely to have issues with attention (27.5% with clinical elevations, as measured by the ADHD-IV Rating Scale), whereas hyperactivity did not purport to be as significant an issue (2.5% with clinical elevations) (Figure 10-1).

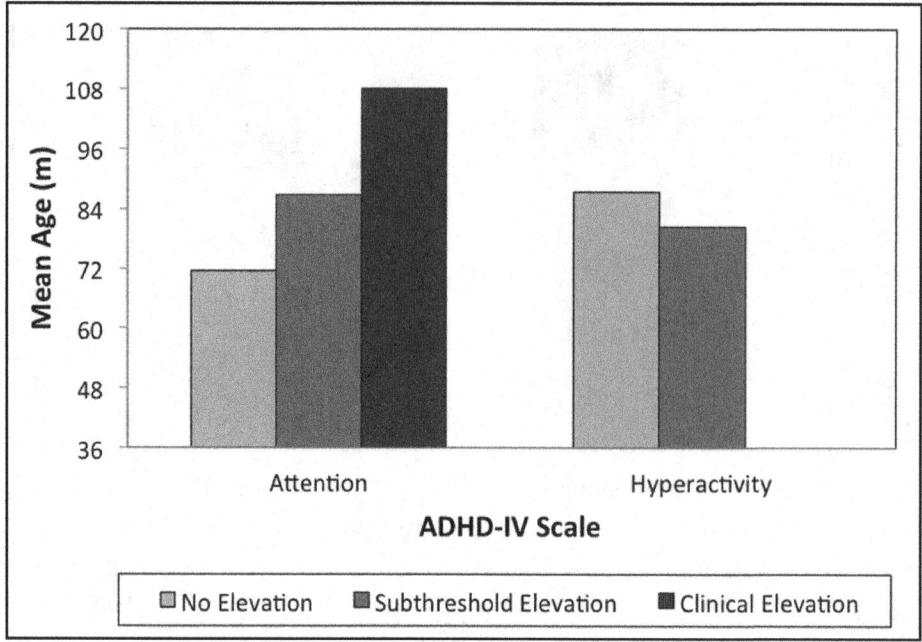

Figure 10-2. Average age of participants classified as having no elevation (< 80th percentile), subthreshold elevation (80th to 90th percentile), and clinical elevation (≥ 93rd percentile) on the Attention and Hyperactivity scales of the ADHD-IV.

FAMILY FOCUS BOX
Key concept: Children with a history of stroke and ADHD symptoms should be screened for other psychiatric/learning problems.
Tools: Several emotional/behavioral screening measures are available (parent and self-report) that can be used with the help of a consulting psychologist.
Next steps: If there are concerns for additional diagnoses, refer to a mental health professional for further assessment. Referral to a neuropsychologist may also be warranted for a more thorough evaluation of cognitive/behavioral strengths and weaknesses.

When examining the effects of various demographic (age, sex) and medical (stroke type, stroke laterality and anatomical location, stroke size, comorbid epilepsy) variables on attention outcomes in children with PAIS, this study also found that age and lesion size were significant predictors of outcome.[34] First, children with clinical elevations on the ADHD-IV Attention scale were significantly older than children with no elevations (Figure 10-2). With respect to stroke size, children with both subthreshold and clinical elevations on the ADHD-IV Attention scale had larger strokes than children with no elevations.

The findings of these studies raise several important issues. First and foremost, all children with a history of stroke should be screened for symptoms of ADHD. In addition, although factors like gender or family history of ADHD should be considered, in the case of ped stroke, these factors may have less importance. Finally, although these issues can be discussed with a child's medical physician, it is also often helpful to involve a mental health professional, such as a neuropsychologist, when there are

concerns about a child's thinking or attention skills. A neuropsychologist is a specialist in the field of psychology who has expertise in understanding brain–behavior relationships. This individual can help work with the team to better understand and evaluate the child's attention difficulties and can help make recommendations for the child's school, home, and community functioning.

These findings also suggest that there are high rates of other comorbidities in children with a history of stroke and ADHD. This is not a surprising finding, as children with a history of idiopathic ADHD also have high rates of these same comorbid disorders, as well as specific learning disorders.[35]

Evidenced-Based Treatments for Attention Deficit Hyperactivity Disorder Symptoms

As a result of the findings from the Multimodal Treatment Study of ADHD,[36] most clinicians agree that using multiple treatments in combination is the best approach for treating ADHD. There are several areas for targeting treatment for individuals with this condition. The key components include 1) parent training, including education of child and parent on diagnosis, symptoms and treatment, and teaching effective behavioral management techniques; 2) consideration of medications, including psychostimulants and nonstimulants; and 3) educational supports.

Parent Training

Parents are an integral part of this treatment plan, and models of parent training and counseling are described in the writings of Russell Barkley.[35] Most parent training methods include a combination of counseling and education about ADHD and teaching specific behavioral management techniques. This training can be administered in one-to-one or group settings. Research has shown that interventions not only improve the child's behavior, but also other aspects of the family's environment, including reducing parenting stress and increasing parents' self-esteem.[37] Experts in the field have stated that there is reason to be "cautiously optimistic" about the efficacy of parent training interventions for children with ADHD, although they caution that the field needs more controlled studies in this area to judge and compare particular interventions.[37]

Education

The first step in treating ADHD is to educate the child and caregivers about the disorder. This includes common symptoms, how the diagnosis is made, and reviewing various treatment options (described further later). Many parent training/counseling programs include an initial session focused on education.

Behavior Management

With behavior modification, parents, teachers, and children learn specific techniques and skills from a therapist or an educator experienced in the approach, that will help improve children's behavior. This is one of the most crucial elements of treating children with ADHD, as these techniques help children and parents learn to cope with the symptoms. The basics of behavior management include understanding the *ABCs of behavior*. This refers to understanding the A (antecedents) of a behavior, that is, what is happening before the problem behavior; B (behavior), the behavior itself that you are trying to target; and C (consequence), the things that happen after the behavior. Barkley's parent training model includes teaching several behavior management techniques such as skills to improve positive attending skills and child compliance, establishing a home point/token system, using time-out appropriately, and managing behavior in public places. Regardless of the behavior being targeted, it is important that any intervention include the following:

- Define the problem and set a goal: Clear definition of the problem behavior (eg, Johnny calls out in

class 10 to 15 times/day) and a goal for improvement (Johnny will call out in class fewer than 10 times/day).

- Consistency: It is also important for interventions to be consistent across settings, that is, across different teachers and at home with each caregiver. Change tends to be gradual, and it is important to realize that these interventions may take time to work (there may actually be a spike in the problem behavior at first).

Medication

Stimulant medications are the most common psychotropic drugs used to treat ADHD. Use of these medications to treat behavioral disturbances dates back to the 1930s, and there are now hundreds of randomized controlled studies on the effects of stimulants on the core symptoms of ADHD.[38] Several different stimulant medications are available on the market with different release preparations (immediate, intermediate, or extended release). The National Institute of Mental Health conducted a major research study (the largest medication study for ADHD), called the Multimodal Treatment Study of Children with ADHD,[36] involving 579 children with ADHD-combined type. Each child received 1 of 4 possible treatments over a 14-month period: 1) medication management (which was carefully monitored and tailored); 2) behavioral treatment; 3) combination of the 2; or 4) usual community care. Results of this study revealed that children who received medication alone or medication and behavioral treatments had the best improvements in their ADHD symptoms. The combined behavior/medication treatment group also had the highest proportion of children showing positive response regarding improvement in oppositional symptoms and other areas of functioning (eg, academics).

Although stimulant medications are highly effective for treating ADHD symptoms, about 30% of affected individuals cannot tolerate and/or do not respond to stimulant medications. Thus, there are other alternative medication options with a noradrenergic mechanism of action that may be helpful in treating ADHD symptoms. Following several controlled trials, the Food and Drug Administration (FDA) approved the first nonstimulant medication for treatment of ADHD in children and adults: Strattera (atomoxetine). Strattera is a specific norepinephrine reuptake inhibitor and may be an appropriate alternative to stimulant medication. There is also one other class of drugs that has been FDA approved to treat ADHD symptoms: the alpha-2 adrenergic agonists (ie, guanfacine and clonidine).

Despite the positive effects of medication on ameliorating ADHD symptoms in children, caution should be taken in extrapolating prior study results to children with a history of ADHD symptoms presumed to be secondary to stroke. Most medication studies have all been completed

---

FAMILY FOCUS BOX

Key concept: Evidence-based treatments for ADHD

Consider:

- Parent training—including education about ADHD and teaching behavioral management strategies
- Medication—stimulant or nonstimulant (Strattera)
- Educational interventions—to address learning/cognitive, behavior, and social skills

Who can help? Mental health professionals may include psychologists, neuropsychologists, psychiatrists, social worker, licensed school counselor and/or educational team from school.

Next steps: Ask your physician (neurologist, rehabilitation doctor, and/or pediatrician) about where you should start.

---

with purely developmental cases of ADHD (ie, no known neurological disorders), and thus medications may not have the same efficacy in children whose ADHD symptoms are presumed secondary to neurological injury. However, there are some promising pilot studies in children with traumatic brain injury and sickle cell disease that suggest stimulant treatments may be helpful in treating children with neurological conditions.[39,40] Further research with children with stroke and other neurological conditions is clearly needed to better understand the efficacy of medication in treating ADHD symptoms. In addition, treatment with stimulant medications may not be an option for some patients with a history of stroke, as they may have an underlying medical issue that is a contraindication to treatment with a stimulant. Thus, it is important that the treating physician is aware of the individual patient's comprehensive medical/developmental history, and that he or she considers all of the risks and benefits of treatment and the full range of treatment options.

School/Educational Supports

Many supports can be provided for a child with a history of stroke and ADHD symptoms in the educational setting. Accommodations can be focused on both the cognitive and behavioral symptoms of ADHD. These kinds of accommodations are often included in a child's individualized education program (IEP). Please see Table 10-1 for examples of some of the accommodations that may address the behavioral aspects of ADHD symptoms.

Rewards, punishments, and feedback must be swift and immediate in order to be effective. Parents may wish to request a consultation from the school's behavioral specialist to assist in putting appropriate accommodations into place. The specialist can also conduct a functional behavioral analysis in the classroom, an assessment method in which data are collected on a carefully defined target behavior (eg, the child getting out of his or her chair), the antecedents and consequences of that behavior, and generation of hypotheses about the function of the target behavior.

Once these data are collected, they can help the child's team create an intervention to reduce the problem behavior.

Many classroom supports may be helpful in addressing the cognitive symptoms of ADHD, such as difficulties with attention and executive functioning. Please see Table 10-2 for some examples.

Children with ADHD may also have difficulties with social skills. Thus, additional goals in the child's IEP may include targeting social behaviors such as how to enter a peer group, be a good sport, accept consequences, and be appropriately assertive.[41]

Anxiety/Mood Disorders

Although much of the focus has been on behavioral problems following pediatric stroke, children are also at risk for internalizing disorders including anxiety and depression. As mentioned in the prior section, anxiety and mood disorders are the second and third most common psychiatric disorders following ADHD and are often diagnosed as comorbid conditions.

Anxiety Disorders

Although anxiety is a common reaction to life stressors, it becomes problematic when the intensity and duration affect one's functioning and QOL.[42] There are many different types of anxiety disorders, which include diagnoses such as specific phobia (eg, fear of a particular thing), generalized anxiety disorder, social phobia, obsessive compulsive disorder, separation anxiety, agoraphobia without panic, panic disorder with agoraphobia, and posttraumatic stress disorder (PTSD). The most commonly reported anxiety disorders in childhood stroke are reported to be social phobia, specific phobia, and separation anxiety disorders.[7]

The cause for anxiety symptoms in children with a history of stroke is likely a combination of biological, family/genetic, and other environmental factors. In childhood stroke, the child/adolescent is likely to be quite aware of a change in their health status and feel stress about the new

---

TABLE 10-1. EXAMPLE ACCOMMODATIONS TO ADDRESS ATTENTION DEFICIT HYPERACTIVITY DISORDER-ASSOCIATED BEHAVIORS IN THE CLASSROOM

- Seat student in a place that will minimize distractions—for some this may be front and center, near the teacher, and away from distractions (eg, door, window).
- Have a special signal (eg, teacher's hand on the desk) to redirect the student to task.
- Discuss the behavior in private rather than calling him or her out in front of the class.
- Have student sit next to a well-behaved role model.
- Increase the distance between desks, if possible.
- For younger students, mark an area with tape around his or her desk in which he or she can move freely.
- Create an incentive/reward-based system for on-task and nonimpulsive behaviors (eg, raise hands).
- Create a home-school note so that parents get daily feedback on their child's behavior in school.

TABLE 10-2. EXAMPLE ACCOMMODATIONS TO ADDRESS ATTENTION DEFICIT HYPERACTIVITY DISORDER-ASSOCIATED COGNITIVE DIFFICULTIES IN THE CLASSROOM

- Develop an effective organizational system for keeping track of assignments/materials (eg, planner, electronic organizer).
- Identify a coach or mentor who can meet with the student daily (or several times a day) to help keep him or her organized.
- Provide critical instructions verbally and in writing so that the student does not have to hold multiple pieces of information in mind.
- Encourage/teach self-monitoring techniques, such as always double-checking work before it is handed in.
- For children with slowed processing speed or sluggish cognitive tempo, consider allowing extended time for in-class and homework assignments
- Teach students how to stay organized by techniques such as making to-do lists, writing an outline, keeping a calendar, budgeting time, and approaching new/novel tasks.

---

medical, physical, cognitive, and psychological sequelae of the stroke. Children with ongoing physical symptoms (eg, headaches, sensory symptoms, transient ischemic attacks) may be at particular risk for anxiety, as their somatic symptoms related to these secondary issues may trigger panic attacks and other anxiety symptoms. Children may ruminate about their symptoms and worry that they are having another stroke. These particular issues are less of a concern for children with perinatal stroke or stroke during infancy, as these children are not aware of life before the stroke and typically do not have conditions that are likely to recur. In contrast, the parents of children who have a perinatal stroke are often at greater risk for anxiety and symptoms of PTSD. Often, these parents are excited and anticipating becoming new parents and quickly (in the first few days of life) learn that their child has experienced a stroke. In these cases, it is extremely important to monitor the parents' adjustment and coping, both in the short run and throughout the first few years of development. In these cases, a psychologist or social worker in the follow-up program may be a valuable resource to the parents so that they can learn to cope with the diagnosis and move forward with supporting their child's development in a positive way.

Difficulties coping with a chronic medical condition can contribute to the phenomenon of pediatric medical traumatic stress (PMTS). PMTS has received increasing recognition and is defined as:

> [A] set of psychological and physiological responses of children and their families to pain, injury, serious illness, medical procedures, and invasive or frightening treatment experiences. These responses may include symptoms of arousal, re-experiencing, and/or avoidance. They may vary in intensity, but are related to the subjective experience of the event, and can become disruptive to functioning.[43]

These symptoms can include diagnosable disorders, such as PTSD, but also a range of stress symptoms resulting from potentially traumatic experiences.[44] Thus, it is important for mental health professionals working with pediatric

---

FAMILY FOCUS BOX

Key concept: PMTS

What is it? Stress/anxiety symptoms that result from potentially traumatic medical experiences, such as hospitalization for a stroke.

Next steps: If red flags emerge, let your doctor know and ask for a consultation with a psychologist, social worker, or a child life specialist.

Parents may also experience symptoms of medical traumatic stress and should be provided with support and resources if these symptoms interfere with their own mental health or ability to parent their child.

---

patients to identify events that might lead to PMTS and to try to intervene to prevent the symptoms or ameliorate them when they occur.[45] In addition to recognizing medical traumatic stress in the patient, it is very important that physicians and other professionals recognize when other family members are experiencing traumatic stress so that the social worker or psychologist can work with the family to help manage the stressors.

Anxiety symptoms may also be secondary to the biological consequences of pediatric stroke. Studies examining the neurobiology of individuals with anxiety disorders (without comorbid neurological disorders) have found alterations in a diverse range of neurochemical systems and altered functioning of neural networks between the amygdala and prefrontal cortex and in the interior insula.[46] Although the neurobiology of anxiety in pediatric stroke has not been studied, prior research in children with acquired brain injury has suggested that difficulties with affective regulation may be related to damage in the dorsal frontal lobes and frontal white matter systems.[47] Additional research is warranted in order to better understand the underlying neurobiological and psychosocial factors that contribute to anxiety in children with pediatric stroke.

Mood Disorders

Despite very limited research in pediatric stroke, there is a large body of literature examining mood disorders following adult stroke. Poststroke depression is extremely common in adults, occurring in approximately one-third of all adult stroke survivors.[48] Mood disorders have been found to be the third most common psychiatric disorder following neonatal/childhood stroke (21% of stroke cases) and included most often DSM-IV diagnoses of major depression and mood disorder, not otherwise specified.[7]

In the case of mood and anxiety disorders, there is always a question of the relative contribution of environment vs biology. This is particularly true for childhood-onset stroke (as opposed to neonatal stroke) in which the child may perceive him- or herself as different than they were prior to the stroke. In studies with adults, several psychosocial factors have been studied and found to play a role in the development of poststroke depression. For example, the absence of family support has been found to be a strong determinant

of acute depression reactions.[49] These researchers have also found that 1 year poststroke, the persistence of few social contacts is the main psychosocial factor associated with poststroke depression. However, others have highlighted that although the literature points to a relationship between social contacts and depression, the relationship is ambiguous (ie, having reduced social contacts may be the cause of the depression).[50]

Although understanding adult stroke may be helpful, it is important to point out the limitations in applying this information to pediatric stroke. Children with stroke may have very different medical and environmental risk factors. For example, it is rare that a child has the absence of family support following a stroke; in fact, in many cases the family support is increased when a child is critically ill. Children also have a different social environment. They are typically in school and are still in the role of being taken care of, and are not typically a caretaker themselves.

Adult stroke researchers have also postulated several biological mechanisms that lead to poststroke depression including disruption of biogenic amine neurotransmission and release of proinflammatory cytokines.[50] The biogenic amine hypothesis[51] postulates that ischemic lesions may interrupt the biogenic amine-containing axons that ascend from the brainstem to the cerebral cortex leading to decreased production of serotonin and norepinephrine in limbic structures in the frontal and temporal lobes, as well as the basal ganglia. There has been some support for this hypothesis. Alternatively, the proinflammatory cytokine hypothesis purports that proinflammatory cytokines that are involved in the initiation and amplification of the inflammatory response following ischemia may also result in depressogenic properties. Several studies have attempted to evaluate the relationship between lesion location and depressive symptoms—again with mixed results. Several studies have postulated a relationship between poststroke depression severity and proximity of the lesion to the left frontal pole. However, studies examining left anterior vs posterior lesions have been quite mixed. It has been suggested that these different findings may be related to the way depression is measured and at what point in recovery it is being measured.[50] For example, it may be that biological factors (such as reduced serotonin and norepinephrine) may play a more important role during the acute recovery phase and that psychosocial factors/difficulties adjusting to the impact of the stroke may lead to later-onset depression.

Again, although it is important to consider these adult studies, there may be some limitations in applying all of these findings to children. Most notably, strokes in the adult population occur at a time when brain development is largely complete. In contrast, children's brains are still actively developing, and the biological impact of the stroke may be quite different depending on the child's age at the time of the stroke and where they are in terms of a particular skill development. This is particularly relevant for perinatal stroke, as children in this group have been shown to have remarkable plasticity for other cognitive functions (eg, language reorganization), making it difficult to extrapolate from adult studies. In addition, adults are more likely to have underlying cardiovascular disease and small vessel vascular disease as the mechanism behind their stroke. Thus, adults often have microvascular lesions that predate a larger stroke. The vascular depression hypothesis has also been postulated.[52] This hypothesis purports that a single lesion, or the accumulation of many small ischemic lesions, can disrupt prefrontal systems that are important for mood control. Support for this hypothesis comes from the high comorbidity of depression, vascular disease, and vascular risk factors.

Apathy Versus Depression

Although mood and affect often coincide and reflect one another, it has been long recognized that individuals with neurological disorders may have dissociations of mood and affect. Mood is best understood as the internal state of mind or emotional state of a person, and affect is the behavior or external manifestation of mood and emotions.[53] Affect often includes facial expressions, tone of voice, and body language. Individuals with acquired brain injuries show increased rates of apathy (disturbance in motivation). These individuals may present with a depressed affect, but may not have corresponding changes in mood. In a meta-analysis of adult studies, poststroke apathy was found to occur in 36% of individuals with stroke.[54] Although poststroke apathy has not been studied in pediatric stroke, studies of children with other acquired neurological disorders have found that apathy is often present following pediatric traumatic brain injury. One study found that 14% of children with severe traumatic brain injury in their sample had apathy as part of their reported personality change.[55] Another group studied 81 children with traumatic brain injury and found that parents who reported high levels of distress in the care of their children were specifically concerned about several factors including apathy, the child's poor school performance, lack of friends, and inability to control angry feelings.[56]

Evidence-Based Treatments for Mood and Anxiety

Although there are limited data for treating mood and anxiety in children with medical illnesses (and none published in pediatric stroke), treatments can be extrapolated from the large body of work supporting empirically based treatments for children with these disorders.

Psychotherapy

Cognitive-behavioral therapy (CBT) is a form of psychotherapy in which the goal is to help the individual recognize cognitively distorted thoughts, reality-test these thoughts, and teach the individual skills to challenge these irrational thoughts and replace them with more rational ones. A 2006 review of the available meta-analyses found large effect sizes for CBT to treat both anxiety and depression in children.[57]

One large meta-analysis (13 studies) found that the remission rate for anxiety disorders was 56% in children who received CBT vs 28.8% in the control groups.[58] Although research is more limited in medical populations, CBT has been used in several studies to treat anxiety in children with medical disorders. It has been most studied in pediatric cancer treatment, but also in disorders such as sickle cell disease, diabetes, inflammatory bowel disease, and several other conditions with results indicated treatment effectiveness.

In addition to CBT methods to treat depression, research has found that interpersonal therapy (IPT) has well-established efficacy for adolescent depression.[59] Similar to CBT, IPT is a form of psychotherapy that is time-limited and present-focused. In IPT, the therapist creates a treatment alliance in which the therapist empathically engages the patient, helps the patient to feel understood, arouses affect, presents a clear rationale and treatment ritual, and yields successful experiences.[60] IPT is founded on 2 major principles: 1) depression is a medical illness (not the patient's fault) and is treatable; and 2) mood and life situations are related (ie, there is a practical link between the 2).

There are several additional issues to consider when utilizing CBT techniques in children with complex medical issues.[44] These include 1) initial distress reaction to the diagnosis, 2) anxiety and pain during treatment, 3) disease-related chronic pain, 4) coexisting psychological distress, 5) adherence to medical regimen, and 6) provision of social skills for the introduction of school and life after (or with) the disease. Several of these issues are relevant to the pediatric stroke population. For example, children may have to deal with chronic headaches, may need to follow medication and therapy regimens, and may have to reintegrate into school and/or the community following their initial diagnoses/hospitalizations. Children with disorders that

```
┌─────────────────────────────────────────────────────────────────────────────┐
│                              FAMILY FOCUS BOX                                  │
├─────────────────────────────────────────────────────────────────────────────┤
│ Key concept: Evidence-based treatments for mood and anxiety issues            │
│ Consider:                                                                      │
│                                                                               │
│  ▪ Psychotherapy: Most effective techniques include                           │
│                                                                               │
│     □ CBT for depression and anxiety                                          │
│                                                                               │
│     □ IPT for adolescent depression                                           │
│                                                                               │
│  ▪ Medication: SSRIs such as Prozac are most commonly used, but there are     │
│    other options as well.                                                      │
│ Who can help? Mental health professionals may include psychologists,          │
│ neuropsychologists, psychiatrists, social workers, or licensed counselors.    │
│ Next steps: Ask your physician (neurologist, rehabilitation doctor, and/or     │
│ pediatrician) about where you should start. If you are considering medication, │
│ a medical doctor, such as a psychiatrist or neurologist, should be involved in │
│ the decision-making process.                                                   │
└─────────────────────────────────────────────────────────────────────────────┘
```

have the potential for stroke recurrence may be at higher risk for anxiety given the uncertainty of their future medical status. Another important aspect of CBT in individuals with acquired brain injuries may be to assist the child/adolescent to have insight into his or her areas of strength and weakness (ie, improving self-awareness). With improved self-awareness, children may be able to better address their areas of weakness and accept help in the areas that they need it most.

Medication

The most commonly used medications to treat childhood mood and anxiety are selective serotonin reuptake inhibitors (SSRIs). These medications have been found to be effective in reducing anxiety and depression in children and adolescents.[61,62] Fluoxetine (Prozac) is the only FDA-approved SSRI for children and adolescents ages 6 and older, although other medications are often used in clinical practice. However, data are somewhat limited on the efficacy of these medications in children/adolescents with comorbid medical disorders.

Several other kinds of medications have been used to treat anxiety in children with chronic medical conditions. In conjunction with distraction techniques, benzodiazepines are frequently used in low doses during medical procedures to reduce anxiety. However, classes of medications other than SSRIs have not been as well studied in pediatric patients. Whenever medication is being considered, it is very important to involve the key individuals in making the decision, including the child, his or her parents, the treating physician (often the neurologist), and a mental health provider. In more complex cases, it is often helpful to refer the child to a psychiatrist for managing these medications. In the most ideal situation, the psychiatrist can work with the child's neurologist to optimize his or her medical care.

It is also very important to consider all of the medications that a child with stroke is taking in order to assess for drug–drug interactions and to ensure that other medications he or she is taking are not causing or exacerbating mood and anxiety symptoms. For example, several antiepileptic drugs (AEDs) can have emotional/behavioral side effects. In a 2012 review of the impact of AEDs on behavior, the authors note that AEDs are a "heterogeneous group of drugs with different underlying mechanisms that can differentially affect children's behavior."[63] For example, AEDs with GABAergic mechanisms may trigger symptoms of depression, anxiety, and irritability,[64] whereas those with stimulating or activating effects might trigger ADHD symptoms, irritability, mania, and psychosis.[65] Thus, it is important for physicians and families to work closely together to obtain the best risk/benefit ratio for treating different aspects of the child's medical condition. In addition, patients will benefit from physicians collaborating with the patient's other mental health professionals. For example, the child's regular psychotherapist, school counselor, or neuropsychologist may be able to provide the psychiatrist with additional information that could be helpful in deciding the best combination of treatments for a particular patient.

OTHER FACTORS TO CONSIDER

Impact of Emotional-Behavioral Difficulties on Interventions

All of the previously mentioned behavioral and emotional difficulties have the potential to affect a child's ability to engage in other therapies and interventions. For example, if a child is impulsive, easily frustrated by his or her limitations, or depressed, he or she may have difficulty engaging in physical or occupational therapy tasks that challenge or focus on his or her areas of weakness. In these situations, we recommend close consultation with the team's mental health professionals, which may include a psychologist,

INTERDISCIPLINARY TEAM FOCUS BOX

Key concept: Strategies to manage behavioral challenges in other therapies (eg, occupational therapy, physical therapy, speech-language)

Techniques:

- Behavioral momentum: A technique in which a person is given a task with which he or she is more likely to comply immediately before being presented with a task that is more problematic. That is, people tend to keep going in the behavioral direction they are already heading. Care providers can help set the stage by helping patients achieve small successes then build on the momentum and work on harder tasks.
  - Step 1: Assess the difficulty level of different tasks.
    - Easy: Any task the patient can perform accurately (ie, minimum of 80% accuracy) and fluently.
    - Moderate: Tasks in which patients are accurate but not yet fluent (may be slower).
    - Difficult: Tasks in which patients are neither accurate nor fluent (ie, less than 50% accuracy).
  - Step 2: Sequence together tasks (building blocks). Mini-tasks can be sequenced together within one lesson for the day. For example, patients may be given 2 or 3 easy tasks, followed by 1 or 2 moderate tasks, and ending with a difficult task.
- Preparing for change: Patients with stroke may have difficulty with changes in routine or unexpected events/people. Try to prepare the child well in advance for any changes (eg, a substitute therapist, change in usual routine), and watch them more closely in times of change.
- Control antecedents: By definition, children with inhibitory control difficulties struggle to consider potential consequences of their actions in the moment, even though they may demonstrate appropriate knowledge of consequences. Therefore, behavioral programs geared toward controlling stimuli that precede or lead to impulsivity are likely to be more successful than those that focus on the consequences that follow an impulsive action.
- Breaks/rewards/positive reinforcement: It is important to determine the right amount of time to expect patients to work before giving a break. With more challenging tasks, breaks will likely need to be sooner.
- Teach self-talk scripts: There are many self-talk scripts that children can learn to evaluate a particular situation. Several scripts that may be helpful in a therapy situation might include the following:
  - Big deal/little deal: This script helps children evaluate a situation and take a step back to see what is important and what is not important. This is often a helpful script for children who melt down or get frustrated over small things.
  - Hard to do/easy to do: This script is important for children with stroke who often encounter tasks that are difficult for them and need to learn strategies to cope with these challenges.
  - Ready/not ready: This script may be particularly important for children who are impulsive and need to stop and think of a plan before starting a task.[66]

For more information on these scripts, please visit http://www.projectlearnet.org/tutorials/sr_ef_routines.html

neuropsychologist, or social worker. Please see later in this chapter for some common behavioral strategies/techniques to consider when working with children with behavioral challenges and low frustration tolerance.[66]

Relationship Between Impairments in Executive Functioning and Psychological Functioning

As is reviewed in Chapter 9 of this book, problems with executive functioning (EF) are common in children with a history of pediatric stroke. The term *executive functioning* covers a broad range of both cognitive and behavioral skills. In the behavioral realm, skills such as a child's ability to inhibit impulses, regulate his or her emotions, and be flexible in new situations are all part of the executive skill set. Previous research has found that both teachers and parents reported elevated levels of concern with the behavioral aspects of EF in children with a history of stroke (parent Behavioral Regulation Index T score = 59.11, teacher Behavioral Regulation Index T score = 61.15).[67] The authors also reported that children with larger lesions (encompassing more than 25% of brain matter) had the most negative impact on EF, even though these large lesions were not in the frontal cortex. Thus, once a lesion crosses a particular threshold, the influence of the lesion location may be less predictive of outcome and the amount of brain damage may be of utmost importance. These authors suggest that larger lesions have more potential to disrupt the critical neural pathways and networks that rapidly develop during childhood that support efficient EF skills. Executive skills are implicated in social-emotional processes, such as modulation of emotions, personal and social decision making, perspective taking, affect, and social self-awareness. Thus, deficits in this area have the potential to affect learning/cognition, and behavioral and social functioning.

Relationship Between Language Impairment and Psychological Functioning

Children with a history of stroke sometimes present with delays in language development. This is particularly relevant for children with perinatal stroke or those whose stroke occurred before/during the prime years of language acquisition. Developmental language disorders occur in 20% to 25% of children with history of perinatal stroke, independent of site of lesion.[1] Children with language delays are often frustrated by their communication difficulties and may act out these frustrations with behavioral difficulties. In these cases, the function of a negative behavior (eg, hitting, biting, tantrums) may be to communicate with the caregiver. In children with language delays, it is important to consider both therapeutic interventions (ie, speech-language therapy and other early intervention services) and teaching caregivers effective behavioral management strategies for helping the young child manage these frustrations.

Language impairment may also affect psychological health in older children and adolescents. Children with a history of stroke with greater communication difficulties have been shown to have poorer psychological health on a QOL measure.[16] Language difficulties following a stroke are common and may include deficits in word finding, expressive language, receptive language, and other motor aspects of speech production (see Chapter 8). In older

children/adolescents, those with a left hemisphere stroke are at highest risk for acquired language deficits (ie, aphasia). In these cases, the child/adolescent may experience high levels of frustration and sadness when he or she is unable to fully communicate with others. These language difficulties also often affect his or her academic skills and placement in school, which in turn may worsen feelings of sadness, anger about his or her diagnosis, and lower self-esteem. Although psychotherapy may provide some benefit, this can also be a challenge, as many therapy techniques require a minimum level of expressive and receptive language to participate. In these cases, it will be important for mental health providers to work in conjunction with the speech-language therapist to best support the child's recovery.

Relationship Between Impairments in Social Competence and Psychological Functioning

Chapter 9 in this book includes a thorough review of the literature on social cognition and social skills outcomes following pediatric stroke. As was noted in that chapter, there is evidence from questionnaire measures and behavioral studies that children with a history of pediatric stroke have more social impairments than controls,[68] difficulties with aspects of social information processing, and lower levels of socialization on QOL measures.[18,69]

Given that children go to school and live in a very social world, one could hypothesize an interaction effect between social skills difficulties and other mental health concerns in this population. For example, children with ADHD have high rates of difficulty in social relationships due to several factors, including reduced knowledge of social skills and the ability to act appropriately.[35] Weaknesses in self-regulation and self-monitoring also likely contribute to social skills difficulties in children with comorbid ADHD, so these can also be the targets of treatment. Thus, children with perinatal stroke and ADHD symptoms may be at higher risk for social difficulties, and it is important to ascertain where/how the breakdown occurs in order to properly plan interventions. In addition, decreased peer relationships and successful friendships have been shown to be related to increased symptoms of anxiety and depression.

CASE STUDIES

Case #1: Patient KM; Difficulties With Behavior and Learning

Reason for Referral

KM is an 8-year-old, left-handed male with a history of left hemisphere perinatal stroke associated with right-side hemiparesis. He was referred for neuropsychological assessment due to concerns regarding learning difficulties, poor frustration tolerance, problems with attention, and social skill difficulties.

Background

- KM was born at 40 weeks' gestation via vaginal delivery. No prenatal or postnatal complications noted.
- Birth weight = 7 lbs, 9 oz
- Early left hand preference observed at 4 to 6 months along with slowed head growth.
- Brain magnetic resonance imaging at ~age 1 revealed large remote stroke involving left middle cerebral artery territory.
- Moderate right-sided weakness
- Developed seizures at age 4, continues to have seizures (3 to 5/year), treated with Trileptal (oxcarbazepine).
- Family history: brother with learning disability, mother with ADHD

Evaluation Results

- Strengths (age appropriate or better): KM demonstrated strengths in verbal intelligence, basic visual perception, rote memory/learning, left-sided motor skills, gross motor skills/athletic ability, and social motivation.
- Weaknesses: KM demonstrated weaknesses in nonverbal reasoning, speed of processing, attention, EF, academic skills, and many aspects of behavioral/social functioning. In particular, he struggled to focus in class, stay organized, and monitor his behavior and emotional reactions. KM was motivated to have friends, but tended to annoy other children by touching them, getting in their faces, and struggling to read their social cues. As a result of the findings, KM was diagnosed with ADHD—combined presentation and specific learning disability, with impairments in reading and math.

Behavioral and Emotional Recommendations

- Management of ADHD symptoms: Recommended that parents consider treatment options for his ADHD symptoms, including learning more about behavioral interventions or consideration of pharmacological management. Recommended a parent group focused on education and behavioral strategies.
- Behavior management interventions: Recommended a combination of individual and family support/parent training to help set up behavioral strategies in the home to address noncompliance, frustration tolerance, and dysregulated behaviors. Recommended that the patient learn cognitive-behavioral strategies to manage his increasing anxiety in new situations and perseverative/rigid thinking.
- Social skills interventions: Recommended interventions to address KM's emerging social skills difficulties. K may benefit from small group treatment where he could learn new skills and practice them in a safe environment with other children.
- Academic programming: Recommended continuing KM's current IEP in order to support his academic and emotional/behavioral development. The focus of the cognitive/academic support for KM was in systematic remediation of math skills, reading and related skills (ie, decoding, fluency, writing), as well as assisting his attention and executive control systems. He also needed to develop consistent systematic problem-solving routines for task setup (working memory, planning, and organization) and completion.
- Follow-up neuropsychological evaluation in 2 to 3 years.

(continued)

CASE STUDIES (CONTINUED)

Case #2: Patient CL; Difficulties With Anxiety

Reason for Referral

CL is a 16-year-old, right-handed female with history of sickle cell disease and recent right hemisphere stroke (3 months prior to referral). She has returned close to baseline in terms of neurological recovery, but has developed increased moodiness and difficulties concentrating. She was referred for a neuropsychological consultation in the stroke clinic to further investigate these concerns.

Background

- Normal pregnancy/delivery
- Diagnosed with sickle cell disease after birth.
- Medically stable until stroke 3 months ago.
- Family stressors: Rocky relationship with her father who has recently moved away.
- Lives with mother, grandmother, and one younger sibling.
- No prior history of academic concerns.
- No report of any new cognitive symptoms. Upon further questioning, patient has not had any new problems at school. Problems with concentration occur in conjunction with other increased symptoms of anxiety.

Assessment

CL became very tearful during the assessment and reported significant fears about her future and the possibility of stroke recurrence. She reported that she does not discuss these fears with anyone, as she tends to be a more shy, reserved person and doesn't want to burden her family members with her fears. She reports having a few friends at school, but that she has always been a bit more of an outsider and doesn't talk with her peers about her medical issues. She also stated that she would like to talk more with other adolescents with sickle cell disease. She denied any suicidal thoughts or intentions. Her family members felt concern about her increased anxiety/mood symptoms and had taken her to a counselor. She had only been seeing the counselor once a month and had mostly discussed her relationship with her father.

Recommendations

- Increased frequency of mental health therapy (once/week) given CL's ongoing symptoms and difficulty coping with stroke and complex family situation.
- Connect with support services for adolescents with sickle cell disease. A referral was given to the local chapter of the Sickle Cell Disease Association of America.
- Recommended close monitoring of CL's school performance upon returning to school in the fall. If any concerns with thinking arise (eg, attention, visual-spatial processing, memory problems), she may benefit from a neuropsychological evaluation to document her cognitive strengths and weaknesses following this recent stroke.

SUMMARY

Behavioral and emotional problems are relatively common in children with a history of both perinatal and childhood stroke. The most prevalent diagnoses include ADHD, anxiety disorders, and mood disorders, with comorbidity being a very common occurrence. Thus, it is very important that all health professionals who work with pediatric patients are aware of these issues, ask the right questions, and consult with specialized mental health professionals when they see a red flag in their patients. Fortunately, several treatments can be helpful to children and their families with these conditions, including both medication options and behavior management or psychotherapy techniques. Treating these behavioral and emotional symptoms is critical for improving the long-term outcome and QOL for pediatric stroke survivors and their families.

REFERENCES

1. Kirton A, deVeber G. Life after perinatal stroke. *Stroke.* 2013;44(11):3265-3271. doi:10.1161/STROKEAHA.113.000739.

2. deVeber G, MacGregor D, Curtis R, Mayank S. Neurologic outcome in survivors of childhood arterial ischemic stroke and sinovenous thrombosis. *J Child Neurol.* 2000;15(5):316-324.

3. Kirton A, deVeber G, Pontigon A, Macgregor D, Shroff M. Presumed perinatal ischemic stroke: vascular classification predicts outcomes. *Ann Neurol.* 2008;63(4):436-443.

4. Steinlin M, Roellin K, Schroth G. Long-term follow-up after stroke in childhood. *J Pediatr.* 2004;163(4-5):245-250.

5. Ganesan V, Hogan A, Shack N, Gordon A, Isaacs E, Kirkham FJ. Outcome after ischaemic stroke in childhood. *Dev Med Child Neurol.* 2000;42(7):455-461. doi:10.1017/S0012162200000852.

6. Lee J, Croen L, Lindan C, et al. Predictors of outcome in perinatal arterial stroke: a population-based study. *Ann Neurol.* 2005;58(2):303-308.

7. Max JE, Mathews K, Lansing AE, et al. Psychiatric disorders after childhood stroke. *J Am Acad Child Adolesc Psychiatry.* 2002;41(5):555-562. doi:10.1097/00004583-200205000-00013.

8. Duncan PW, Samsa GP, Weinberger M, et al. Health status of individuals with mild stroke. *Stroke.* 1997;28(4):740-745.

9. Carod-Artal J, Egido J, Gonzalez J, Varela de Seijas E. Quality of life among stroke survivors evaluated 1 year after stroke: experience of a stroke unit. *Stroke.* 2000;31(12):2995-3000.

10. Matza L, Swensen A, Flood E, Secnik K, Leidy N. Assessment of health-related quality of life in children: a review of conceptual, methodological, and regulatory issues. *Value Health.* 2004;7(1):79-92.

11. Muller-Nordhorn J, Nolte C, Rossnagel K, et al. The use of the 12-item short-form health status instrument in a longitudinal study of patients with stroke and transient ischaemic attack. *Neuroepidemiology.* 2005;24(4):196-202.

12. Suenkeler I, Nowak M, Misselwitz B, et al. Timecourse of health-related quality of life as determined 3, 6 and 12 months after stroke. Relationship to neurological deficit, disability and depression. *J Neurol.* 2002;249(9):1160-1167.

13. Centers for Disease Control and Prevention. Health-related quality of life (HRQOL). http://www.cdc.gov/hrqol/concept.htm. Published March 7, 2011. Accessed May 12, 2016.

14. Cnossen MH, Aarsen FK, Van Den Akker SLJ, et al. Paediatric arterial ischaemic stroke: functional outcome and risk factors. *Dev Med Child Neurol.* 2010;52(4):394-399. doi:10.1111/j.1469-8749.2009.03580.x

15. Friefeld S, Yeboah O, Jones JE, deVeber G. Health-related quality of life and its relationship to neurological outcome in child survivors of stroke. *CNS Spectr.* 2004;9(6):465-475.

16. Gordon A, Ganesan V, Towell A, Kirkham F. Functional outcome following stroke in children. *J Child Neurol.* 2002;17(6):429-434.

17. Neuner B, von Mackensen S, Krumpel A, et al. Health-related quality of life in children and adolescents with stroke, self-reports, and parent/proxies reports: cross-sectional investigation. *Ann Neurol.* 2011;70(1):70-78.

18. O'Keeffe F, Ganesan V, King J, Murphy T. Quality-of-life and psychosocial outcome following childhood arterial ischaemic stroke. *Brain Inj.* 2012;26(9):1072-1083.

19. Smith SE, Vargas G, Cucchiara AJ, Zelonis SJ, Beslow LA. Hemiparesis and epilepsy are associated with worse reported health status following unilateral stroke in children. *Pediatr Neurol.* 2015;52(4):428-434. doi:10.1016/j.pediatrneurol.2014.11.016.

20. Friefeld SJ, Westmacott R, MacGregor D, deVeber GA. Predictors of quality of life in pediatric survivors of arterial ischemic stroke and cerebral sinovenous thrombosis. *J Child Neurol.* 2011;26(9):1186-1192. doi:10.1177/0883073811408609.

21. Johnson A, DeMatt E, Salorio C. Predictors of outcome following acquired brain injury in children. *Dev Disabil Res Rev.* 2009;15(2):124-132.

22. Yeates K, Swift E, Taylor H, et al. Short- and long-term social outcomes following pediatric traumatic brain injury. *J Int Neuropsychol Soc.* 2004;10(3):412-426.

23. Max J, Mathews K, Manes F, et al. Attention deficit hyperactivity disorder and neurocognitive correlates after childhood stroke. *J Int Neuropsychol Soc.* 2003;9(6):815-829.

24. American Psychiatric Association. *Diagnostic and Statistical Manual of Mental Disorders,* 5th ed. Washington, DC: American Psychiatric Publishing; 2013.

25. Muir-Broaddus JE, Rosenstein LD, Medina DE, Soderberg C. Neuropsychological test performance of children with ADHD relative to test norms and parent behavioral ratings. *Arch Clin Neuropsychol.* 2002;17(7):671-689. doi:10.1016/S0887-6177(01)00170-6.

26. Gerring JP, Brady KD, Chen A, et al. Premorbid prevalence of ADHD and development of secondary ADHD after closed head injury. *J Am Acad Child Adolesc Psychiatry.* 1998;37(6):647-654. doi:10.1097/00004583-199806000-00015.

27. Gerring J, Brady KD, Chen A, et al. Neuroimaging variables related to development of secondary attention deficit hyperactivity disorder after closed head injury in children and adolescents. *Brain Inj.* 2000;14(3):205-218. doi:10.1080/026990500120682.

28. Herskovits EH, Megalooikonomou V, Davatzikos C, Chen A, Bryan RN, Gerring JP. Is the spatial distribution of brain lesions associated with closed-head injury predictive of subsequent development of attention-deficit/hyperactivity disorder? Analysis with brain-image database. *Radiology.* 1999;213(2):389-394. doi:10.1148/radiology.213.2.r99nv45389.

29. Max JE, Arndt S, Castillo CS, et al. Attention-deficit hyperactivity symptomatology after traumatic brain injury: a prospective study. *J Am Acad Child Adolesc Psychiatry.* 1998;37(8):841-847. doi:10.1097/00004583-199808000-00014.

30. Max JE, Lansing AE, Koele SL, et al. Attention deficit hyperactivity disorder in children and adolescents following traumatic brain injury. *Dev Neuropsychol.* 2004;25(1-2):159-177. doi:10.1080/87565641.2004.9651926.

31. Alderson RM, Mullins LL. Theoretical and clinical implications of using an ADHD framework to understand attention, concentration, and executive functioning deficits in pediatric cancer survivors. *Pediatr Blood Cancer.* 2011;57(1):4-5. doi:10.1002/pbc.23061.

32. Everts R, Pavlovic J, Kaufmann F, et al. Cognitive functioning, behavior, and quality of life after stroke in childhood. *Child Neuropsychol.* 2008;14(4):323-338. .

33. Bosenbark DD, Krivitzky L, Ichord R, Jastrzab L, Billinghurst L. Attention and executive functioning profiles in children following perinatal arterial ischemic stroke. *Child Neuropsychol.* 2016;1-18. doi: 10.1080/09297049.2016.1225708

34. Bosenbark DD, Krivitzky L, Ichord R, Jastrzab L, Billinghurst L. Clinical predictors of attention and executive functioning outcomes in children after perinatal arterial ischemic stroke. *Pediatr Neurol.* 2017;69:79-86. doi: 10.1016/j.pediatrneurol.2017.01.014.

35. Barkley RA. *Attention-Deficit Hyperactivity Disorder: A Handbook for Diagnosis and Treatment,* 3rd ed. New York, NY: The Guilford Press; 2005.

36. Jensen PS, Hinshaw SP, Swanson JM, et al. Findings from the NIMH Multimodal Treatment Study of ADHD (MTA): implications and applications for primary care providers. *J Dev Behav Pediatr.* 2001;22(1):60-73. doi:10.1097/00004703-200102000-00008.

37. Anastopoulos AD, Rhoads LH, Farley SE. Counseling and training parents. In: Barkley RA, ed. *Attention-Deficit Hyperactivity Disorder: A Handbook for Diagnosis and Treatment*, 3rd ed. New York, NY: The Guilford Press; 2005:453-479.

38. Connor D. Stimulants. In: Barkley RA, ed. *Attention-Deficit Hyperactivity Disorder: A Handbook for Diagnosis and Treatment*, 3rd ed. New York, NY: The Guilford Press; 2005:608-647.

39. Daly B, Kral MC, Brown RT, et al. Ameliorating attention problems in children with sickle cell disease: a pilot study of methylphenidate. *J Dev Behav Pediatr.* 2012;33(3):244-251. doi:10.1097/DBP.0b013e31824ba1b5.

40. Nikles CJ, McKinlay L, Mitchell GK, et al. Aggregated n-of-1 trials of central nervous system stimulants versus placebo for paediatric traumatic brain injury—a pilot study. *Trials.* 2014;15:54. doi:10.1186/1745-6215-15-54.

41. Pfiffner LJ, Barkley RA, DuPaul GJ. Treatment of ADHD in school settings. In: Barkley RA, ed. *Attention-Deficit Hyperactivity Disorder: A Handbook for Diagnosis and Treatment*, 3rd ed. New York, NY: The Guilford Press; 2005:547-589.

42. Pao M, Bosk A. Anxiety in medically ill children/adolescents. *Depress Anxiety.* 2011;28(1):40-49.

43. National Child Traumatic Stress Network. Medical trauma. www.nctsn.org/trauma-types/medical-trauma. Accessed May 12, 2016.

44. Kazak A, Schneider S, Kassam-Adams N. Pediatric medical traumatic stress. In: Roberts MC, Steele RG, eds. *Handbook of Pediatric Psychology*, 4th ed. New York: The Guilford Press; 2010:201-215.

45. Wu YP, Aylward BS, Roberts MC. Cross-cutting issues in pediatric psychology. In: Roberts MC, Steele RG, eds, *Handbook of Pediatric Psychology*, 4th ed. New York: The Guilford Press; 2010:32-45.

46. Mathew S, Price R, Charney D. Recent advances in the neurobiology of anxiety disorders: implications for novel therapeutics. *J Med Genet.* 2008;148C:89-98.

47. Max J, Keatley E, Wilde E, et al. Anxiety disorders in children and adolescents in the first six months after traumatic brain injury. *J Neuropsychiatry.* 2011;23(1):29-39.

48. Hackett M, Anderson C. Predictors of depression after stroke: a systematic review of observational studies. *Stroke.* 2005;36(10):2296-2301.

49. Astrom M, Adolfsson R, Asplund K. Major depression in stroke patients. A 3-year longitudinal study. *Stroke.* 1993;24(7):976-982.

50. Santos M, Kovari E, Gold G, et al. The neuroanatomical model of post-stroke depression: towards a change of focus?. *J Neurol Sci.* August 2009:1-2.

51. Robinson R, Bloom F. Pharmacological treatment following experimental cerebral infarction: implications for understanding psychological symptoms of human stroke. *Biol Psychiatry.* 1977;12(5):669-680.

52. Alexopoulos GS, Meyers BS, Young RC, Campbell S, Silbersweig D, Charlson M. "Vascular depression" hypothesis. *Arch Gen Psychiatry.* 1997;54(10):915-922. doi:10.1001/archpsyc.1997.01830220033006.

53. Sohlberg MM, Mateer CA. *Cognitive Rehabilitation: An Integrative Neuropsychological Approach*, 2nd ed. New York, NY: The Guilford Press; 2001.

54. Caeiro L, Ferro JM, Costa J. Apathy secondary to stroke: a systematic review and meta-analysis. *Cerebrovasc Dis.* 2013;35(1):23-39. doi:10.1159/000346076.

55. Max J, Robertson B, Lansing A. The phenomenology of personality change due to traumatic brain injury in children and adolescents. *J Neuropsychiatry.* 2001;13(2):161-170.

56. Prigatano G, Gray J. Parental concerns and distress after paediatric traumatic brain injury: a qualitative study. *Brain Inj.* 2007;21(7):721-729.

57. Butler A, Chapman J, Forman E, Beck A. The empirical status of cognitive-behavioral therapy: a review of meta-analyses. *Clin Psychol Rev.* 2006;26(1):17-31. doi:10.1016/j.cpr.2005.07.003.

58. James A, Soler A, Weatherall R. Cognitive behavioural therapy for anxiety disorders in children and adolescents. *Cochrane Database Syst Rev.* 2005;(4):CD004690. doi:10.1002/14651858.CD004690.pub2.

59. David-Ferdon C, Kaslow NJ. Evidence-based psychosocial treatments for child and adolescent depression. *J Clin Child Adolesc Psychol.* 2008;37(1):62-104. doi:10.1080/15374410701817865.

60. Markowitz JC, Weissman MM. Interpersonal psychotherapy: principles and applications. *World Psychiatry.* 2004;3(3):136-139.

61. Ipser J, Stein D, Hawkridge S, Hoppe L. Pharmacotherapy for anxiety disorders in children and adolescents. *Cochrane Database Syst Rev.* 2009; 8;(3):CD005170. doi: 10.1002/14651858.CD005170.pub2

62. Smiga SM, Elliott GR. Psychopharmacology of depression in children and adolescents. *Pediatr Clin North Am.* 2011;58(1):155-171. doi:10.1016/j.pcl.2010.11.007.

63. Caplan R. Psychopathology in pediatric epilepsy: role of antiepileptic drugs. *Front Neurol.* 2012;3:163.

64. Mula M, Sander J. Negative effects of antiepileptic drugs on mood in patients with epilepsy. *Drug Saf.* 2007;30(7):555-567.

65. Mula M, Monaco F. Antiepileptic drugs and psychopathology of epilepsy: an update. *Epileptic Disord.* 2009;11(1):1-9.

66. Ylvisaker M. Tutorial: Self regulation/executive functioning routines after TBI. *LEARNet.* http://www.projectlearnet.org/tutorials/sr_ef_routines.html. Published November 1, 2007. Accessed May 12, 2016.

67. Long B, Anderson V, Jacobs R, et al. Executive function following child stroke: the impact of lesion size. *Dev Neuropsychol.* 2011;36(8):971-987. doi:10.1080/87565641.2011.581537.

68. Trauner DA, Panyard-Davis JL, Ballantyne AO. Behavioral differences in school age children after perinatal stroke. *Assessment.* 1996;3(3):265-276. doi:10.1177/1073191196003003007.

69. Hurvitz E, Warschausky S, Berg M, Tsai S, Roth EJ. Long-term functional outcome of pediatric stroke survivors. *Top Stroke Rehabil.* 2004;11(2):51-59. doi:10.1310/CL09-U2QA-9M5A-ANG2.

SUGGESTED READINGS

General Parenting/Behavior Management

Clark L. *SOS: Help for Parents*, 3rd ed. Bowling Green, KY: SOS Programs & Parents Press; 2005.

Greene R. *The Explosive Child: A New Approach for Understanding and Parenting Easily Frustrated, Chronically Inflexible Children.* 5th ed., rev ed. New York, NY: Harper Paperbacks; 2014.

Phelan TW. *1-2-3 Magic: Effective Discipline for Children 2-12*, 4th ed. Glen Ellyn, IL: Parentmagic, Inc; 2010.

Attention Deficit Hyperactivity Disorder

Barkley R. *Taking Charge of ADHD: The Complete, Authoritative Guide for Parents.*

Flick G. *Power Parenting for Children with ADD/ADHD: A Practical Parent's Guide for Managing Difficult Behaviors.* New York, NY: The Guilford Press; 2013.

Hallowell EM, Ratey J. *Driven to Distraction: Understanding and Coping with Attention Deficit Disorder from Childhood to Adulthood.* New York, NY: Anchor Books; 1994.

Lougy RA, DeRuvo SL, Rosenthal D. *Teaching Young Children With ADHD: Successful Strategies and Practical Interventions for PreK-3.* Thousand Oaks, CA: Corwin; 2007.

Rief S. *The ADHD Book of Lists: A Practical Guide for Helping Children and Teens with Attention Deficit Disorders.* San Francisco, CA: Jossey-Bass; 2003.

Rief S. *How to Reach and Teach ADD/ADHD Children: Practical Techniques, Strategies, and Interventions.* San Francisco, CA: Jossey-Bass; 2005.

Roberts E. *The ADHD Parenting Handbook.* Lanham, MD: Taylor Trade Publishing; 1994.

Executive Functioning

Cooper-Kahn J, Dietzel L. *Late, Lost, and Unprepared: A Parents' Guide to Helping Children with Executive Functioning.* Bethesda, MD: Woodbine House Inc;2008.

Dawson P, Guare R. *Smart but Scattered: The Revolutionary "Executive Skills" Approach to Helping Kids Reach Their Potential.* New York, NY: Guilford Press; 2009.

Anxiety and Depression

Biegel G. *The Stress Reduction Workbook for Teens: Mindfulness Skills to Help You Deal with Stress.* Oakland, CA: Instant Help Books; 2009.

Chansky T. *Freeing Your Child from Anxiety: Powerful, Practical Solutions to Overcome Your Child's Fears, Worries, and Phobias.* New York, NY: Broadway Books; 2004.

Chansky T. *Freeing Your Child from Negative Thinking: Powerful, Practical Strategies to Build a Lifetime of Resilience, Flexibility, and Happiness.* Cambridge, MA: Da Capo Press; 2008.

Huebner D. *What to Do When You Worry Too Much: A Kid's Guide to Overcoming Anxiety.* Washington, DC: Magination Press; 2006.

Rapee R, Wignall A, Spence S, Lyneham H. *Helping Your Anxious Child: A Step-by-Step Guide for Parents.* Oakland, CA: New Harbinger Publications Inc; 2008.

Serani D. *Depression and Your Child: A Guide for Parents and Caregivers.* Lanham, MD: Rowan & Littlefield; 2013.

Tompkins M, Martinez KA. *My Anxious Mind: A Teen's Guide to Managing Anxiety and Panic.* Washington, DC: Magination Press; 2010.

Zucker B. *Anxiety-Free Kids: An Interactive Guide for Parents and Children.* Austin, TX: Prufrock Press; 2008.

Social Skills

Frankel F. *Friends Forever: How Parents Can Help Their Kids Make and Keep Good Friends.* San Francisco, CA: Jossey-Bass; 2010.

Nowicki S, Duke MP. *Helping the Child Who Doesn't Fit In.* Atlanta, GA: Peachtree Publishers; 1992.

SUGGESTED WEBSITES

Children and Adults with Attention Deficit/Hyperactivity Disorder (CHADD): www.chadd.org

Children's Hemiplegia and Stroke Association (CHASA): www.chasa.org

LEARNet: A Resource for Teachers, Clinicians, Parents, and Students by the Brain Injury Association of New York State: www.projectlearnet.org.

National Institute of Mental Health: www.nimh.nih.gov/health/topics/child-and-adolescent-mental-health/index.shtml

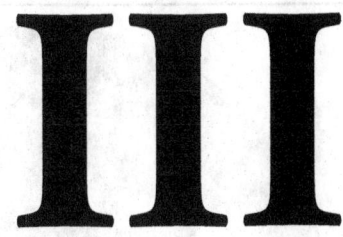

The Child's Environment
Family and Community

Kim Nixon-Cave, PT, PhD, PCS

MATTHEW'S STORY: A GIFT FROM GOD
Matthew Gabriel, meaning gift from God, but who knew what a gift I received. Born at 35 weeks with a complex congenital heart defect, he underwent a lifesaving 7-hour open-heart operation, and during the surgery he had a stroke. He was only 2 days old.
I was stunned and speechless; yes, I knew the risks, but to actually hear that it happened to my baby was life changing—forever.
Matthew suffered a perioperative left frontal lobe stroke. His first pediatric stroke team visit was the most memorable. He was 6 months old at the time; he should have had deficits—big ones—but no one could find any. Because of his young age and prematurity, his little brain rerouted itself, meaning all of the things the left frontal lobe are responsible for were taken over by another part of the brain—simply amazing.
I won't say that it was ever easy: most days include a challenge; some days are overwhelming. He has his struggles—more than any child should. He knows he's different, he knows he has to work harder than his peers, learning and school take much more work and repetition for him, and some days, as his mom, it's painful to watch him. A day never goes by that I don't wish it was me and not him; if I could only change that. He never passes up a challenge and has learned to compensate in ways I never thought possible. I am in awe just watching him grow and learn. We have learned to live every day to the fullest and enjoy the little things in life; they are by far the most important.
Matthew will soon be 9 years old. If you didn't know him, you wouldn't have a clue he has such a medical history—he has truly defied the odds. He has no idea the inspiration he is, especially to me. He has taught me so much about life, love, and perseverance. I am blessed to be his caretaker and honored to be his mom. Life has been a journey, life is still a journey…one of hope, love, and great possibilities…a gift from God.

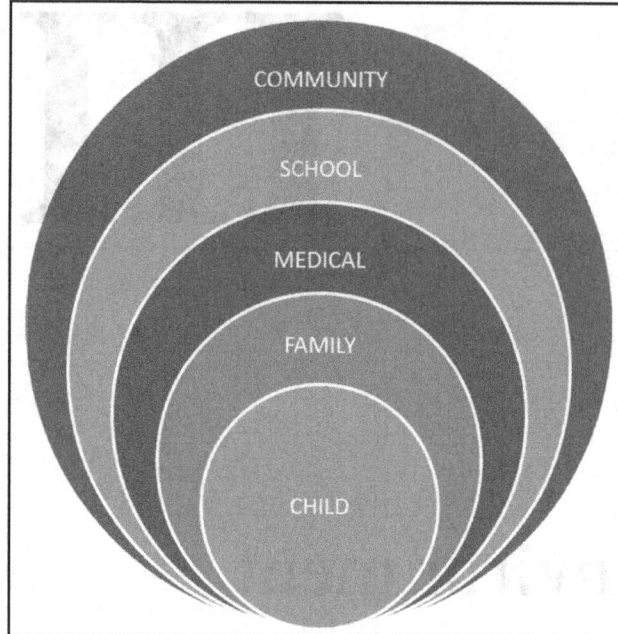

Figure III-1. The child being the focus and at the center of each level of the environment from a biopsychosiasl perspective.

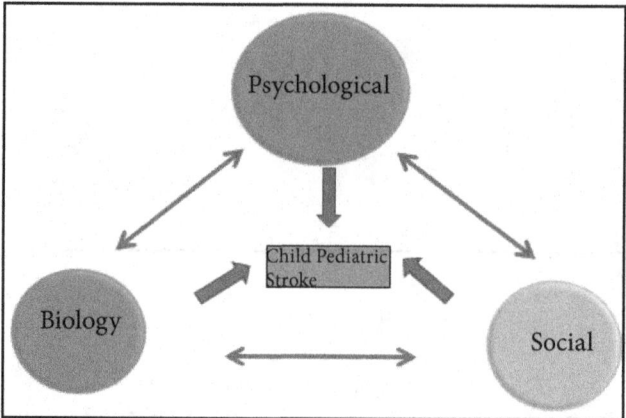

Figure III-2. Components of the biopsychosocial model and how they interact and impact the individual who is experiencing an illness or chronic condition.

INTRODUCTION

An infant or child who suffers a pediatric stroke faces many unique challenges. These challenges are also faced by everyone who is involved in the care of the child, especially the parents, caregivers, and immediate family. This section of the book focuses on these challenges, which include acquiring the appropriate care and support needed for the child to function in the community and allow him or her to return to home and school. The chapters in this section provide professionals working with a child and family following a pediatric stroke with information and resources to facilitate and support a successful outcome following a stroke as the child returns home and returns to daily routines. The chapters will consider the psychological and social factors that affect the child and his or her family following a stroke and what the child may need from a biopsychosocial perspective.

Figure III-1 frames the format for this section, addressing not just the medical diagnosis of the pediatric stroke, but all of the other contributing factors from a biopsychosocial perspective. The child, who is the central focus, is surrounded by immediate and extended support systems ranging from family support to community programs that serve the needs of the child. Individuals who work with a child or infant and his or her family following a stroke need to remember that it is important to make the child the central focus of every decision. Each chapter in this section will focus on a different aspect of the support system and will be presented within the child's biopsychosocial environment. Chapter 11 will focus on the child's family and

environment, exploring and discussing the issues that the child and family may face as a result of the pediatric stroke. Chapter 12 will focus on the educational needs of a child following a stroke, as well as on the federal and state laws that support entry or re-entry into an educational setting in spite of some possible major deficits. Finally, Chapter 13 will focus on advocacy and resources in the community, as well as medical resources that the child and family may need to access in order to support successful outcomes in the home environment following a stroke.

THE BIOPSYCHOSOCIAL MODEL OF HEALTH AND ILLNESS

As previously stated, this section is presented from a biopsychosocial perspective of health and illness, considering the biological, psychosocial, and social factors that affect the child and his or her family following a stroke. The biopsychosocial model of looking at causes and manifestation of health was developed by George Engel in the late 1970s in an attempt to move from the traditional biomedical model, which focuses on the disease and not the individual, to a model that focuses more on the person and the environment.[1] Instead of looking at the disease of the individual, the biopsychosocial model addresses the interaction between the individual's genetic makeup (biology), psychology (mental health and personality), and social or sociocultural aspects that contribute to a person's health or illness.[2] According to Engle, the biological, psychological, and social factors are all involved in the causes, manifestations, and outcomes of health and illness.[3] The biopsychosocial model of health implies that the treatment of disease processes requires a interprofessional team of medical professionals, social workers, and rehabilitation, behavioral, and educational specialists to address the biological, psychological, and social influences on the individual's functioning. The model facilitates teamwork and adds a preventative component to facilitate a successful outcome for the patient. Figure III-2 illustrates how the components of the biopsychosocial model interact and affect the individual who is experiencing an illness or chronic condition, such as a pediatric stroke. Each component of the biopsychosocial model will be described here briefly.

Biological Component

The biological component is the physical insult that results from a major medical event, such as a stroke. The pathophysiology and medical event of a pediatric stroke have been described in detail in Section I of this text in terms of etiology, types, and resulting impairments. As a quick review, a stroke occurs when blood flow to an area of the brain is blocked or interrupted, either by a blood clot or a broken blood vessel. When either of these things happens, brain cells begin to die and brain damage can occur.[4] A stroke can lead to mild to significant impairments that directly affect the child's ability to function within his or her environment or to develop the typical cognitive, motor, or affective skills and/or progress through a normal developmental sequence. Many resulting impairments can affect the child's overall development and ability to interact with peers and family and to participate in typical childhood activities. There are various types of pediatric stroke, including arterial ischemic stroke, cerebral sinovenous thrombosis and intracranial hemorrhage, and each has a different biological impact.[5] For detailed information regarding the pathophysiology of pediatric stroke, refer to Section I of the text. The biological aspect is reviewed here as a component of the biopsychosocial model of health and illness and how it may affect the psychological and social aspects of the child.

Psychological Component

The psychological component of health and illness from the biopsychosocial perspective considers the potential psychological causes of health problems and the resulting psychological issues that result from an illness or disease process such as a stroke.[1,6] The psychological impairments can affect the child's ability to interact within his or her environment or to return to typical childhood activities, such as play and/or school, that can directly affect habitation or rehabilitation. The psychological issues associated with an illness or disease can also indirectly affect the parents and family as they deal with having a child who has suffered a stroke.[1,6] Parents not only need to process the concept that their child has a health condition or illness that is typically associated with older individuals, but they also have to learn how to explain it to friends and family who question even the diagnosis of a stroke in a child. They also have to inform the school and the child's peers about the stroke and that the child may be different in many ways from other children or is different from how he or she was before. Parents are faced with these challenges, along with having a child who will need to face life with very different experiences from most of his or her peers, which can affect everyone psychologically. Viewing the child and parents from the biopsychosocial model makes it possible to see the psychological impact on the child, parent, and family following a stroke in relationship to the biological illness and the social impact, which can lead to a more complete understanding of the individual and not just the neurological event. A research study that examined the impact on parents and families of raising a child with perinatal stroke concluded that mothers of the children typically adapted well; however, mothers who had children with a moderate to severe stroke appeared to have a higher risk of psychological concerns or issues compared to those who had children with a mild to moderate stroke.[7]

Social Component

Finally, the social component of the biopsychosocial model addresses the social, cultural, and environmental factors of the child and family, including how cultural values and beliefs, socioeconomic status, religion, technology, and community can affect the child and family.[1,3] When individuals face a significant challenge, or when someone they love faces a challenge, such as an illness or stroke, they rely on their social and cultural values and beliefs to help them deal with the situation. Professionals working with individuals with serious health conditions such as a stroke should focus on being culturally competent. Cultural competency for a health care professional includes being able to understand the values and beliefs of the patient and family, as well as being able to communicate effectively. A culturally competent professional should create an environment of respect and mutual trust that demonstrates the value of diversity and celebrates differences.[8] The individual's internal and external environment plays a major role and can affect the outcome and all decisions made by the individual and his or her family.

THE BIOPSYCHOSOCIAL MODEL OF HEALTH AND ILLNESS AND INTERNATIONAL CLASSIFICATION OF FUNCTIONING, DISABILITY AND HEALTH—CHILDREN AND YOUTH

The concept of the biopsychosocial perspective of a child following a stroke from a rehabilitation perspective is best illustrated using the *International Classification of*

BOX III-1

DIMENSIONS OF THE INTERNATIONAL CLASSIFICATION OF FUNCTIONING, DISABILITY AND HEALTH WITH DESCRIPTIONS[9,10]

Health Condition

- Body functions are the physiological functions of body systems (including psychological functions).

- Body structures are anatomical parts of the body such as organs, limbs, and their components.

- Impairments are problems in body function or structure, such as a significant deviation or loss.

Activity

- The execution of a task or action by an individual

- Activity limitations are difficulties an individual may have in executing activities.

Participation

- The involvement in a life situation

- Participation restrictions are problems an individual may experience in involvement in life situations.

Environmental/Personal Factors

- The makeup of the physical, social, cultural, and attitudinal environment in which people live and conduct their lives.

Functioning, Disability and Health—Children and Youth (ICF-CY), a classification focused on health and health-related issues from a biopsychosocial approach, which was described in the introduction of this book.[9] Using ICF-CY supports the biopsychosocial model by allowing health care professionals caring for the infant or child to focus on the impact of the stroke, looking at the child's ability to function within his or her environment while dealing with resulting impairments. The ICF-CY allows for the child to be viewed within their environment, which can be a dynamic and interactive dimension of the individual, while attempting to meet the medical, therapeutic, and educational needs of the child and family.[9] The ICF-CY can assist providers, administrators, policy makers, and parents in documenting children and youth characteristics that are important for promoting growth, health, and development.[10] Box III-1, shows the components of the ICF-CY, which reflects the interactive relationship between health conditions and contextual factors, with a shift from terms that focus on the disease or illness to terms that focus on the individual.

In working with a child following a pediatric stroke from a therapeutic perspective, the ICF-CY fits the goal of this section to examine and provide support to the child and the family. The integrative approach of the ICF-CY classification system can be used for any individual with a health condition, regardless of the severity.[9] It recognizes the complex and multidimensional phenomenon of an individual's health condition or disability and acknowledges the impact of both individual features and social factors as important to consider in the understanding of disability while focusing on function and intervention.[11] The ICF-CY views the individual from a holistic perspective, focuses on function, and views the disability within the context of the environment. It recognizes the ongoing influence of the environment on the individual level of functioning and the associated understanding that disability could be prevented or reduced. Based on these principles and concepts, the ICF-CY provides a conceptual framework to act as a guide for a holistic and interdisciplinary approach to assessment and intervention for not just rehabilitation, but also for education. Figure III-3 illustrates how a pediatric diagnosis, such as a pediatric stroke, fits into the ICF-CY classification system.[10,12]

Family-Centered Care From a Biopsychosocial Perspective

When looked at from a biopsychosocial perspective, the ICF-CY allows a focus on the child and his or her environment, which involves the family, including the context in which the child grows and develops and in the case of child status poststroke recovers.[9-11] If the family is recognized as an important component of the child's recovery, professionals should practice family-centered care. Family-centered care is defined as[13]:

[A]n approach to the planning, delivery, and evaluation of health care that is grounded in mutually beneficial partnerships among health care providers, patients, and families. Family-centered care assures the health and well-being of patients and their families through a respectful family-professional partnership.

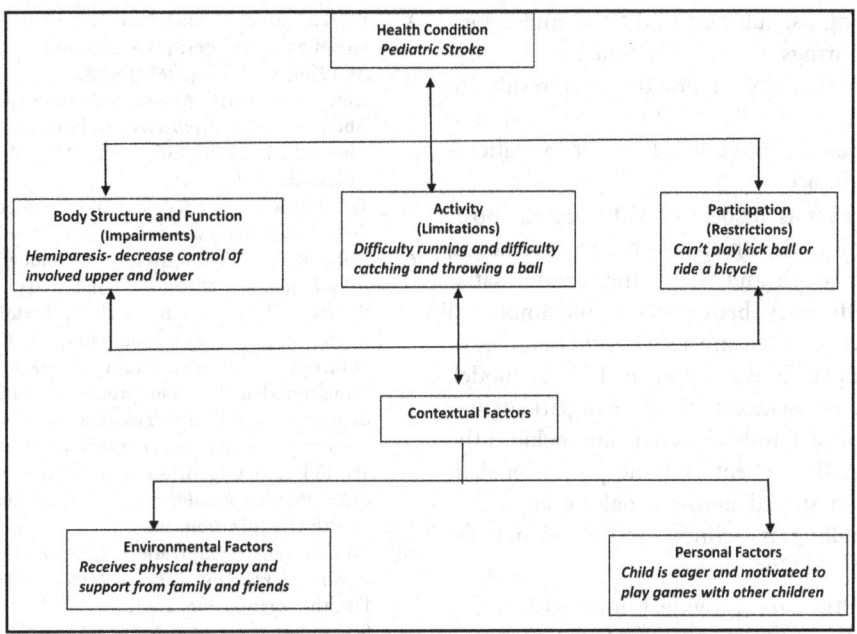

Figure III-3. ICF model showing family-centered care from a biopsychosocial perspective.

Box III-2

The Institute for Patient- and Family-Centered Care (IPFCC) defines patient- and family-centered care as:

- "[A]n approach to the planning, delivery, and evaluation of health care that is grounded in mutually beneficial partnerships among health care providers, patients, and families."[13]

- Patient- and family-centered practitioners recognize the vital role that families play in ensuring the health and well-being of infants, children, adolescents, and family members of all ages. They acknowledge that emotional, social, and developmental supports are integral components of health care. They promote the health and well-being of individuals and families and restore dignity and control to them.

- Patient- and family-centered care is an approach to health care that shapes policies, programs, facility design, and staff day-to-day interactions. It leads to better health outcomes and wiser allocation of resources, and greater patient and family satisfaction.

The IPFCC identifies 4 core concepts to patient- and family-centered care: *respect and dignity, information sharing, participation, and collaboration*[13]:

1. "Respect and dignity. Health care practitioners listen to and honor patient and family perspectives and choices. Patient and family knowledge, values, beliefs and cultural backgrounds are incorporated into the planning and delivery of care.

2. "Information sharing. Health care practitioners communicate and share complete and unbiased information with patients and families in ways that are affirming and useful. Patients and families receive timely, complete, and accurate information in order to effectively participate in care and decision making.

3. "Participation. Patients and families are encouraged and supported in participating in care and decision making at the level they choose.

4. "Collaboration. Patients and families are also included on an institution-wide basis. Health care leaders collaborate with patients and families in policy and program development, implementation, and evaluation; in health care facility design; and in professional education, as well as in the delivery of care."

It honors the strengths, cultures, traditions, and expertise that everyone brings to this relationship. Family-centered care is the standard of practice that results in high-quality services.[13,14] See Box III-2 for a description of family-centered care as outlined by the Institute for Patient- and Family-Centered Care.[13]

Family-centered care is associated with several positive outcomes for children with special health care needs, including improved health and well-being, greater satisfaction, improved efficiency, better access, and improved communication.[15] Lastly, to ensure a successful outcome of care for the patient and effectively apply the ICF-CY model, family-centered care is essential to the care of patients following a stroke. Because family-centered care includes the relationship between the patient and the professional, it is important to use a shared decision-making approach. Sharing decision making is defined by the Agency for Healthcare Research and Quality[16] as:

[W]hen [a health care provider] and patient (including family members and caregivers) work together to make a health care decision that is best for the patient.

[T]he optimal decision takes into account evidence-based information about available options, the provider's knowledge and expertise, and the patient's values and preferences.

Shared decision making and family-centered care allows patients and families to make informed decisions about their care and to collaborate with professionals, which improves the patient's experience of care, as well as adherence and outcomes, and which, in some cases, lowers health care cost and stress on the family.[17]

REFERENCES

1. Engel G. The need for a new medical model: a challenge for biomedicine. *Science.* 1977;196(4286):129-136.
2. Boundless. The biopsychosocial model of health and illness. *Boundless Psychology.* www.boundless.com/psychology/textbooks/boundless-psychology-textbook/stress-and-health-psychology-17/introduction-to-health-psychology-85/the-biopsychosocial-model-of-health-and-illness-326-12861/. Published September 20, 2016. Accessed March 30, 2017.
3. Borrell-Carrio F, Suchman A, Epstein R. The biopsychosocial model 25 years later: principles, practice, and scientific inquiry. *Ann Fam Med.* 2004;2(6):576-582.
4. American Heart Association/American Stroke Association. About Stroke. http://www.strokeassociation.org/STROKEORG/AboutStroke/About-Stroke_UCM_308529_SubHomePage.jsp. Accessed April 1, 2016.
5. Tsze DValente J. Pediatric stroke: a review. *Emerg Med Int.* 2011. doi:10.1155/2011/734506.
6. Adler R. Engel's biopsychosocial model is still relevant today. *J Psychosom Res.* 2009;67(2009):607-611.
7. Bernister T, Brooks B, Dyck R, Kirton A. Parent and family impact of raising a child with perinatal stroke. *BMC Pediatr.* 2014;14:182. doi: 10.1186/1471-2431-14-182
8. Campinha-Bacote J. The process of cultural competence in the delivery of healthcare services: a model of care. *J Transcult Nurs.* 2016;13(3):181-184. doi:10.1177/10459602013003003.
9. World Health Organization. *ICF: The International Classification of Functioning, Disability and Health.* Geneva, Switzerland: World Health Organization; 2001.
10. World Health Organization. *ICF: The International Classification of Functioning, Disability and Health.* Geneva, Switzerland: World Health Organization; 2007.
11. Schneidert M, Hurst R, Miller J, Üstün B. The role of environment in the International Classification of Functioning, Disability and Health (ICF). *Disabil Rehabil.* 2003;25(11-12):588-595. doi: 10.1080/0963828031000137090.
12. Simeonsson R, Leonardi M, Lollar D, Bjorck-Akesson E, Hollenweger J, Martinuzzi A. Applying the International Classification of Functioning, Disability and Health (ICF) to measure childhood disability. *Disabil Rehabil.* 2003;25(11-12):602-610. doi:10.1080/0963828031000137117.
13. Institute for Patient- and Family-Centered Care. http://www.ipfcc.org/. Accessed November 18, 2016.
14. Definitions and Principles of Family-Centered Care. http://www.familyvoices.org/admin/work_family_centered/files/FCCare.pdf. Updated February 2017. Accessed March 30, 2017.
15. Kuhlthau KA, Bloom S, Van Cleave J, et al. Evidence for family-centered care for children with special health care needs: a systematic review. *Acad Pediatr.* 2011;11(2):136-143.
16. Agency for Healthcare Research & Quality. The SHARE approach. http://www.ahrq.gov/professionals/education/curriculum-tools/shareddecisionmaking/index.html. Accessed February 16, 2016.
17. HealthIT National Learning Consortium. *Shared Decision Making.* https://www.healthit.gov/sites/default/files/nlc_shared_decision_making_fact_sheet.pdf. Published December 2013. Accessed February 16, 2016.

The Family and Child's Environment in Children With Stroke

Lois J. Robbins, DSW, LSW and Kim Nixon-Cave, PT, PhD, PCS

This chapter focuses on the family and environment, specifically the parents of a child following a stroke. From the biopsychosocial *International Classification of Functioning, Disability and Health* (ICF) perspective, the focus is on the environmental and social aspect of the impact of stroke on the child and his or her family.

FACING PEDIATRIC STROKE

Pediatric stroke can occur at any point in an infant, child, teen, or young adult's life. Although almost always a shock, the family's reaction to the diagnosis may be affected by the time of the diagnosis and other conditions the child may have endured. When a stroke is detected in utero, for instance, the family has time to adjust to the diagnosis and to begin preparing for the challenges ahead. The parents need to adjust to the fact that their child may be different from what they expected or planned. This experience is described in "Welcome to Holland," a parent's essay to expectant parents who have been informed that the healthy baby that they were expecting will not arrive.[1]

WELCOME TO HOLLAND

©1987 by Emily Perl Kingsley.
All rights reserved.
Reprinted by permission of the author.

I am often asked to describe the experience of raising a child with a disability—to try to help people who have not shared that unique experience to understand it, to imagine how it would feel. It's like this...

When you're going to have a baby, it's like planning a fabulous vacation trip—to Italy. You buy a bunch of guide books and make your wonderful plans. The Coliseum. The Michelangelo David. The gondolas in Venice. You may learn some handy phrases in Italian. It's all very exciting.

After months of eager anticipation, the day finally arrives. You pack your bags and off you go. Several hours later, the plane lands. The flight attendant comes in and says, "Welcome to Holland."

"Holland?!?" you say. "What do you mean Holland?? I signed up for Italy! I'm supposed to be in Italy. All my life I've dreamed of going to Italy."

But there's been a change in the flight plan. They've landed in Holland and there you must stay.

Atkinson HL, Nixon-Cave K, Smith SE, eds.
Pediatric Stroke Rehabilitation: An Interprofessional and Collaborative Approach (pp 211-225).© 2018 Taylor & Francis Group.

The important thing is that they haven't taken you to a horrible, disgusting, filthy place, full of pestilence, famine and disease. It's just a different place.

So you must go out and buy new guide books. And you must learn a whole new language. And you will meet a whole new group of people you would never have met.

It's just a <u>different</u> place. It's slower-paced than Italy, less flashy than Italy. But after you've been there for a while and you catch your breath, you look around…and you begin to notice that Holland has windmills…and Holland has tulips. Holland even has Rembrandts.

But everyone you know is busy coming and going from Italy…and they're all bragging about what a wonderful time they had there. And for the rest of your life, you will say "Yes, that's where I was supposed to go. That's what I had planned."

And the pain of that will never, ever, ever, ever go away… because the loss of that dream is a very significant loss.

But…if you spend your life mourning the fact that you didn't get to Italy, you may never be free to enjoy the very special, the very lovely things…about Holland.

When a stroke occurs at the time of birth, the child may need to be transported to a different hospital or a pediatric facility that can better care for the infant while the mother remains in the hospital where the baby was delivered. The other parent may find him- or herself going back and forth between the 2 locations in order to see both the baby and the mother. When the stroke occurs at an older age, there are rarely any known preexisting conditions that raise the likelihood of a stroke occurring. Sometimes there is a known, albeit small, risk of a stroke occurring in connection to another condition, such as sickle cell disease or surgery. When a child suffers a stroke, his or her life and that of the family can change in an instant. Pediatric strokes often strike quickly and without warning. One minute a child is his or her usual self, and the next second something is notably amiss. For example, a youngster may be happily playing a game and then is hit by an object. If a stroke occurs, the symptoms may necessitate a trip to the emergency department. One concern is that the emergency room frontline staff will not consider stroke a possible diagnosis for an infant or child. Additionally, if symptoms resolve as quickly as they occurred, the patient may be sent home only to have symptoms redevelop later. In both of these scenarios, crucial time is lost.

PARENTAL REACTION TO THE DIAGNOSIS OF A CHILD WITH A SERIOUS MEDICAL CONDITION

Because limited information is available for the child and family facing the diagnosis of pediatric stroke, it can be useful to consult research on families with children with other medical conditions and/or disabilities. Research from Norberg[2] addressed the emotional concerns of parents who have pediatric cancer patients and found that most parents experienced a crisis when their child was diagnosed with cancer. Research from Cameron et al[3] addressed the emotions of mothers when they became a parent to a child with special needs. Even after many years, the mothers could vividly describe the sadness, anger, frustration, loss, disbelief, and guilt, as well as the feelings of isolation they felt when given the diagnosis. According to these findings, the mothers' sense of loss of the "normal" child was similar to experiencing the death of a child. The experience is not necessarily similar for all parents. Carpenter and Towers[4] stated: "In families of children with disabilities, mothers and fathers can react differently to the news that their child has a disability or special need." In a study that looked at children newly diagnosed with cancer, the researchers found that the mother is usually the key to maintaining the family as an intact unit.[5] The mother tends to hold everyone together, and as a result mothers can be more susceptible to stress and may suffer posttraumatic stress syndrome as a result.[5] The mother may develop anxiety, depression, and other psychological responses. For fathers, for instance, the birth of their child with a disability is a challenge that allows them to display aspects of their personality not previously acknowledged.[4] Fathers can be prone to behaviors atypical for them, such as antisocial behaviors like substance abuse or drinking.[5] The birth of a child with special needs may transform parents in unexpected ways. Research conducted by Lehman et al[6] found that parents can show signs of posttraumatic stress disorder as a result of their child experiencing a stroke.

REACTION TO A DIAGNOSIS OF PEDIATRIC STROKE

In working with parents and caregivers, keep in mind that the overwhelming majority of people have never heard of stroke occurring in children, and as a result the parents may face special challenges in dealing with others who are unfamiliar with the diagnosis. If a child breaks his or her leg, there is a well-known set of procedures to deal with the diagnosis and provide information and education to the parents and caregivers about the diagnosis and how to deal with it. This is not the case with the diagnosis of pediatric stroke. Parents are unsure how to react when faced with the diagnosis. The initial reaction may be a feeling of shock and terror; however, a common reaction is to question whether the child will live or die. Another major concern is what the future might hold for the child who had once been "normal" and now faces an uncertain journey. Shapiro[7] noted that although similar experiences can generate very different outcomes, different experiences might generate similar results.

In order to gain some insight into how people may react and cope with the stroke diagnosis, researchers have studied how the fathers of pediatric stroke survivors of various ages reacted to the experience.[5,6] As part of a doctoral dissertation, the researcher interviewed 13 fathers whose children were seen in the Pediatric Stroke Program at a large pediatric hospital.[8] All but 3 of the fathers had been expecting to raise normal, healthy children. One of these children with other medical issues came into the family through kinship care adoption; the other 2 families knew that their children had suffered a stroke in utero. For one father and his wife, the physicians informed the couple that the baby's ability to survive at birth was in question. These parents developed a plan before the birth of the baby regarding to what extent they were willing to accept medical interventions. The dad indicated[9]:

> I was sad. It was more of holding it together to find out what the situation was. We didn't know. We knew there was hydrocephalus. They figured it out that it had something to do with the stroke. And at that point it was month to month until he was delivered. We had prepared for the fact that if he did not breathe on his own that we were going to try and keep him breathing long enough that everybody could spend a moment with him. We didn't want any kind of ventilation system started because if it wasn't meant to be, it wasn't meant to be. We didn't want to subject him to a life that was a burden to him, to live that way. So we actually had a priest there.

Most parents do not have time to adjust because they expected the birth of a typical child or because the stroke happened suddenly to an older child. Parents can display a variety of reactions to their child being diagnosed as having a stroke, the most common of which are discussed in the next section.

BOX 11-1

COMMON PARENTAL REACTIONS TO A DIAGNOSIS OF PEDIATRIC STROKE

- Shock and disbelief
- Uncertainty
- Panic and anxiety
- Heartbreak and sadness
- Helplessness
- Questioning God
- Why did this happen?

COMMON PARENTAL REACTIONS TO A DIAGNOSIS OF PEDIATRIC STROKE

Parents can have many different reactions to their child being diagnosed with a stroke. Box 11-1 lists the most common ones, each of which will be discussed briefly.

Shock and Disbelief

When given the diagnosis of pediatric stroke, most parents and family members are in a state of shock and disbelief. One reason for this reaction is that the overwhelming majority of people have never heard of children having a stroke. Most people believe that strokes happen to the elderly. In a study looking at the parents of pediatric patients diagnosed with a stroke, one father, when asked, reported that he was in shock because "I didn't know babies could have strokes. Nothing I ever thought about; nothing that happened on either side of the family. It was unbelievable. I couldn't believe what I was hearing."[6] Another contributing factor to this reaction may be that the parents receive the diagnosis for their child in the unexpected setting of the neonatal or pediatric intensive care unit.[9]

Uncertainty

When facing a diagnosis of pediatric stroke, uncertainty is a huge factor in what the parents feel and how they react when given the information that their child has had a stroke. The uncertainty ranges from not knowing if the child will survive to what life will be like for their child and how, as parents, they will deal with the situation. Initially families may question whether the child will live and, if so, what their quality of life will be. Once the child is out of the initial critical period, no longer needing the intensive care environment, the uncertain impact of the stroke also raises many questions. A stroke can cause a continuum of problems and concerns that may be temporary or permanent and lasting for indefinite periods. Often health care professionals, including physicians and therapists, can only offer a best guess as to how the stroke will affect the child's future functioning. Parents must continue to wonder about the impact of the stroke on the future quality of life of the child, as well as the impact on the entire family. This uncertainty often causes significant stress for both the stroke survivor and the family.

Panic and Anxiety

Parents can experience both panic and anxiety when hearing that a child has suffered a stroke, no matter when the stroke occurs. The diagnosis feels unbelievable and comes with immense angst. If the parent is not physically with the child when the stroke occurs, there is an added level of panic and anxiety. Not only are parents concerned about the implications of the stroke, but they also need to figure out how to get to the hospital as quickly as possible. Panic and anxiety continue even after the initial assessment is made that the child will survive. Families may panic if the child displays any symptoms of the original stroke or any other unusual and potentially critical signs. Such ongoing uncertainty may lead to continued feelings of panic and anxiety.

Heartbreak and Sadness

Many parents experience a natural sense of sadness.[9] They feel heartbroken for the image of a youngster growing up without obstacles in his or her way. One parent in the study expressed the sadness of losing the child he or she had been hoping to raise.[9] The parent stated:

> I was saddened with the fact that there were issues, probably feeling sorry for myself as much as for him. He was legally blind. He wouldn't be able to drive a car or all of those things you want to teach your children. The milestones you look forward to…

The parent of a 3-year-old boy with an arteriovenous malformation (AVM), a tangled mass of arteries and veins that affects the circulatory system, expressed the following when his wife was about to give birth to their third son[9]:

> I was a dreamer, dreamed about traveling the world and surfing with my kids and doing all these amazing things. Now, how am I going to do that? We didn't know if he would recover. If he wouldn't recover…I kind of shut my brain off at this point and worked myself up into a meltdown basically. The whole time we never left the hospital, we never left his side.

In addition to being concerned for the child who had just survived a stroke, the parents expressed concerns that future siblings could be born with an AVM resulting in a

stroke. The strain of even happy events, such as the birth of another child, adds stressors for many parents who have a child who has survived a stroke.

Helplessness

Feelings of helplessness arise when hearing that a child has experienced a stroke. Parents usually feel that they are able to protect their children from harm, yet they could do nothing to prevent the stroke. Angst occurs as a result of the inability to make the nightmare go away. For many, praying is the only option.[3,4] Many parents of children with special needs and/or disabilities feel a similar sense of helplessness.[3,4] Therefore, it is critical that all options are made available to families of children with special needs, including support groups, educational information, therapy, mindfulness programs, and compassion in the community.

Questioning God

According to research, most Americans have some religious or spiritual beliefs. In trying times, parents often find it difficult to reconcile their belief in a divine power with the reality of what has happened to their son or daughter. In the study of fathers, one father reflected the following sentiment: "A lot of people told me to turn to religion, which I couldn't do. The way I was thinking at the time was how could God let something like this happen? How could any power let something like this happen?"[9] Whereas some people will question God, others may feel a sense of comfort in the belief that God will take care of the child and the family. For those involved in faith communities, both clergy and lay members can offer practical and emotional support. Often congregants will offer to provide meals, escort other children to their activities, collect needed funds for the family, and offer prayers for the recovery of the child.

Why Did This Happen?

It is human nature to wonder why a serious illness or injury occurs to oneself or a loved one. Everyone wants to understand why their child has had a stroke. Some people will ask the question from a spiritual or an existential view. Others will want to know a concrete cause of the stroke. Unfortunately, there are often no good answers. Even with advanced technology, medical personnel may not be able to determine the cause of a stroke in a previously healthy child. This can create anxiety because parents may feel unsure whether another stroke will occur. Parents often become hypervigilant and overprotective after the child suffers a stroke in the hopes of preventing another one or at least of being aware of the symptoms if they occur. Many become preoccupied by the fear that another stroke may occur and afraid of letting the child out of their sight. Some patients are put on specific medication to decrease the chance of recurrence of stroke, while other patients have restrictions on physical activities to decrease the chance of recurrence. Both medications and activity limitations may be discontinued after a time if a child does well. As time passes and no new medical concerns are found, parents may find themselves relaxing, at least slightly.

THEORETICAL CONCEPTS

This section addresses theories of ambiguous loss, grief and sorrow, and boundary ambiguity, in addition to looking at long-held Western beliefs, such as the assumptive world concept. It is hoped that these constructs, used frequently in both psychology and social work, will offer a new stance to those who are unfamiliar with these conceptual theories.

In order to gain an understanding of why a child suffered a stroke, parents may find it useful to examine different belief systems about suffering and loss. Western belief and philosophical systems focus on finding the truth and individual rights, whereas the Eastern belief and philosophical systems focus more on accepting the truth as given and are more interested in finding the balance in life and addressing social responsibility.[10] In order to gain an understanding of what has happened to disrupt one's Western beliefs, it may be useful to examine theoretical concepts. Eastern philosophies are often dissimilar to those ideas of people living in countries aligning with Western thought.[10] For example, Buddhism features specific teachings about suffering and why things happen in life, and Buddhist philosophy is concerned with basic human suffering and ways to alleviate such suffering.[11] Chan et al[12] expressed the Buddhist belief that human beings are meant to be confronted by all experiences in life, no matter whether those experiences are good or bad, and furthermore, all kinds of experiences simply happen in life, and one should not take good fortune for granted or deny bad experiences.

Assumptive World

For those who were taught that "good" things will happen to those who are "good" people, a diagnosis of pediatric stroke can be not only devastating, but can also shake previous beliefs.

Beder[13] described the concept of the assumptive world as one where assumptions or core beliefs provide a way to see the world as a place that functions to ground, secure, stabilize, and orient people. This sense of how the world works is shattered in the face of trauma because tragic losses invalidate the assumptive world[14] on which we rely as our "taken-for-granted senses of security, predictability, trust, and optimism are profoundly and perhaps permanently undercut by traumatic experience."[15] The security once found in the beliefs is no longer present. The world

can no longer be seen as a safe place with good and caring people who have at least some control over what happens to them and their loved ones.[12] For many parents, the world no longer makes sense when something devastating happens to their child.

Ambiguous Loss

Pauline Boss' theory of *ambiguous loss* has implications for those facing pediatric stroke. Boss defined ambiguous loss as a circumstance where a loved one is physically present while psychologically absent, or where a loved one is psychologically present but physically absent because the physical status is unclear. It is not known if the loved one is dead or alive, dying, or in remission.[16,17] Both types of ambiguous loss lead to suffering that differs from a clear-cut, ordinary loss.[16] Boss described the following attributes: "ambiguous loss is unclear loss; ambiguous loss is traumatic loss; ambiguous loss is a relational disorder; ambiguous loss is externally caused (eg, illness, war), not by individual pathology; and, ambiguous loss is an uncanny loss—confusing and incomprehensible."[18] Boss and her colleagues found several areas of ambiguity that may contribute to family distress. These include the following[18]:

- A lack of clarity in diagnosis
- Difficulty in predicting outcomes
- Day-to-day changes in functioning of the ill person that affect family relationships
- The fact that the ill individual may give an outward appearance of health, thus raising expectations for his or her behavior and functioning within the family
- Fear that important emotional relationships will be affected by the illness.

Boss[16,18] stated that ambiguous loss might traumatize and be traumatic because the pain can be so incomprehensible and immobilizing that coping is blocked. Denial of the loss may sometimes provide a temporary respite from the reality of a potential loss. It may sometimes be beneficial when it allows the family to maintain its optimism and hope; however, it may also render people powerless in dealing with the situation at hand.[16] Finding meaning, or being able to make sense out of what is happening is especially difficult with ambiguous loss. Viktor Frankl[19] believed that there is no meaning without hope and no hope without meaning. In cases of ambiguous loss, people may move from hope to hopelessness and then back again to hope. This uncertainty is confusing and can cause tension, stress, and torment that can lead to personal and family problems. These conflicts occur not because of any inherent deficit of the person experiencing the loss, but rather because the situation is out of their control or because other constraints block the coping and grieving processes. People can feel helpless and are therefore more susceptible to anxiety and depression.[8,16]

Boundary Ambiguity

Whereas ambiguous loss is a situation in which information is unclear or unavailable, boundary ambiguity may be a family's response to the ambiguous loss. For example, a parent of a child with special needs may feel like a medical provider rather than a mother or father.[20] Boundary ambiguity "has been defined as a state in which family members are uncertain in their perception about who is in or out of the family and who is performing what roles and tasks within the family system."[21] For parents of children with chronic illness, boundary ambiguity can lead to psychological distress.[20]

Stages of Grief and Loss

A variety of theories deal with coping with the loss of a loved one or the loss of the person he or she once was. Some of the major tenets of concepts expounding this topic have changed over time. In the 1960s and 1970s, Elizabeth Kübler-Ross[22] proposed one of the most famous theories by describing how people deal with significant loss in stages. She identified 5 stages of emotional response to the death of a significant person: denial, anger, bargaining, depression, and acceptance. Although these stages suggest a sequential progression through the various stages of grief where one comes to feel acceptance or resolution at the end, Kübler-Ross acknowledged that individuals may go back and forth between stages.

Several researchers more recently proposed that such time-bound theories of grief are inappropriate[22] when attempting to help ease the grief and sadness that may afflict parents facing the loss of the "perfect" child. When parents are faced with raising a child with a chronic illness and/or disability, the theory of chronic sorrow may be more appropriate. Chronic sorrow is a way to explain the reaction to an ongoing living loss that is permanent, progressive, persistent, and cyclical. It is a way not to pathologize the feelings of parental grief and sadness. Olshansky stated that chronic sorrow is a normal psychological reaction rather than a neurotic response.

Many studies support the paradigm shift away from the time-oriented theories of grief and toward the concept of chronic sorrow.[5] Similar to Olshansky, Teel described chronic sorrow as a "reoccurring sadness, interwoven with period[s] of neutrality, satisfaction, and happiness; a parental reaction to chronic illness which suggests functional adaptation to, but not acceptance of, the child's condition"[23] Copley and Bodensteiner[24] elaborated on the theory of chronic sorrow after working with parents of children with disabilities. They identified 2 phases of parental feelings of loss: the first phase includes the impact, denial, and grief and is experienced as a cycle of highs and lows; in the second phase, parents begin to use appropriate coping strategies when resolving crises and adapting to their new life situation. Although emotional turmoil continues, it is less intense in this second phase. Even though the sorrow may fade over time, the sorrow never ends. Copley and Bodensteiner acknowledged, however, that because of the ongoing nature of the loss, some parents of children with disabilities are never able to move on to phase two and remain in phase one.[23] As the person with the chronic illness or disability remains in the physical environment, family members are constantly reminded of the loss. Although there may be adaptations and adjustments, and even some times of happiness, many continue to experience periodic and recurrent sadness. Therefore, where there is a "disruption in the relationship, consideration of bereavement theory does not necessarily contribute to an understanding of response to loss—loss that is ongoing."[25]

Realizing the New Normal

When a child suffers a stroke, changes often occur that affect not only the stroke survivor, but also those who are a part of his or her world. Often physical, social, and emotional adaptions and modifications need to transpire in order to meet the changed needs of the individual and his or her family. These changes may need to occur not only in the home, but also in the educational system, and perhaps the entire community. For the survivor and his or her family, previous plans for the future may no longer be realistic after the stroke. For instance, alternate blueprints may need to be drawn up for the high school superstar who was being recruited to play Division I football and was offered a football scholarship prior to the stroke. The stroke survivor may not have the same attributes that he had before the stroke; the family is now a different unit as well. They may no longer be the family who lives down the street, but may be identified by the community as the family whose child suffered a stroke. Siblings may be "branded" as the brother or sister of the kid who now has issues. There is often a heightened level of stress, increased responsibility for all family members, and changed identity and dynamics for the entire family.

Dreams Altered/Dreams Denied

Parents, young adults, and even children often have hopes for what they want their future to be. When a stroke occurs, this dream may no longer be possible, perhaps because new physical limitations make the dream unrealistic. Furthermore, families may need to remain close to medical care, thereby limiting their living and housing options. The financial toll created by providing therapies and medical care and the loss of parental income due to the need to be a caregiver to a recovering child also affects whether the child and family can follow a dream.

Change in Identity

In the instant that the child has a stroke, changes occur for all those close to that child. They may no longer be able to identify with the "normal" American family. After the initial period when there may be a question of survival, many parents face the task of determining where to obtain treatment for their child and how to pay for the care, and they may start to wonder what the future holds. In the adult stroke world, "stroke brings about a crisis in family systems as well as in patients themselves due to its sudden onset. Stroke results in physical and cognitive impairments, communication deficits, and depression for the patient."[26] Many pediatric stroke survivors are left with cognitive and emotional deficits.

When children experience stroke, parents need to deal with myriad new challenges, including issues with medical insurance and obtaining therapies, deciding what advice to follow, educational changes, emotional labiality, change in family structure, dealing with a condition that almost no one has even heard about, dreams altered/dreams denied, searching for the cure, hypervigilance, and deciding who can or should know. But most of all, the question remains, what will the future bring for my child?

Caregiver Burden

Families of a child who has suffered a stroke have many challenges. Often one parent might need to quit his or her job to become a full-time caregiver to the pediatric stroke survivor. This loss of an income has huge implications because there will most likely be an increase in expenses in caring for the youngster. There are often many therapy and doctors' appointments. Especially in the beginning, parents are often nervous to leave the child even for a second, for if the cause of the initial stroke is not known, the parents are concerned that another stroke may occur. The toll of becoming a caregiver may be both physically and emotionally exhausting. It may be difficult to determine the line between being the child's caregiver and the child's mother or father, thereby creating a feeling of boundary ambiguity.

RELATIONSHIPS WITHIN AND OUTSIDE THE FAMILY

The relationships with all those in the family may change after a child has suffered a stroke. Changes within the family structure may continue well into the future as the impact of a stroke may linger and affect the child and his or her family, for "the real and potential losses associated with chronic illness can be viewed as a continuum covering an indefinite period of time."[27] Family dynamics may change and continue to be altered as time passes. Parents may disagree on recommended therapies or best school placements. Siblings may need to increase their share of helping with household chores or not be able to participate in activities that were taken for granted before their brother's or sister's stroke. There will most likely be both financial and time constraints for all family members. Although this may be an extreme time of relational stress, it must also be noted that many new and/or stronger bond connections can be formed within the family unit as well as the opportunity to meet and form friendships and alliances with others.

Relationships Between the Parents or Partners

As Lazarus[28] points out, "coping with an ongoing source of stress can increase tension or conflict between partners." Although a devastating event can create a chasm between parents, many parents of pediatric stroke survivors report that they grew closer to their spouse or partner. Some parents felt it was the 2 of them and their child against the world.[9] The child's recovery becomes a shared goal. For many parents holding their family together while meeting the needs of all their children becomes the primary mission. Squabbles that may have once been part of the couple's everyday life may disappear as both parents must now focus their energies on what has become their new priority. Parents often realize that they play unique and important roles in this new and unexpected life.

Role of Mothers

Although both mothers and fathers of chronically ill children have to manage to cope with a variety of stressors related to the child's care, several researchers believe that mothers, as the traditional and primary caregivers, are more heavily burdened, both socially and psychologically, than fathers of children with chronic illness.[29] In addition to coping each day with the child's needs, mothers are often the parent responsible for the day-to-day requirements of the family, whether or not the mother works outside of the house. The prolonged care of the child with special needs has been shown to have adverse effects on her physical, emotional, and social well-being. Depression, guilt, distress, and high levels of worry have been documented in mothers caring for a child with a chronic illness. Mothers with fewer social resources reported a greater sense of burden and loneliness from being the child's primary caregiver.[9,29] It is therefore imperative that mothers spend time taking care of themselves. The analogy of the instruction for airline travelers to put the oxygen mask on oneself before assisting others is often presented.

FAMILY FOCUS BOX
A SIBLING'S STORY

Hello. My name is Tyler, and I am the brother of a stroke survivor. My brother was born 8 years ago with a serious heart defect. At 2 days old he had to have an emergency open-heart surgery to repair the defect. During the long operation, he suffered a stroke on the left frontal lobe of his brain. As a family, we knew that life was going to have to change and that it was going to be a major life adjustment.

Being the oldest, I have more responsibilities than my younger siblings. Having a little brother with disabilities has made me learn things I never thought I would have to learn and do things I never thought I would have to do. One thing I have learned is how to give him feeds through a feeding pump. As he has grown older he is beginning to eat more by mouth and is being weaned off of the feeding tube, but still receives one feed a day.

I think that the past 8 years have made us all stronger as a family and have pulled us closer together. My brother has come a long way since he was younger. He runs and plays, yet we all know what he has been through and what it has put us through as a family. We have come through so much and know there is still more to come, but we will do what we have done before and that is to persevere as a family. We know that if we try to go through this alone we are weak, but when we go through it together, we are strong.

Role of Fathers

Fathers are an important part of the care team when a child suffers a stroke. Like mothers, fathers also need to be aware of the importance of self-care so that they may become a vital caregiver for their child. Compared to years past, many of today's fathers are more involved in parenting. Fathers of children with a chronic health condition often transcend the "traditional male stereotype and embrace the opportunity for a more intimate and involved style of parenting."[30] These dads have reported being deeply affected by their child's diagnosis and needs, expressing feelings of guilt, sadness, anger, and anxiety. Many adopted a protective stance for both their child and the child's mother, and were more meaningfully involved with the child and family.[30]

Stroke Survivor

In a study by Robbins,[9] parents reported that their relationship with their son or daughter grew stronger after the stroke and expressed appreciation for the hard work that their child needed to do to regain skills. Fathers revealed that they became more sensitive and sympathetic toward their child. Mothers described a special closeness with their child that may not have occurred if the child had not suffered a stroke.

Siblings

Immediate and extended family members also experience difficulty when someone in the family is diagnosed with a stroke or a serious medical condition. Siblings of pediatric stroke survivors are affected on a daily basis. They not only have to cope with the changes caused by a stroke to their brother or sister, but they must also adapt to the now unequal distribution of their parents' attention, time, and resources.

Throughout their lives, brothers and sisters share most of the experiences that parents of children with special needs describe including isolation, a need for information, concerns about the future, and caregiving demands. Brothers and sisters also face issues that are uniquely theirs, including resentment, peer issues, embarrassment and pressure to achieve.[31]

IMPACT OF CULTURE, RELIGION, AND SPIRITUALITY

Myriad factors come into play in life after pediatric stroke. As noted earlier, various ethnic and religious groups have different views of suffering. Some groups are more focused on the community rather than the individual. Some communities have a religious figure who will guide decisions, and families may defer to that elder for decisions about medical care. Sometimes the faith community may be at odds with the family of the stroke survivor. One family in the study by Robbins[9] reported that their religious community did not believe in medical treatments, so they not only needed to go against their long-held religious beliefs to obtain treatment for their critically ill child, but in doing so they also forever altered their relationship with their church family.

Reconciling Beliefs

Views on culture, religion, and spirituality typically converge when trying to reconcile one's belief system with the reality of the child's diagnosis. As stated earlier, many people assume that there is a logical reason why things happen. Many involved in the life and care of the pediatric stroke survivor must begin to integrate their former beliefs with a worldview that no longer makes sense. It is important for the stroke survivor and his or her loved ones to come to terms with what they have learned—that in reality, it is a chaotic world.

Use of Belief Systems to Help Cope With Grief/Loss

Some families have a strong belief in a higher being—in God or a divine presence—that helps them cope with their child's stroke and gives them faith that God will protect their child and family. Others believe that everything is under God's will and therefore one must accept what has happened. Still others believe that suffering is a part of life.

COPING STRATEGIES

If your child or grandchild has had a stroke, how do you begin to cope with the reality of an often life-changing diagnosis? Some people are more adept at coping with unforeseen devastation; most will have a difficult time. Fathers who were part of the study by Robbins[9] delineated strategies that they found useful and that may be helpful for others. One of the goals of the study was to identify approaches that assisted these fathers on their journey, because most of them began at a point of not knowing how they would cope with the news of the diagnosis. Strategies that were most prominent are highlighted in the following paragraphs.

Spirituality/Religion/Prayer

A sense of spirituality may be a huge comfort to parents in coping with the stroke diagnosis for their child. Participating in rituals or prayer may be especially useful during a stressful time. Reaching out and receiving support from those in one's faith community may be helpful.

Taking One Day at a Time

Many parents, once the initial shock has worn off, cope with the situation by taking time in small measures and not looking too far into the future. This can be a helpful coping mechanism until the patient and family are more confident about the child's recovery. Some parents will continue to live day by day, especially if the child is at risk for another stroke or the child has a tough recovery or comorbidities.

Getting More Information

Although there is very limited information for families of pediatric stroke survivors, most families will try to find all information that is available. In the study by Robbins,[9] one father stated, "All the information I got once the diagnosis was told to us was very helpful. I was trying to become a little more knowledgeable about his current situation, his current status." A parent similarly offered that it was important to try to learn as much possible about pediatric stroke: "Reading and trying to become more familiar with different ways to help him, help him grow, help him cope himself, and I guess it's a way for me to cope."[9] It is important to note that not all information available, especially on the Internet, is correct. Professionals can help guide parents in their search for information about pediatric stroke and direct them to the appropriate resources.

Realizing You Are Not Alone

Although most people have never heard of children suffering from strokes, once it happens to a family, it is important that parents and families reach out and identify others in a similar situation. In the study conducted by Robbins, one parent affirmed[9]:

> As it became more of a reality, you start doing research and realize that you're not the only one out there who has been through it. Talking to caseworkers and other people at the hospital you realize that you're not in it by yourself, which helps along the way.

It is also critical that parents reach out to others, both professionals and nonprofessionals, letting them know how they can assist the child, the parents, and the rest of the family.

Appreciation of the Small Things

Most people involved in the life of a stroke survivor share that they are more appreciative of the small, everyday things that they previously took for granted. This appreciation can go a long way in the coping process and assist the parent and stroke survivor through the process.

Changing Priorities

There is often a rearranging of priorities by parents and different family members. A new sense of what is important is born. The intensity of surviving a serious threat can change how the survivors and their families choose to spend their time and energy. In the study of fathers, one of the fathers stated that his priority was "spending time with him and my other boys. Cherishing every hour, every minute, every second of the day we got to spend together and not really focusing on the future."[9]

Others Have It Much Worse

In talking with parents of children who have suffered a pediatric stroke, you routinely hear these parents comment on how happy or blessed they feel when seeing the difficult conditions other children and families face. Once a child begins the recovery phase and family members observe some regaining of lost skills, parents are extremely thankful that their child's condition is "not that bad." They will notice how their child is faring in comparison to the child in the next bed or the next room. Walking the halls at a hospital, rehabilitation center, or the outpatient building, parents see many children who are clearly extremely disabled due to their medical condition. A parent staying at the Ronald McDonald House shared the following[9]:

> We were in the lunchroom/dining area at Ronald McDonald and we're talking to some lady. I guess she saw we were new there and she started giving us her cabinet and all the food she had in the cabinet. She said, "Oh we're going home," and we said, "Congratulations." She said, "No you don't understand. My daughter has 8 weeks to live" or something like that. It was such a sad story. She had an inoperable brain tumor at the base of her brain.

Network of Support

Another coping strategy can occur from reaching out to various networks for support. These networks can be found in long-standing friendships, work relationships, family, religious affiliations, and so on. Although some of these supports can come from people and organizations to which the parents may have had a relationship prior to the stroke, other support networks can come from part of the new world and network that the patient and parents are now entering.

Specific Organizations

In looking for new networks of supports, it is important to know there are a number of organizations that can be helpful. These groups and organizations can help families adjust to their new identity as a family with a stroke survivor. Some of the organizations specific to brain injury and stroke are provided in Chapter 13. Other organizations may also be found in a hospital or rehabilitation setting, a school setting, within the community, or on the Internet.

Counseling/Speaking With Others

Professional counseling is often recommended for those facing a devastating event. Speaking with a mental health therapist, usually a social worker or a psychologist, can be a useful step in the coping process. If medication is warranted, parents or caregivers may be referred to a psychiatrist. These types of mental health services can be found by contacting the insurance provider and health care professionals to obtain a list of providers. It is important for the parents to form a positive therapeutic relationship with the therapists, but unfortunately, the first or second therapist might not be a good fit. Parents should be encouraged not to give up; a second, third, or even fourth therapist may need to be tried in order to find the therapeutic alliance that is most effective for coping with the loss of one's old life.

Child Getting Stronger

As the child gets better and skills return, parents generally show an increasing sense of hope. The improvement in the child's level of functioning is a major source of the parents' and family's ability to cope. Even when the child is still in the hospital, even small improvements in the child's condition helps the parent begin to cope with the diagnosis. Parents are comforted as their child regains skills. One father stated, "Once we came home I coped with it by working with him and helping him get stronger."[9] Another parent indicated, "Her therapy helps; she's getting a little bit stronger, but she's still young. But seeing her progress, I think that's helped along the way."[9] Additionally, a parent said, "Over time he started getting better. It's treatable. We'll just try to get him the right treatment. Right now I'm happier than ever because I see him running around."[9]

Accepting the Situation

At some point, it is necessary for the family to accept the situation and adjust to the circumstances and the reality they face. This state of acceptance is sometimes referred to as the new normal. This acceptance may be a significant step in coping with the idea that the child is now identified forever as a stroke survivor. Giving up the what ifs and dealing with the current situation while maintaining hope is an important step toward adapting to the life everyone now faces.

ADAPTATION AND RESILIENCY

Human beings are truly amazing in their abilities to rebound from disasters. This resiliency is especially strong in children. The spirit of individuals allows for recovery that they may have never thought possible. As the tongue-in-cheek message goes, "when given lemons, make lemonade." However, the child and the parents may have to change expectations of the life they assumed they would lead. Within those changed expectations and beliefs, a new and perhaps better sense of life's purpose may arise. It is important to focus on the resiliency of the child and the family as they begin the new phases in their lives.

Treating the Child as Normally as Possible

It is crucial for all involved to treat the stroke survivor as normally as possible. If, for example, children in the household are expected to complete chores, the stroke survivor should have appropriate jobs assigned with clear and delineated expectations. Appropriate praise and rewards are acceptable for the hard work a stroke survivor may demonstrate in therapy, just as praise and rewards are acceptable for other children who show great achievement. It is important to work with the child's team to define what the child can and cannot do in everyday situations. For all involved, it is necessary not to overindulge the stroke survivor simply because he or she is a stroke survivor. This is often especially hard for grandparents or extended family to grasp. Although during the initial period all the attention needs to be focused on the stroke survivor, while trying to follow a path of normalcy, all children in the family should be given equal attention.

Making Meaning

In order to move on, pediatric stroke survivors and their parents must find meaning in life, even if initially finding meaning must be delayed. Some find a spiritual meaning. Others may acknowledge that life is sometimes unfair, but this is the reality of life as we know it. Others look to positive things that have happened because they are involved with the pediatric stroke community. This may be seen as nuclear families becoming closer, a shy mother coming into her own by advocating for her child and others who have suffered a stroke, or increasing the number of positive relationships by meeting people they never would have met if not for the commonality of loving a pediatric stroke survivor.

Posttraumatic Growth

When tragedy occurs, sometimes amazing things develop. Many people find it necessary to make peace with the pain by finding meaning in the loss of a typically developing child or by finding some good that can come from the tragedy. Many foundations and charities advocate to assist individuals who may be afflicted with a similar loss. For instance, one father of a stroke survivor established an

organization to raise awareness and funds for pediatric stroke. Another family started a charity that helps high school football players improve their ball playing skills while learning about and raising funds for their daughter's condition. At each charity event, their daughter speaks about her experience in suffering a pediatric stroke, and a book about her is sold to raise funds and awareness about pediatric stroke Another parent has spoken about pediatric stroke before Congress many times. She and her daughter reach out to those in the political and general community who may be interested or able to help advocate for issues important for pediatric stroke prevention and for those who have survived the diagnosis.

Accepting the Situation: The New Normal

Amazingly sometimes even though the dreams are denied, new dreams become realities. These new futures may be more meaningful to the patient and his or her family. Two examples, both involving young men dreaming of careers in sports, come to mind. One young man suffered a life-altering stroke at the age of 15. He had been training with a college coach and planned to make the Olympic ice hockey team in a few years. He was famous in his town for his athletic abilities, and for years it looked like he would be able to conquer the world by excelling in ice hockey. He had been given a scholarship to an elite private boarding school. One day, his mother came home and found him on the floor. He had suffered a stroke, probably the result of a dissection (tear in an artery) caused by being hit by a hockey puck. He was rushed to the hospital and underwent emergency surgery. Everyone was thankful that he survived; however, the stroke ended his dreams of becoming a famous ice hockey player and all the perks that accompany that career. He spent 55 days in the intensive care unit and then the better part of a year in a pediatric rehabilitation hospital. He now attends a local college and is doing well. His future career may be uncertain, but he has provided inspiration and hope for many people and other young stroke survivors.

Another example involves a young man who was recruited to play Division I football and dreamed of the chance for a career in the NFL. He hoped that his football skills would earn him a scholarship to college, because family financial resources were limited. During the summer between his junior and senior years of high school, however, he suffered a stroke due to a pontine cavernoma and was given only a 50% chance of surviving. The physician who was part of his palliative care team is now his mentor as he begins college with plans to become a doctor. Three years after the stroke, he can no longer pursue his prestroke dream, but he has stated that his new dream is even better. While continuing to face physical challenges, he has developed a new sense of self and become a positive face for pediatric stroke. He often talks to other survivors and their families and gives them encouragement and hope. He has met and impressed a congressman who is working on a national level to increase funding for neuroscience research, including pediatric stroke. He has developed leadership skills and self-esteem and been given opportunities that would not have happened without suffering his stroke. His parents, who had been divorced at the time of his stroke, have even gotten back together. Dealing with his medical crisis created a new sense of what is important for his entire family.

Like this young man and his family, many families report reassessing their priorities after a pediatric stroke. Many of the fathers in the study by Robbins[9] stated that work is no longer a top priority, and they now spend much more time with their children and wives. They enjoy being with their families and cherish the everyday moments in their lives. A pediatric stroke may cause people to reprioritize simple joys and allow them to relish what they have instead of always wanting something more or different.

WHEN THE CHILD RETURNS HOME POST (INITIAL) STROKE

There is often a sense of reassurance while the child is still in the hospital or rehabilitation facility that if something goes wrong, medical staff are right there to provide the necessary care. Going home can be scary for the child and especially for the parents because medical support will no longer be so immediately available. In addition, when families spend most of their time at the hospital to be with the stroke survivor, they often find it easier to ignore mundane everyday tasks than when they are home. Returning home may be a very stressful time because the family needs to take on the everyday responsibilities of working outside of the home and running the household, as well as caring for the young stroke survivor. The following information may help parents and caregivers as they prepare to take their child home following a stroke.

Re-Entering the Community

In addition to the physical challenges, there will be emotional and social challenges for both the child and the family. When returning home, the child may be tired, and it is important to educate the parents about limiting the number of visitors, as well as the length of the visit. Parents must consider that it may be difficult for the child to follow conversations among multiple friends. It is recommended that only 1 or 2 friends visit at a time in the beginning and that the time limit (30 to 60 minutes) is set prior to the visit.

Once the child leaves the rehab facility or program, there may be some disappointment as the child/family acknowledges the new normal. Children and parents should be encouraged to access mental health services in order to deal with the loss of how things were supposed to be and the reality of how things are now. The therapy may not need to be extensive, but it is important to see a psychologist or social worker in the beginning and to revisit the therapist if new concerns arise. The insurance company will have a list of in-network providers. If medication may be beneficial, a psychiatrist can help make that determination.

Home Modifications

If the stroke survivor has been left with physical challenges, the family home may need structural and environmental modifications. Often the child's rehabilitation physical therapist can be instrumental in assisting the family in determining what is required. A child's second floor bedroom may need to be modified or moved. If the child needs to be discharged to home in a wheelchair, structural modifications to the family home may be needed. A ramp may be needed in order for the child to overcome steps at the entry to home. The bathroom may need modifications to be wheelchair accessible. Some items for modification, such as a shower chair or a toilet seat to raise the level and make it easier for the child to transfer to use the toilet, are relatively inexpensive.

As soon as the child begins the rehabilitation process, parents should talk with the rehabilitation team about what accommodations the child might need upon returning to the family home. Insurance companies will often pay for some of the necessary home modifications. However, both the process of getting the approval from the insurance company and having the work done can be daunting, and parents will need support from professionals to navigate the system.

Safety/Child Care Concerns

Many families put a baby monitor in the child's room in order to hear if the child needs assistance. This can also be a useful strategy for parents who are concerned that the child may have another stroke.

Networks of Support

It is important to utilize your networks, family, friends, and communities, such as neighbors and church communities. Often faith communities or neighbors will arrange to take care of everyday tasks in order to provide the parent time to deal with the complexities of bringing the child home after this serious medical event and subsequent course of care. Family and friends can provide meals, take other children to their activities, pick up needed items, or just be available to listen to the parents and/or caregivers. Just as parents would provide these helpful activities for their friends and family in need, parents need to allow them to provide these items for them. People want to help in time of crisis, and this gives friends and family concrete tasks to perform to support the family.

Invisible Disability Issues

Depending on the nature of the stroke, some children are left with no visible signs of change, although the child may be left with intellectual and/or emotional challenges. Without a visible disability people may question if the child actually had a medical diagnosis, especially because very few people have ever heard of children having strokes. It is important that parents educate family and friends about their child's diagnosis and subsequent impairments and limitations. This information will directly and indirectly allow family and friends to have a better understanding of the stroke diagnosis, as well as be in a better position to support the parents and the child.

Recreation

Following a stroke, children should engage in physical activities that facilitate their continued rehabilitation and improved function. It is extremely important to ask the child's physician and the rest of the health care team about activities the child may safely participate in following the stroke. For example, when a stroke has occurred, there may be limitations for all contact sports. After a period of time when the child has not shown any further concerns, the restriction may be lifted and some contact activities may be allowed.

From the ICF perspective, the focus is on the child's activity and his or her ability to participate in life activities. Adaptive sports and general play can be important components of the recovery of a child following a stroke. It is important to assess the tasks that the child can achieve and identify the ones that present limitations. This assists the child and parents in determining what assistance the child needs with different tasks for daily activities. Assessing the child's level of activity and ability to participate in daily activities from an ICF perspective helps identify which activities the child can participate in and at what level both in play and the educational environment.

LEGAL/FINANCIAL IMPLICATIONS

Unfortunately many additional issues face the stroke survivor and his or her family that have little to do with the functional recovery from the stroke. However, these items are of utmost importance and may need to be addressed at multiple times throughout the life of the child. Although legal and financial matters are other sources of stress for families, families may be able to receive valuable assistance from local, state, and federal agencies for the disabled, such as a qualified social worker, educational consultant, patient advocate, and/or lawyer. It is important that parents begin the legal and financial processes as soon as possible.

Legal and Guardianship Issues

Although it is hoped that all children will have sufficient recoveries so that at the age of 18 they are able to handle their own legal, financial, and medical decisions, some pediatric stroke survivors may not be able to do so. It is important for parents to confer with legal counsel in order to make sure all needed documents are in place. Parents may need to obtain a medical and/or financial power of attorney for their child. For example, if the parent or caregiver does not have power of attorney and the child receives a monthly check from the government due to his or her disability, the child has the right to spend it as he or she wishes upon reaching the age of 18. Similarly, if the child is over 18 years of age and needs to be taken to an emergency room, the parents and/or caregiver may not be allowed to provide input into the medical care of the child.

Parental Employment

Sometimes it is necessary for one or both parents to stop working in order to care for the child who has suffered a pediatric stroke. In most cases parents are eligible to take a continuous or intermittent leave under the Family Medical Leave Act. Although the employer will hold the job for when they return, they do not receive a paycheck during this time.

Special Needs Trusts

In order to protect assets for the child, parents should investigate setting up a special needs trust. This process should be done under the guidance of a lawyer. If the stroke survivor has financial resources, funds from governmental sources such as Social Security Income (SSI) and Medical Assistance (MA) may not be received. A special needs trust is designed to protect money and various assets that may remain with the stroke survivor until needed.

NAVIGATING THE HEALTH CARE SYSTEM

Unfortunately for those living in the United States and most other countries, navigating the health care system can be a nightmare. Some families have described this as a new full-time job. Some insurance companies provide special case managers to assist parents with complex medical issues. These managers can be quite helpful in navigating the various procedures and processes. In addition, parents must always be alert for any changes in health care benefits.

Insurance

It is important that parents understand what their insurance policy or policies do and do not cover. Parents should review their policy during any open enrollment period to consider changing their policy and/or health care provider(s). If the child is receiving SSI from the government, it is essential to support the parents through the process and encourage them to complete any requested forms in a timely manner. Children receiving SSI are automatically eligible for MA. However, parents need to be aware that the requirements for continued SSI and MA change once the child reaches the age of maturity, age 18. By age 17.5, parents should be investigating whether the child will continue to qualify for SSI and MA benefits.

Medical Home

For individuals who need to see multiple specialists, it is useful to have one medical provider and his or her team oversee and coordinate their care. A medical home is a fairly new concept in health care that allows for all therapists, teachers, and other medical providers to coordinate a patient's care with one provider. Please remember that the parent and child will continue to be very important members of any team.

TRANSITION TO ADULTHOOD OR PREPARING TO LEAVE HOME

The transition to adulthood is a scary time for both the stroke survivor and his or her family. The educational system should be involved to smooth the transition. In addition, some groups run workshops and/or provide individual guidance for this new phase of life. These are often based in hospitals, rehabilitation units, agencies (governmental and others), and school districts. It is important to start early in this process. For students entering high school, now is the time to begin!

Preparing to Enter the Work Force

States have specific agencies that assist people with special needs and/or disabilities in finding and maintaining employment. Although the name of the agency may differ by state (for example, it is the Office of Vocational Rehabilitation in Pennsylvania and it is the Division of Vocational Rehabilitation in New Jersey), the vocational rehabilitation agency offers a variety of services and resources. The parents and the child should register with the state agency for employment by the time the child is entering the final year of high school.

It is also important to know what accommodations an employer must agree to in accordance with the Americans with Disabilities Act (ADA). The ADA prohibits discrimination against people with disabilities.

College Supports

If your child is attending college outside of the home area, a neurologist and any other needed providers should be found as part of the college selection process. The child's pediatric neurologist may continue to be involved, but a local neurologist is necessary for any emergencies. If the child has an unusual medical condition, he or she may need to attend college in an area with a major medical center.

Parents should be aware that those teens who plan to attend college should give written permission for their parents to be notified if they need health care services. Parents of college students may be surprised to learn that once a child is over the age of 18 years, all of the services provided to the child are confidential. Parents only receive the bill. In addition, the college student should carry the business card for his or her pediatric physician and a note stating that they are a pediatric stroke survivor and listing any crucial medical information, including how to contact the parents and physician.

Unfortunately, the symptoms of stroke are sometimes similar to other causes. For example, if a person enters the emergency room with slurred speech and/or an uneven gait, emergency room personnel may jump to the false conclusion that the student may have taken drugs.

Going to college is an exciting and scary time for most people, and pediatric stroke survivors must consider taking special precautions. Although it is hoped that no student engages in drinking or drugs, these behaviors can be especially problematic for stroke survivors. Depending on the type of stroke, the use of birth control pills may be contraindicated.

By law, all colleges must provide services for students with special needs and have a specific office for students who have disabilities or require special support while in college. Parents and students should make sure to connect with a staff member in this office when considering various colleges. It is helpful to bring any medical information, individualized education program, or 504 plans. Unlike elementary, middle, and high school, it is up to college students to self-identify their needs and request the services that they may need.

SUMMARY

Although a pediatric stroke can deeply alter the life course of the survivor and those who love him or her, it can also bring about unexpected positive consequences. Many individuals develop a new appreciation for their loved ones, a reprioritization of items of importance, a sense of accomplishment and increased self-esteem, and an expansion of their world. They may, over time, come to find that it is not the devastating event that most people believe it is when they first received the diagnosis.

REFERENCES

1. Kingsley EP. Welcome to Holland. 1987.
2. Norberg A. Burnout in mothers and fathers of children surviving brain tumour. *J Clin Psychol Med Settings.* 2007;14(2):130-137.
3. Cameron S, Snowdon A, Orr R. Emotions experienced by mothers of children with developmental disabilities. *Child Health Care.* 1992;21:96-102.
4. Carpenter B, Towers C. Recognizing fathers: the needs of fathers with children with disabilities. *Support Learn.* 2008; 23(3):118-125. doi:10.1111/j.1467-9604.2008.00382.x.
5. Sahler OJ, Varni JW, Fairclough DL, et al. Problem-solving skills training for mothers of children with newly diagnosed cancer: a randomized trial. *J Dev Behav Pediatr.* 2002;23(2):77-86.
6. Lehman LL, Maletsky K, Islam, F, Rivkin MJ, Mrakotsky C. A pilot study: parents show evidence of PTSD while children display anxiety following childhood stroke. *Stroke.* 2015;46:(Suppl 1).
7. Shapiro E. Whose recovery, of what? Relationships and environments promoting grief and growth. *Death Studies.* 2008;32(1):40-58.
8. Children's Hospital of Philadelphia. Pediatric stroke program. http://www.chop.edu/stroke. Accessed March 30, 2017.
9. Robbins L. Hearing his story: a qualitative study of fathers of pediatric stroke survivors. http://repository.upenn.edu/cgi/viewcontent.cgi?article=1054&context=edissertations_sp2. Published March 28, 2014. Accessed March 30, 2017.
10. Difference Between Eastern Religions and Western Religions. http://www.differencebetween.net/miscellaneous/religion-miscellaneous/difference-between-eastern-religions-and-western-religions/. Accessed March 30, 2017.
11. Turner K. Mindfulness: the present moment in clinical social work. *Clin Soc Work J.* 2016;37:95-103.
12. Chan C, Ng S, Ho R, Chow A. East meets west: applying Eastern spirituality in clinical practice. *J Clin Nurs.* 2006;15:822-832.
13. Beder J. Loss of the assumptive word: how we deal with death and loss. *Omega.* 2004;50:255-265.
14. Janoff-Bulman R, Berg M. *Disillusionment and the Creation of Values: From Traumatic Losses to Existential Gains in Perspectives on Loss. Harvey.* Philadelphia, PA: Brunner/Mazel; 1998.
15. Neimeyer R, Prigerson H, Davies B. Mourning and meaning. *Am Behav Sci.* 2002;46:235-251.
16. Boss P. *Ambiguous Loss: Learning to Live with Unresolved Grief.* Cambridge, MA: Harvard University Press; 1999.
17. O'Brien M. Ambiguous loss in families of children with autism spectrum disorders. *Family Relations.* 2007;56:135-146.
18. Boss P. The trauma and complicated grief of ambiguous loss. *Pastoral Psychol.* 2010;59:137-145.
19. Frankl V. *Man's Search For Meaning,* 3rd ed. New York, NY: Simon & Schuster; 1984.
20. Berge J, Holm K. Boundary ambiguity in parents with chronically ill children: integrating theory and research. *Fam Relat.* 2007;56:125-134.
21. Boss P, Greenberg J. Family boundary ambiguity: a new variable in family stress theory. *Family Process.* 1984;58:535-546.
22. Kübler-Ross E. *On Death and Dying.* New York, NY: Macmillan; 1969.
23. Lowes Lyne P. Chronic sorrow in parents of children with newly diagnosed diabetes: a review of the literature and discussion of the implication for nursing practice. *J Adv Nurs.* 2000;32:41-48.
24. Copley M, Bodensteiner J. Chronic sorrow in families of disabled children. *J Child Neurol.* 1987;2:67-70.
25. Teel C. Chronic sorrow: analysis of the concept. *J Adv Nurs.* 1991;16:1311-1319.
26. Kim J, Moon S. Needs of family caregivers caring for stroke patients. *Soc Work Health Care.* 2007;45:81-97.
27. Moulton P. Chronic illness, grief, and the family. *J Community Health Nurs.* 1984;1:75-88.
28. Lazarus R. *Stress and Emotion: A New Synthesis.* New York: Springer Publishing Company, Inc.; 1999.
29. Florian V, Krulik T. Loneliness and social support of mothers of chronically ill children. *Soc Sci Med.* 1991;32:1291-1296.
30. McNeill T. Fathers of children with a chronic health condition: beyond gender stereotypes. *Men Masc.* 2007;9:409-424.
31. Conway S, Meyer D. Developing support for siblings of young people with disabilities. *Support Learn.* 2008;23:113-117.

SUGGESTED WEBSITES

Brain Injury Association of America: www.biausa.org (BIAUSA has local chapters and support groups.)

Children's Hemiplegia and Stroke Association (CHASA): www.chasa.org (CHASA has local organizations and activities.)

International Alliance for Pediatric Stroke (IAPS): www.iapediatricstroke.org/home.aspx

12

Educational Needs of a Child/Adolescent Following a Stroke

Elisa Olson D'Achille, MEd and Juliana Bloom, PhD

After the initial shock of finding out that a child has had a stroke, school will probably not be the first thing on a parent's mind. But before long, parents of school-aged children may find that returning to the normal activities of school will be something the child is ready to do. It is important for the child to have opportunities to learn and spend time with peers, and both the parent and child will likely want to return to a normal routine. However, changes in the child's functioning, including physical and cognitive differences, will need to be taken into account. There may be a need for modifications and resources within the school that are necessary to accommodate the needs of the child so they can successfully return to school and access their education.[1]

THE MEDICAL ENVIRONMENT VERSUS THE EDUCATIONAL ENVIRONMENT

In order to navigate the educational system, one must first understand how school environments differ from medical environments. A medical team will focus on maximizing the recovery of the child and how to support the child, family, and school through that process. A school's focus will be on the child's ability to access their education during this particular school year and what supports will be necessary in order to achieve that goal. Accessing one's education includes being able to navigate the school environment and participate in the curriculum, but does not include maximizing a child's potential. Thus, the goals for any child in the hospital, rehabilitation center, or when

participating in outpatient therapy will differ from the goals put into place within a school.

EDUCATIONAL LAWS AND PROCESSES

One must understand the laws that govern school districts as they provide education for children with special needs, including children who have had strokes. The most notable laws include the Individuals with Disabilities Education Act (IDEA) and Section 504 of the Rehabilitation Act.[2]

Individualized Education Program

IDEA is the cornerstone of special education and states that children with disabilities must be given a *free and appropriate public education* (FAPE) at the public expense.[2] All students must also be educated in the *least restrictive environment*. Furthermore, this law requires the student to be included within the regular education classroom for as much of the school day as possible. If the child's stroke has led to cognitive or physical problems that make it hard for him or her to learn, he or she may qualify for an individualized education program (IEP) under the special education category "Other Health Impaired." An IEP that includes the goals and supports, including specially designed instruction, needed to participate in school is developed.[2]

The team that develops the IEP includes teachers, therapists, guidance counselor, representative from the local education agency, special education coordinator, and any

Atkinson HL, Nixon-Cave K, Smith SE, eds.
Pediatric Stroke Rehabilitation: An Interprofessional and Collaborative Approach (pp 227-245).© 2018 Taylor & Francis Group.

individual who can add information to support the team. It is important for parents to be part of the educational team responsible for developing the IEP. Students who are 14 years of age or older are encouraged to be part of the process as well. The process also allows for parents to bring outside advocates as they see appropriate. The IEP outlines the services and supports that the student needs in the school setting. It must be updated within 1 year or as frequently as requested by any team member. An IEP is a legally enforceable document bound by due process that allows the parents the rights and legal recourse under the law if the IEP is not being followed. Other school services that a child may qualify for under IDEA include physical, occupational, and speech therapy, counseling, and transportation and health services (such as administration of medications); although some districts provide these services under a 504 plan.[2]

504 Plan

Section 504 of the Rehabilitation Act is a law outlawing discrimination in public schools. A 504 plan also addresses a student's unique learning needs as a result of a disability, primarily through accommodations. However, it does not provide the specially designed instruction that is provided through an IEP and is served through regular education rather than special education. Children who do not qualify for an IEP may qualify for a 504 plan. A 504 plan can be helpful when a child has difficulty with a specific area (eg, the student cannot participate in physical education) but does not need any changes within his or her classroom. When a headache or seizure plan is a necessary part of a child's school plan, those details can be outlined in a 504 plan.[3]

Parents, as well as older children, should be involved in every step of any evaluation process as well as the IEP/504 plan. Parents will be asked for their input as well. There are a great number of rights for the family and processes in place for when the school and the family cannot agree on the proper placement and related services.

Revising the 504 Plan or Individualized Education Program

By law the IEP or 504 plan must be updated once/year with a full meeting of the entire IEP team. However, a school plan is a fluid document and changes can be made at any time. Any member of the IEP team, including the parent or guardian, has the right to request a change be made at any time and as often as needed. If the parent/guardian is making this request, then it is best to be made in writing and should include the date, child's name, and a signature. A full team meeting is not required every time a change is made, but parents/guardians are required to receive a copy of the changes and can request a new copy of the complete updated plan.[2,4]

Any number of changes may be needed throughout the school year. Weaknesses and deficits after a pediatric stroke can sometimes improve over time as recovery from initial injury occurs. Some of the deficits of a stroke will take months to return, others can take years, and some deficits may be permanent.[5] As a result, the modifications and accommodations necessary to access a child's education will need to be reconsidered and changed accordingly.

The difficulties and solutions will change throughout the school years depending on the age and grade level of the child. A student with weakness in their dominant hand may need their homework written down for them throughout elementary school, but in middle and high school when the homework is available on the teacher's website, it is more appropriate for them to receive a copy of class notes. Throughout a child's education, the curriculum for that school year needs to be considered when planning to meet the needs of the student at the appropriate level.

Extended School Year

Extended school year (commonly referred to as *ESY services*) are eligible to students who regress in skills or take so long to recoup skills after summer break that it interferes with the child's ability to participate in the curriculum after a break. The ESY program helps children maintain their educational skills throughout a long school break and to avoid losing valuable classroom time recovering the skills they had already mastered the previous school year. Other related services provided in the IEP may be provided during the ESY if the child has lost skills before over long school breaks. Most states require students be observed and tested before and after long holiday breaks to determine if there is a regression in skills and if these skills are not quickly recouped.[1]

An ESY program does not mimic a typical school day. The programs generally include shorter sessions and are not provided throughout the entire school break. The exact standards for eligibility for ESY are governed by each state board of education.[1]

Special Education Law Resources

Information and resources concerning special education services and laws are available on a state-by-state basis. The Education Justice website (www.educationjustice.org/index.html) offers links to law centers in every state. Education law centers provide resources and advocates for families trying to navigate the special education system. Educational resources and advocates vary greatly state by state and can change depending on the current available funding from each particular state department of education.

THE TRANSITION BACK TO SCHOOL

The process and timing of a child returning to school after a stroke will vary greatly based on the severity of the deficits and extensiveness of the school modifications needed. It is important for parents to keep the school informed throughout the recovery process so school staff will be aware of what adaptations or supports may be needed. Medical care plans, classroom modifications, equipment, length of the school day, and transportation are just some areas to be considered before a child can safely and effectively return to school. The collaboration and input between parents, school staff, medical providers, and therapists is necessary to ensure a smooth transition.

Keeping in touch with friends while out of school can also assist the child in settling back into their new normal and reduce any anxiety or fear when it is time to return to the classroom. It can be helpful when teachers encourage classmates to make cards or send a video from the class while kids are still in the hospital. Once they are home, parents can arrange for the kids to use technology such as Facetime (Apple) or Skype to help the child keep in touch with peers when missing school. Reintegrating into the social aspects of school is just as important for recovery as returning to the assignments, homework, and tests.

Each of the following sections highlights the topics that will need to be addressed when planning for a child to return to school after a stroke.

Medical Clearance

The medical team following a stroke patient will provide guidelines as to when the child is medically stable and safe to return to school. In order for any medical professionals to correspond with a child's school team, the parents or guardian must sign a permission to release information form for all to speak and share information. Hospitals and medical offices will provide the family with a release of information form, and schools will also require their own release forms for the families to consent before any information can be exchanged. These forms will need to be updated once/year. Generally, schools will require documentation stating the child is cleared medically before returning to the school.

The School Meeting

Communication between medical team, school team, and the family is imperative to ensure that everyone involved has the most updated information. Because a stroke is not the most common problem teachers see in the classroom, it is helpful for parents to meet with the child's school team (teachers, therapists, aide, guidance counselor, principal) to provide a brief explanation of the reason for the stroke (if known), the rehabilitation that the child has been or is currently participating in, and the plan for further recovery. The school should be aware of what physician appointments and therapy plans and appointments have already been scheduled. Someone at school should be designated as the contact person to receive any updated information that can affect the current school plan. It is important for school personnel to expect that in the first few months after a child has suffered a stroke there will be big fluctuations in the child's progress and recovery. These changes will need to be continuously reflected in the school plan.[6] It can be helpful for educators to be provided with references from the child's medical team and other pediatric stroke resources listed at the end of this chapter.

Child Study or School Team Evaluations

Many children who have had strokes have unique motor and learning challenges and will require special education services in school. Some children may require a different classroom or need certain accommodations within the classroom. Each child is unique and will need his or her own individual plan. The needs of a child will vary greatly between children and also as a function of a particular child's age and development. As children grow and develop, the demands and expectations in school expand and so will the modifications needed for each child to access his or her education. For example, students in first grade are not required to organize the details of completing a long-term, multistep project, so supports for executive functioning skills will need to be added to the child's education plan as the demands for those areas increase. The focus of any special education plan between preschool and college will vary greatly, and this is the same for a student who has a history of stroke.

Formalized neuropsychological or psychoeducational evaluations to determine an individual child's cognitive capacity and academic skills inform the IEPs that will need to be developed before a child with a brain injury can safely and successfully return to school. A neuropsychologist or school psychologist will administer standardized tests to evaluate intelligence, academic skills, learning, memory, attention, and how any deficits from the stroke will affect a student's ability to participate in the classroom. These neuropsychological evaluations will help determine the child's current skills and ability and make recommendations regarding instruction and accommodations. The school will review these reports and determine if a 504 plan or IEP is necessary. These evaluations are essential for the IEP team to determine an appropriate classroom placement and what modifications will need to be made for the student to access the school curriculum. Stroke survivors will often need to be evaluated by a physical, occupational, speech, and/or vision therapist to determine what other accommodations are needed in the classroom. If deficits are found that will affect a child's ability to access the curriculum, therapy will be included in the IEP. The therapy provider will be part of the IEP team, and goals will be written and updated at the yearly meetings. The frequency and duration of therapies will be determined by the therapist in collaboration with the IEP team. Therapy sessions are provided outside the classroom, either one on one with the therapist or with a few other students who generally have the same goals, or the therapist will be in the classroom to address the immediate needs during class.

Homebound Instruction

Once a child is able to complete some form of schoolwork, parents may request the start of homebound instructional services. Most schools require a note signed by a physician to initiate home instruction and the reason why attending a traditional school day is not an option. Homebound school services provide a student with a tutor through their school program and options for making up missed work.[6] Many times the tutor will be a teacher from the school.[7]

Homebound instruction generally takes place once/week for one hour/subject area. The laws regulating the length of time, hours/week of home instruction, and which subjects are offered vary from state to state. There are no federal laws that regulate home instruction provided by a school; each state sets their own homebound instruction regulations.[8] Homebound instruction is designed to be a temporary solution and is not intended to take the place of a student attending school.

Private School

A private school that receives federal funding cannot discriminate against a child with a disability. If a parent chooses to send their child to a private school that receives federal funding, then the school cannot refuse acceptance of the student. However, they are not required to follow the IEP or provide special education services. A private school receiving federal funds is required to make "reasonable modifications."[9] An example would be extra time between classes for a student with a physical weakness, a frequency modulation (FM) system for a student with a hearing disability, or extra time for a student with slowed processing speeds. These reasonable modifications are generally at low cost and do not involve modifying the curriculum or hiring additional staff.

A private school that does not receive any federal funding does have the right to pick and choose who attends the institution. Private schools are not required to provide a FAPE to all students and therefore do not have to provide special education services. Related services, such as speech, physical, and occupational therapy, can be provided by the local school district, but will depend on the funding and cannot be guaranteed. These services can take place at the private school or at the local public school. Generally the special education services offered in a private school are going to be less than what can be offered in the public school due to the limited resources and funding.[2]

The exclusion to this law is when an IEP team determines that a private school placement is more appropriate than the local public school. At that time the local public school pays the private school tuition, and both schools will collaborate and support the IEP and all curriculum modifications listed.[2,4] There are numerous private schools where the curriculum is focused specifically on certain disabilities or learning difficulties. The process of having a child moved to this type of private school at the cost of the local public school can be extensive. Commonly, a child will need to participate in his or her local school district, and only after years of curriculum adjustments and careful documentation that the child is not progressing and the district is not able to meet the educational needs of that child will the district then consider transferring and financing a private school placement.

Gradual School Re-Entry

The initial return to a regular school day after a stroke can be overwhelming and exhausting for a child. A gradual return can make the transition much easier for everyone. Consider the option of having the student return for just 2 to 3 hours at a time initially and gradually working toward a full school day as tolerated. Also, working with the school to designate a quiet place in the nurse's office or guidance office where the child can have the option of resting if needed throughout the day can be helpful.[6] Looking at the class schedule and trying to optimize the few hours the child will be in school is ideal. Attempt to incorporate 2 to 3 core classes into the initial return so the child can be fresh and caught up on the more challenging classes.

Remember that the social aspect of school can be just as important for a child's overall recovery. If possible, include a lunch period so the child can gradually immerse him- or herself back into the social aspects of his or her school life. Increased fatigue after a stroke is to be expected.[10] If there is an increase in headaches or if the child is coming home and sleeping excessively that would be an indication that the length and/or intensity of the school day will need to be reevaluated.

Returning to school requires looking at the big picture. How much homework is expected? If a student is barely able to make it through 3 or 4 hours of classes, it is not reasonable to expect another 1 to 2 hours of homework be completed. Therefore, homework expectations will also need to be modified during this time. Following the cues of the child is the best way to determine what is the optimal plan. It is crucial for parents to be in close communication with teachers and school staff to determine a child's readiness to increase the school day.

Missed Schoolwork

The amount of missed schoolwork that will need to be made up will be determined by the teachers and the school. There are no federal laws mandating the amount of missed work or tests that need to be completed. School districts have their own policies for students making up assignments, quizzes, and tests due to illness. When it is known that a child is going to be absent for multiple days due to an ongoing medical condition, the issue of missed assignments, quizzes, and tests can be addressed in a child's 504 plan or IEP. When a student becomes ill during the school year, often the amount of makeup work will be determined by what the student has already completed and what his or her level of performance was prior to the stroke. Any tests or evaluations required by school districts or by the state will need to be made up. These forms of tests cannot be excused.

Frequent Absences

Missing multiple school days is a reality when a child has chronic or complex medical needs. The law requires that public schools meet the needs of *all* students, even those with chronic illness. When numerous days of school are going to be missed due to illness, procedures, therapies, or physician appointments this issue can be addressed in a 504 plan or a health care plan to ensure a child is not penalized for all the missed time. A health plan can be part of a child's IEP. Each state and local school district mandates the necessary documentation required for students to not be considered truant due to multiple missed school days. The plan for missed school time can include how much of the missed work will be required to be made up and the approved time period for completing the work. When a student will be missing multiple school days communication between teachers, parents, and students (at the appropriate age) is imperative to ensure expectations for completed work and timelines are understood by everyone.

Specialized Transportation

IDEA requires that all students be provided with the same resources.[2] Students who cannot safely access the regular school bus provided by the school district are eligible for specialized transportation services. IDEA requires schools to provide accessible transportation to and from school for every child that is eligible for regular busing services. When specialized transportation is needed, this becomes part of the child's 504 plan or IEP. The plan will address the details of the transportation necessary. Some examples of specialized transportation needs would be an aide on the bus for safety reasons, if any equipment (such as a walker or wheelchair) needs to be transported with the child to and from school, or if a wheelchair lift is required for a child to board the vehicle.

THERAPY SERVICES IN THE EDUCATIONAL ENVIRONMENT

Possible therapies needed for a stroke patient include occupational, physical, and/or speech therapy. Therapies provided through school may also be referred to as *related services* and will be part of a student's IEP.

Outpatient therapy (such as occupational, speech, or physical therapies) and therapy provided in school may differ greatly. A school therapist is required to focus on the child's ability to access the school environment and learning, whereas an outpatient therapist has the goal of improving the child's functioning to premorbid and/or developmentally appropriate levels. For example, for a child receiving occupational therapy in school, the goals may be related to handwriting or different keyboarding options and modifications for making writing more accessible within the classroom. At the same time in outpatient therapy, the child could be working on ways to independently wash his or her hair or different options for buttons and zippers on clothing. Writing is essential to the classroom, so it is a common goal of school-based therapy, but grooming and dressing skills, which are important life skills, do not occur during school hours. A child does need to write to access learning opportunities, but does not need to wash his or her hair or get dressed while at school.

Therapies provided in school can be done within the classroom and are referred to as *push-in services*. Alternatively, the therapist can remove the child from the classroom and work with him or her independently or with a few other students with similar needs, which is referred to as the *pull-out model*. When deciding between pull-out services or push-in classroom support, the team needs to consider the benefit of the services vs the classroom time that is lost. It may not be ideal to pull a child from a class he or she is already struggling or needs remediation in, or to pull an active child from recess time he or she needs. There are times when a family may decline school-based therapies in order for the child to optimize their time in the classroom. Therapists can still be available on a consultative basis to the teacher in case questions or issues arise. Consultative therapy services would still be included in the student's IEP.

Communication between school-based therapists, classroom teachers, parents, and outpatient therapists is crucial. Therapists should be reinforcing what the classroom teacher is doing and helping to modify the current curriculum. Parents should be given a summary of school therapy sessions and ideas or suggestions of what can be done at home to help reinforce the current therapy. When everyone is working toward the same goals and using consistent ideas, progress will be much more consistent.

There may be a time that a child does not qualify for school-based services but may be participating in an outpatient therapy program. This would be when a child can successfully access their school environment and learning but may need rehabilitation towards more global or self-care skills not affecting their ability to learn.

SPECIAL MEDICAL NEEDS OF THE CHILD WHILE AT SCHOOL

Medical Care Plan

The medical team will also need to provide the school with any restrictions that the child is required to follow. For example, if a child is not permitted to participate in any contact sports, the physician will need to provide a letter containing a brief explanation with the stated restriction. Schools typically require updated physicians' notes once every school year. Many stroke patients may also suffer from headaches or seizures. These conditions may interfere with the child's school day, and school staff will need to be prepared for how to handle these occurrences. A formalized health plan will need to be generated by the child's medical team to provide the school with the necessary guidelines of how to safely handle these conditions and situations if they arise during the school day. The plan would address if and when any medications should be administered, when the child's parents should be called, or when a child should be sent home or back to class.

Medication or Nursing Care Needed at School

When a child requires the administration of medication during the school day, the school staff are responsible for safely following the procedures outlined by the child's physician. Schools require a signed order or letter of medical necessity from the prescribing doctor for a medication to be given in school. School nursing guidelines vary from state to state. When the medical needs go beyond what the school nurse can safely provide, the child's health care provider will need to guide the parents and school staff as to what other medical support options are available. Each state sets their own guidelines as to what level of medical support is required by the school vs by the patient's health care benefits. Nursing needs are also included in a student's 504 plan or IEP.

EDUCATIONAL SERVICES: EARLY INTERVENTION TO COLLEGE

Infants and Toddlers

Pediatric stroke survivors may be eligible to receive early intervention services through Part C of IDEA. IDEA Part C provides support services to children with disabilities, and their families, from birth until their third birthday, when the child is delayed in physical, cognitive, or communication skills or due to a medical condition they are at risk for developmental delays. Children who have suffered a stroke are at risk for developing delays across all these areas. The requirement for qualifying for services is mandated by each state. Standardized testing and measurement procedures will determine eligibility and frequency of services offered by the early intervention (EI) service provider. Each state determines if fees will be charged for early intervention services, and charges are determined on a sliding scale according to the household income of parents or guardians. The main idea of early intervention is to assist the family or caregivers with optimizing the child's natural environment so he or she is provided the best opportunity for growth and development. Providing the family with the tools and resources for children to meet the developmental milestones will ensure they are best prepared for school.

Some states consider the diagnosis of a stroke enough of a risk for developing delays and will qualify the child for early intervention services even without obvious delays. Children with a stroke may take longer to learn to walk and talk, and an EI therapist will provide therapy in the child's natural environment to ensure everything is being done to stimulate proper development. The natural environment may include the child's home, daycare setting, or within the community (such as a park) and will include any family members present during the scheduled therapy time. These programs support the family in providing their child with the best opportunity for development and school readiness. An EI therapist could be a physical, occupational, speech, or vision therapist to concentrate on the specific delays or deficits. A special instructor or teacher could be recommended, just like a therapist, when there are concerns regarding a child's learning or cognitive function.[11]

Parents can request an evaluation by contacting their community EI provider, or the pediatrician can assist the family with providing this contact information. A current list of all EI providers in each state can be found at http://ectacenter.org/contact/contactsurl.asp?gc=101.

Once an evaluation is requested, a service coordinator will be assigned and becomes the main contact person for the family. When a pediatric stroke survivor requests an EI evaluation, it can be helpful to provide the evaluator with any paperwork or summaries from physician appointments, therapy sessions, or hospital reports to ensure the evaluators have the most up-to-date medical history. Once the evaluation is complete and services are recommended, the service coordinator will arrange a meeting to plan for the child's services. This meeting will include the service coordinator, parents/guardians, evaluators, and the therapists who will be responsible for providing the services and any other family members or advocates that the family would like to support or assist with the planning. The individualized plan is called the individualized family service plan (IFSP) and will include the child's history, family concerns and goals, evaluations, plan for services, expected goals of service, duration of services, location of services (eg, child's home, daycare, park), fees if determined by the state, and scheduled reviews. The IFSP will be reviewed every 6 months and updated at least once/year. Every update will include a meeting of the full team. The IFSP needs to be agreed upon and signed by the parents or guardians. The family has the right to disagree or decline proposed services at any time. If consent is not given, then the child cannot receive the proposed services.[12]

Outpatient therapy services are another option for a young child who has had a stroke to provide support with the goal of ensuring the child is meeting developmental milestones. These services may be offered at a hospital, rehabilitation center, or other outpatient therapy facility. The benefit of EI is that the therapist comes into the child's natural environment and the child will be more likely to participate in activities where he or she is most comfortable and with his or her own toys. Often, a young child will take a bit of time to come into an unknown facility and warm up to the therapist and effectively participate. The family has the right to decide what therapy option or combination of services is best for their schedules and finances and what works best for the child's personality. At times, a child receiving therapies through his or her insurance as an outpatient may be less expensive, so this option may be chosen rather than EI. Insurance copays for outpatient therapies can sometimes be less than what the state charges for EI services. Families can go through the process of an EI evaluation and turn down the service if they decide outpatient is a better option for their family situation.

Once a child turns 3 years old, he or she is no longer eligible to receive services through the EI system. Approximately 6 to 12 months before the child's third birthday the service coordinator will start discussing this transition process. If eligible for continued services the IFSP will be transitioned to an IEP. Once the child is 3 years old the evaluations and services will now be provided by the local school district and governed by IDEA Part B. The biggest change after the transition is that services will no longer be offered within the natural environment, but rather in a therapeutic facility or the school. Also, there may be a change in eligibility, frequency, and goals of therapies, and

a preschool program may be added to the plan. At this time the focus of therapy goals change from the child's development and the family's needs to the child being ready for school and prepared to fully participate in the classroom.

An example of this change in goals would be if a child was receiving occupational therapy through EI to assist with the fine motor skills needed for feeding, such as scooping with a spoon or using a fork correctly. At the age of 3, the goals will change to focus on the fine motor and pre-handwriting skills needed for school. The goals of the IEP now focus on the child being able to access his or her school environment. If the child no longer qualifies for services, the EI service coordinator will provide the family with any community resources that may be helpful for the child and the family.

Once evaluations are completed by the school district and it is determined that services will be offered, a transition meeting will be scheduled no later than 90 days prior to the child's third birthday. Just like the IFSP meetings, all EI providers, service coordinator, school district evaluators, a representative from any school programs that are being offered, and the parents or other family members the family invites will be part of the transition meeting. One example of a preschool program that may be offered is Head Start, developmental, or private preschools depending on the needs of the child. Just like EI, it is always the right of the parents to decline services or programs offered to the child. Many times a big obstacle with the preschool programs offered through the school system is that they are mostly part time, and working parents cannot accommodate picking up or dropping off a child in the middle of the day. Even if just therapy is offered, parents now have to transport their child to a local school building to participate in therapy.

Elementary School and High School

Throughout the elementary and high school years a child's 504 plan or IEP will continue to grow and change with the increasing demands of the classroom and school curriculum. Each year, both the age expectations for the child and the specific curriculum will need to be considered when making the educational plan. An example of this change would be when a child has visual-spatial deficits but is now taking geometry for the first time. Appropriate modifications will need to be added for that school year to meet the expectations of each class. Another example is a student with hemiplegia who struggles to keep up with the classroom notes. At the high school level, this student will need copies of notes provided for him or her. This modification will be added during the higher grades and would not even be considered for a student in early elementary school.

When a student has an IEP, transition planning becomes part of the educational plan and will be addressed at the yearly IEP meeting starting when the student is 14 years old. At this age, the student will now be invited and able to participate in the IEP meeting every year. Planning for post-high school education, exploring work options, technical school supports, or assisted living arrangements will be addressed by the student's IEP team. Schools can help families navigate what services are available and how to access disability services for a child once they graduate.

COMMON SCHOOL PROBLEMS AND THE NECESSARY ACCOMMODATIONS FOR PEDIATRIC STROKE PATIENTS

The majority of children who have survived stroke experience persistent cognitive difficulties, most commonly with attention, concentration, and speed of processing.[13] Pediatric stroke survivors are also very likely to have academic difficulty and require special education services.[14-15] Special classroom placement, therapies, and specially designed instruction may be necessary for many stroke survivors returning to school. For others, accommodations such as preferential seating, use of a laptop or note taker, extra time on tests, taking tests in a separate room with the provision of breaks, truncated assignments, extra time to complete assignments, voice dictation, and organizational help may prove beneficial. What is appropriate for the student depends on the child's unique needs and may change as he or she recovers, grows, and develops.

Following are outlines of the common problems and possible supportive solutions for students in school after a having a stroke.[16]

DECREASED ATTENTION	
YOU MAY SEE THAT THE STUDENT...	**WHAT CAN YOU DO?**
<ul><li>Makes careless errors</li><li>Has difficulty remaining in the seat</li><li>Seems to forget things</li><li>Loses assignments</li><li>Has difficulty listening to instructions</li><li>Is distractible</li><li>Cannot complete tasks without taking breaks</li><li>Performs inconsistently on tests and quizzes</li><li>Has difficulty following multistep commands</li><li>Needs help from an adult to stay on task</li></ul>	<ul><li>Priority seating<ul><li>Sit student at center-front of the classroom if teacher stays in front of the class.</li><li>For teachers who tend to move around the classroom, efforts should be made to establish eye contact to keep child on task.</li><li>Seat away from windows.</li><li>Seat the child next to peers who have adequate attentional skills.</li></ul></li><li>Have the child's attention before giving instructions.<ul><li>Use verbal and nonverbal cues to direct attention to tasks.</li><li>Say child's name.</li><li>Touch child on his or her shoulder.</li><li>Point to the activity or task.</li><li>Use a phrase (eg, "Listen") or turn off lights when child is expected to attend to instructions.</li></ul></li><li>Provide frequent, regularly scheduled breaks that are routine.</li><li>Directions should be given in 1- or 2-step commands. The shorter, the better. Check to make sure the child has heard and understood the instructions by having the child repeat them back to you.</li><li>Help the child focus attention in conversation and remain on topic by requesting structured verbal output.<ul><li>"Tell me 3 things about the Incas."</li><li>"What are the 2 main points of the story?"</li></ul></li><li>Keep worksheets free from extraneous material. Children with attention problems can become easily overwhelmed with too many problems on a single page. For math computations, have the child circle the final answer.</li><li>Break multi-step directions into short, manageable bits. Give the student one direction at a time and wait for completion before proceeding to the next step.</li></ul>

(continued)

DECREASED ATTENTION (CONTINUED)	
YOU MAY SEE THAT THE STUDENT...	WHAT CAN YOU DO?
	▪ Find ways to draw attention to important aspects of assignments or changes in directions (eg, underline or bold text, highlight with different colors). On math computation sheets, have the child circle the operation sign before beginning the problem. ▪ Block out material by covering or removing from the visual field the material that you visually don't want students to focus on. Remove distracting clutter from the board or screen. ▪ Consider using a timer for students who work well with a beat-the-clock system for work completion.

The Children's Hospital of Philadelphia—Stroke Program. *Transition Packet*. 2014. Philadelphia, PA.

LEARNING AND MEMORY DIFFICULTIES	
YOU MAY SEE THAT THE STUDENT...	WHAT CAN YOU DO?
▪ Forgets things ▪ Gets lost easily ▪ Can't follow more than 1- or 2-step directions ▪ Has trouble telling details from a story ▪ Has difficulty grasping new concepts ▪ Has inconsistent school performance	▪ Teach strategies to assist memory skills. 　□ Chunking information: Reduce the information to be learned into smaller segments (eg, learning a social security number can be chunked into 3 segments and then rehearsed) 　□ Associative learning: Teach mnemonic strategies to recall information based on association. For example, using the phrase Roy G. Biv (red, orange, yellow, green, blue, indigo, and violet) to recall colors of the rainbow. 　□ Rehearsal: Improve recall by rehearsing new information by reciting it out loud or paraphrasing. Writing the material to be remembered may also be helpful. ▪ Reduce the amount of information presented. Only emphasize the essential details. ▪ For rote learned facts (ie, spelling words, math facts, vocabulary), items should be presented in small blocks (4 to 6 units), with rehearsal of the block to mastery prior to the introduction of another block. ▪ Use recognition clues rather than relying on the student's rote memory (ie, providing true/false or multiple choice rather than fill-in-the-blank or essay tests).

(continued)

LEARNING AND MEMORY DIFFICULTIES (CONTINUED)	
YOU MAY SEE THAT THE STUDENT...	WHAT CAN YOU DO?
	■ Repeat, repeat, repeat: Repetition is important.
	■ Use external aids.
	▫ Multicomponent organizational devices: These include devices such as PDAs, memory notebooks, or computers that would allow the child a space to organize, store, and retrieve a relatively significant amount of information. A child should receive training on how to use these devices and be encouraged to use them on a regular basis.
	▫ Simple prospective memory devices: These include simpler tools that remind a child to perform a particular activity at a specific time (eg, calendar, alarm watches).
	■ Enhance meaningfulness: Find ways to relate the content being discussed to the student's prior knowledge.
	▫ Draw parallels to the student's own life.
	▫ Bring in concrete, meaningful examples for students to explore to provide an experiential experience.
	▫ Inform parents about upcoming topics so that they can talk about topics and provide related background activities at home or make a trip to the library.
	■ Before presenting new material, provide the student with a topic for him or her to focus his or her attention on (eg, the main characters of a story, the story setting).
	■ Make sure that the student is attending to the source of information (eg, eye contact is being made, hands are free of materials, the student is looking at the assignment).
	■ Use visualization strategies, experiential learning, and multisensory presentation. For example, if the student is learning about George Washington crossing the Delaware, he or she could hear a story about it, draw a picture about it, and close his or her eyes and imagine what it would feel like to be George Washington. When he or she is later asked to retrieve that information, he or she has multiple pathways (eg, verbal, visual, sensory) by which this information could be retrieved.

(continued)

LEARNING AND MEMORY DIFFICULTIES (CONTINUED)	
YOU MAY SEE THAT THE STUDENT...	**WHAT CAN YOU DO?**
	■ Provide a schedule of daily activities, locations, and materials needed for each class. Use pictorial cues to enhance memory. ■ Daily or weekly communication between teacher and parents is important to ensure that necessary information (which the child may have forgotten) is conveyed. Journals or weekly progress notes are examples of written communication techniques.

The Children's Hospital of Philadelphia—Stroke Program. *Transition Packet.* 2014. Philadelphia, PA.

FINE MOTOR DIFFICULTIES	
YOU MAY SEE THAT THE STUDENT...	**WHAT CAN YOU DO?**
■ Does not anchor the paper while writing ■ Takes a long time to produce written work ■ Has difficulty copying or writing information that is seen ■ Misspells many handwritten words ■ Has sloppy handwriting or drawings	■ Make sure the student's seating is supportive with his or her desk or table at elbow height. ■ Provide opportunities for hand strengthening prior to handwriting tasks. ■ Allow the student to write work on a larger scale to compensate for poor fine motor control. It may also be helpful to provide the student with paper that has boxes on it (ie, graph paper) that would allow him or her to write 1 letter/box. ■ Allow the student to use wide-ruled paper. ■ Allow the student to write on every other line. ■ Allow students to print rather than write in cursive. ■ Realistic and mutually agreed upon expectations for neatness should be established, and care should be taken to avoid pressuring the student to consistently meet standards at the limit of his or her capacity of motor control. ■ If a student has difficulty anchoring a paper, allow him or her to use a clipboard or tape his or her paper to the desk. ■ Allow the student to take a break from paper and pencil tasks. ■ When possible, allow the student to respond verbally when writing is not the focus of instruction. ■ Assignments or other information written on the board should be provided to the student in written form rather than having him or her copy it down.

(continued)

| FINE MOTOR DIFFICULTIES (CONTINUED) ||
YOU MAY SEE THAT THE STUDENT...	WHAT CAN YOU DO?
	▪ Assign the student a note-taking buddy, so that he or she can check her his or her notes against that of another student to ensure there is a full record of information presented in class and he or she is not penalized for the inability to rapidly record information.
	▪ Allow the child to record class lectures or to dictate class assignments.
	▪ Allow the child to type information on a computer instead of writing by hand.
	▪ Provide alternatives to handwritten assignments such as keyboarding, dictation, theatrical presentations, video presentations, or oral reports.
	▪ Assign truncated assignments for writing (ie, having the student copy down only half of the spelling words, then having the others provided for the student to study).

The Children's Hospital of Philadelphia—Stroke Program. *Transition Packet.* 2014. Philadelphia, PA.

| MOBILITY DIFFICULTIES ||
YOU MAY SEE THAT THE STUDENT...	WHAT CAN YOU DO?
▪ Has difficulty getting in and out of chairs or desks	▪ Request a school physical therapy consultation.
▪ Has difficulty navigating the classroom environment	▪ Request evaluation for adaptive gym if needed.
▪ Has difficulty carrying books	▪ Place the desk closer to the board or frequently accessed places in the classroom.
▪ Has difficulty navigating the hallway	▪ Provide an adult 1:1 or peer buddy depending on the level of assistance needed.
▪ Has difficulty on the stairs	▪ Allow elevator access.
▪ Is unsteady on his or her feet or loses balance easily	▪ Provide a second set of books to decrease amount needed to be carried home each night.
▪ Needs help getting on or off transportation	▪ Allow leaving the class a few minutes early to avoid crowded hallways and stairwells.
▪ Demonstrates fatigue over the course of a school day	▪ Consider classroom location and modify if needed and possible.
▪ Has difficulty on uneven surfaces such as playgrounds	▪ Provide needed assistance for transportation, recess, and outings.
▪ Has difficulty keeping up with peers	▪ Consider modified school schedule with team and family if fatigue prevents academic performance.

The Children's Hospital of Philadelphia—Stroke Program. *Transition Packet.* 2014. Philadelphia, PA.

EXECUTIVE FUNCTIONING DIFFICULTIES (ORGANIZATION, PLANNING, INITIATION)	
YOU MAY SEE THAT THE STUDENT...	**WHAT CAN YOU DO?**

• Has difficulty completing long-term projects
• Has good ideas but cannot get them on paper
• Underestimates time needed to finish tasks
• Starts assignments at the last minute
• Turns in written work that is poorly organized
• Has difficulty thinking of alternative ways to complete a task
• Has difficulty getting started with directions or assignments
• Has difficulty getting started on a task despite being able to tell you the instructions
• Does not finish routine tasks without assistance/reminders
	• Help the student to plan out his or her approach for tasks, assignments, and projects. Develop a calendar with a plan for when and how each step will be completed. Have someone frequently review the plan, and the steps required and identify materials needed.
	• Provide incentives for timely completion of work. This may help the student transition from one task to another.
	  ▫ Breaking assignments down into smaller parts will help the student gain a sense of accomplishment and likely decrease feelings of being overwhelmed. Approaching assignments in more manageable chunks will likely reduce the tendency to put off projects until the last minute.
	  ▫ Help the student to develop outlines for reports/essays.

The Children's Hospital of Philadelphia—Stroke Program. *Transition Packet.* 2014. Philadelphia, PA.

REDUCED MENTAL PROCESSING SPEED	
YOU MAY SEE THAT THE STUDENT...	**WHAT CAN YOU DO?**
• Asks for directions to be repeated • Spends more time on tasks/homework than other students • Fatigues easily • Has poor performance on timed tests • Appears confused when instructions are given • Appears inattentive • Does not complete work	• Keep instructions short and simple. Focus on the essential details. • Specify a time commitment for homework (eg, 1 hour/night) or indicate a reduction in the number of problems per assignment that the student is required to complete (eg, 50% of the math problems). • Allow extra time for test taking and assignments. Some students may benefit from taking tests in a quiet resource room rather than among peers. • Allow frequent breaks. • Mix it up: Higher interest with lower interest tasks, less active with more active tasks, and individual with group activities. • Ensure that you have the student's attention (eg, eye contact) before giving instructions. • Classroom assignments should be broken into a sequence of subtasks involving shorter work periods. • The number of concepts introduced during a class period or lesson may need to be reduced.

(continued)

REDUCED MENTAL PROCESSING SPEED (CONTINUED)	
YOU MAY SEE THAT THE STUDENT...	WHAT CAN YOU DO?
	<ul><li>Instructions should be simplified by breaking them down into steps requiring 1 or 2 actions at a time.</li><li>Supplement oral directions with written instructions so that the student has something tangible to refer to if he or she becomes lost.</li><li>Provide student with annotated outline of lectures. Students with processing deficits often have difficulty processing auditory information (ie, teacher's lecture) while trying to keep up with note taking.</li><li>Do not penalize a child who has slowed processing speed for not completing assignments as quickly as his or her peers. If a student requires extra time, allow him or her extra time during study halls or shorten requirements rather than have him or her miss out on a fun activity, such as recess.</li></ul>

The Children's Hospital of Philadelphia—Stroke Program. *Transition Packet.* 2014. Philadelphia, PA.

SENSORY IMPAIRMENTS	
A STUDENT MAY HAVE SENSORY IMPAIRMENTS, SUCH AS VISION OR HEARING DIFFICULTIES, IF HE OR SHE...	WHAT CAN YOU DO?
<ul><li>Complains of headaches</li><li>Complains of double vision</li><li>Appears to be squinting while reading from the board</li><li>Holds reading materials close to his or her face or puts face close to desktop while writing</li><li>Letters are poorly formed or overlapping with each other</li><li>Reads quickly to self but has difficulty answering comprehension questions</li><li>Looks confused when given oral instructions</li><li>Appears to zone out during lectures</li><li>Asks for repetition of instructions</li><li>Speaks loudly</li><li>Notes taken during lectures are spotty and missing essential details</li></ul>	<ul><li>Review concerns with family and/or school nurse to determine if a sensory deficit has already been identified. If these are new concerns, the child may need to have an evaluation.</li></ul> *Vision* <ul><li>Place a ruler under sentences being read for better tracking.</li><li>Adapt worksheets by using larger type (or enlarge on a photocopier) and good contrast between print and background.</li><li>Provide worksheets with fewer items/page.</li><li>Allow student to use all capital letters when spelling to reduce confusion among similar-appearing lowercase letters (eg, d, b, and p)</li><li>Encourage the student to wear an eye patch if he or she experiences double vision or blurriness.</li><li>Position the student in the room according to his or her field cut (ie, left side if child has right visual field cut).</li><li>Place a magnifier over computer monitors.</li></ul>

(continued)

SENSORY IMPAIRMENTS (CONTINUED)	
A STUDENT MAY HAVE SENSORY IMPAIRMENTS SUCH AS VISION OR HEARING DIFFICULTIES IF HE OR SHE...	**WHAT CAN YOU DO?**
	Hearing ■ Seat child in front of the classroom. ■ Use an FM system (microphone attached to the teacher). ■ Record class. ■ Provide student with a copy (either teacher's or classmate's) of class notes to check for missed information. ■ Encourage student to ask for clarification. ■ Check understanding of task instruction by asking the child to repeat them back before beginning a task.

The Children's Hospital of Philadelphia—Stroke Program. *Transition Packet.* 2014. Philadelphia, PA.

SPECIFIC ACADEMIC RECOMMENDATIONS	
YOU MAY HAVE STUDENTS WITH SPECIFIC LEARNING CHALLENGES IF...	**WHAT CAN YOU DO?**
■ Assessments reveal weaknesses in specific academic areas ■ The student shows poor performance on quizzes and homework ■ The student seems unable to keep up with his or her peers during class	■ Review concerns with child's parents and education team. Determine if assessment is needed to clarify the child's current skills and needs. *Math* ■ Allow the student to use a calculator without penalty. ■ Group similar problems together (eg, all addition problems in one section). ■ Provide fewer problems on a worksheet (eg, 4 to 6 problems on a page, rather than 20 to 30). ■ Require fewer problems to attain passing grades. ■ Use graph paper to write problems to help the student keep numbers in columns. ■ Tape a number line to the student's desk. ■ Provide a table of math facts for reference. ■ Use pictures and graphics. ■ Teach the student to break down lengthy word problems into smaller parts. ■ Use visual aids, such as an abacus, blocks, number lines, graphs, and fraction wheels.

(continued)

SPECIFIC ACADEMIC RECOMMENDATIONS (CONTINUED)	
YOU MAY HAVE STUDENTS WITH SPECIFIC LEARNING CHALLENGES IF. . .	**WHAT CAN YOU DO?**
	Reading ■ Highlight key words with a colored marker. ■ Use a lone marker (strip of paper or ruler) to keep place while reading. ■ Ask the student to summarize what he or she has read in short intervals. ■ Use a lower-level test as alternative reading material in subject areas. ■ For classes not specifically teaching reading (eg, science, social studies), allow books on audiotape to accompany written textbooks. Such audiotapes can be obtained free of charge through services such as Reading for the Blind and Dyslexic (www.rfbd.org). The student can utilize the tape during the class by using headphones. ■ Encourage the student to read aloud or subvocalize, rather than silently, to help increase comprehension. ■ Provide the student with a set of textbooks he or she can keep at home to highlight and make notes in. ■ To aid comprehension and retention, provide outlines and periodic review questions during lengthy reading assignments.

The Children's Hospital of Philadelphia—Stroke Program. *Transition Packet.* 2014. Philadelphia, PA.

STUDENT HEALTH CARE PLAN

Student's Full Name: _____

_____

Diagnosis: _____

_____

Treatment Plan: _____

_____

Scheduled Treatments: _____

_____

Potential Side Effects: _____

_____

Limitations or Restrictions: _____

_____

Medical Care Needed in School: _____

_____

Student's Knowledge of His or Her Illness: _____

_____

Information to Share With Staff and Classmates: _____

_____

Siblings in School and Grades: _____

_____

Accommodations and Recommendations: _____

_____

School Re-Entry Plan: _____

_____

The Children's Hospital of Philadelphia—Stroke Program. *Transition Packet.* 2014. Philadelphia, PA.

REFERENCES

1. Wright PW, Wright PD. Extended School Year Services (ESY). *Wrightslaw.* http://www.wrightslaw.com/info/esy.index.htm. Published March 21, 2011. Accessed October 8, 2014.

2. U.S. Department of Education. Individuals with Disabilities Education Act (IDEA) 1997/Services to Parentally Placed Private School Students With Disabilities. http://www2.ed.gov/about/offices/list/oii/nonpublic/idea1.html. Published October 2001. Accessed June 20, 2014.

3. deBettencourt LU. Understanding the difference Between IDEA and Section 504. *Teach Except Child.* 2002;34(3):16-23.

4. U.S. Department of Education. Building the legacy: IDEA. http://idea.ed.gov/explore/view/p/,root,regs,300,D,300%252E324. Accessed October 13, 2014.

5. Dienst J. Children don't have strokes? Just ask Jared. *The New York Times.* http://www.nytimes.com/2010/01/19/health/19stroke.html?pagewanted=all&_r=0. Published January 19, 2010. Accessed March 30, 2017.

6. Pediatric Stroke Program. School packet. *Return to School.* Philadelphia, PA; 2012.

7. Patterson PD. Guidelines for providing homebound instruction to students with disabilities. *Brainline.* http://www.brainline.org/content/2008/10/guidelines-providing-homebound-instruction-students-disabilities_pageall.html. Published October 2008. Accessed April 14, 2014.

8. Wright P. The Wrightslaw way to special education law and advocacy. http://www.wrightslaw.com/blog/?p=8333. Published October 18, 2012. Accessed April 28, 2014.

9. McDonald D. *NCEA Notes.* National Catholic Educational Association; 2013.

10. National Stroke Association. 2014. Retrieved April 2014.

11. U.S. Department of Education. Early intervention program for infants and toddlers with disabilities. http://www2.ed.gov/programs/osepeip/index.html. Published July 2014. Accessed June, 20, 2014.

12. Center for Parent Information and Resources. Writing the IFSP for your child. http://www.parentcenterhub.org/repository/ifsp/. Published March 2014. Accessed October 13, 2014.

13. Smith SB, Sanchez Bloom J, Minniti, N. Cerebrovascular diseases and disorders. In: Armstrong C, Morrow L, eds. *Handbook of Medical Neuropsychology: Applications of Cognitive Neuroscience.* Philadelphia, PA: Springer Press; 2010:101-122.

14. Steinlin MR. Long term follow-up after stroke in childhood. *Eur J Pediatr.* 2004;163:245-250.

15. De Schryver EK-S. Prognosis of ischemic stroke in childhood: a long-term follow-up study. *Dev Med Child Neurol.* 2000;42:313-318.

16. The Children's Hospital of Philadelphia—Stroke Program. *Transition Packet.* 2014. Philadelphia, PA.

13

Prevention to Poststroke Rehabilitation
Lifelong Management, Advocacy, and Resources for Children With Stroke

Kim Nixon-Cave, PT, PhD, PCS and Mary Kay Ballasiotes

This chapter focuses on management of an infant or child following the diagnosis of a pediatric stroke, particularly addressing their needs from a holistic perspective with issues related to lifelong management of possible cognitive and physical impairments, including the role of advocacy community and health care resources that the patients and their families may need over the course of their recovery. There are many challenges for the child and family following a stroke due to the infrequent occurrences of pediatric stroke and the misdiagnosis of children who present with neurological symptoms. These challenges have decreased in recent years due to increasing knowledge about pediatric stroke and increasing diagnostic tools available to care providers.[1] Children who suffer a pediatric stroke can have permanent neurological deficits, including not only hemiparesis or hemiplegia, but also cognitive and sensory impairments, epilepsy, speech or communication disorders, visual disturbances, poor attention, and behavioral problems that could require lifelong management. This patient population will require an interprofessional team with expertise in the management of infants and children diagnosed with pediatric stroke and who are knowledgeable about the etiology, clinical presentation, and clinical management to address the unique nature of the stroke in children.[1,2]

Although there are many known risk factors for stroke in children, no cause is identified among a small percentage. Furthermore, there is limited research on the cause, management, and prevention of stroke in children.[2] It is important that professionals are versed in the evidence and recommendations related to the cause, management, and prevention of pediatric stroke, especially because these children can have lifelong cognitive and motor disabilities as well as an increased likelihood to have a recurrent stroke.[2] Organizations such as American Heart Association (AHA) and American Stroke Association (ASA) have provided guidelines designed to help health care professionals and educators treat and address the needs of infants and children who have suffered a stroke. Professionals must work as a team to provide the best care while considering all options in the treatment of the children.

Patients who have suffered a pediatric stroke will most likely need lifelong management for the lasting effects of the stroke. The *International Classification of Functioning of Children and Youth, Disability and Health* (ICF-CY) classification allows health care rehabilitation professionals to focus on various aspects of the child, including the health condition, body structure, level of function related to the stroke, and any personal and environmental needs that the child may have. In terms of the health conditions, many

Atkinson HL, Nixon-Cave K, Smith SE, eds.
Pediatric Stroke Rehabilitation: An Interprofessional and Collaborative Approach (pp 247-257).© 2018 Taylor & Francis Group.

underlying conditions can lead to a pediatric stroke, including risk factors such as congenital heart disease and sickle cell anemia. The treatment and care of these patients may require many different health care professionals to treat the underlying cause and manifestation of the stroke.[2] The biological component is the physical insult resulting from a brain injury such as a stroke. The ICF-CY helps health care professionals classify the medical event or the health condition of the patient and identify the mild to significant impairments that directly affect the ability to function within the environment or to develop typical cognitive, motor, or affective skills and/or progress through a normal developmental sequence.[3] Several needs must be met when a child is diagnosed with a stroke, the first and most immediate of which is the medical management of the patient followed by rehabilitation or habilitation of the patient.

When children suffer a stroke, they and their families will experience the continuum of care from acute care hospital stay to outpatient services. The medical management generally starts with managing the acute medical needs of the patient and ensuring that any underlying problems are addressed and that the patient is medically stable to begin the rehabilitation or habilitation in order to become functional within his or her environment. These services are provided in the context of a medical health care system that requires multidisciplinary health care professionals to address the various aspects of what each patient and his or her family needs. In the context of the biopsychosocial perspective, these patients and their families require holistic care from the acute care period to discharge home. Patients will need many resources, and their families will need to learn to be advocates for the patient and the care that he or she will need. Most professionals are familiar with the medical management of the pediatric stroke patient as well as the rehabilitation process. However, it is important that professionals fully understand all components of the care and management of patients who have suffered a pediatric stroke, including cost of care and resources needed for the child and family from health care and the community. In a study by Lo et al[4] the authors found that during the first year after diagnosis "the cost of stroke correlates with the extent of physical and functional impairment, so that the cost of stroke care may be considered a proxy for stroke severity. Future outcome studies of pediatric stroke should evaluate social function as well as cognitive and behavioral functions."

In the medical management of stroke, many health care professionals are likely to facilitate the patient's poststroke ability to function within his or her environment. Many services are needed to address the lifelong needs of the pediatric patient with a stroke, and in order to acquire and coordinate this care, parents will need to work with health care professionals, rehabilitation specialists, and social workers. Fortunately, with increasing knowledge of the diagnosis of pediatric stroke, more programs, clinics, and services are available for this patient population. The

professionals involved with the care of infants, young children, and adolescents who have suffered a stroke are listed in Box 13-1.

Each of the professionals who focus on the care of the child following the diagnosis of a stroke plays a role that can contribute to the child's successful functional outcome.[3,5] In each stage of treating a pediatric patient following stroke, the care is based on the needs of the child, as well as on their age. The treatment generally focuses on 3 treatment stages: prevention, therapy immediately after the stroke, and poststroke rehabilitation.[6] In each stage of treatment, the focus is different, and as a result the professionals involved will vary. In the prevention stage, the focus is on preventing a first or recurrent stroke and on treating an individual's underlying risk factors for stroke, such as hypertension, sickle cell anemia, congenital heart disease, atrial fibrillation, and diabetes.[6] In the acute stage, the focus is on stopping the stroke by treating the underlying problem, such as bleeding.[6] In the last stage, the focus is on rehabilitating the individual to regain skills or address impairments that may result from the stroke.[6]

Lastly, this chapter will focus on the environmental and personal factors of the ICF-CY model that affect the quality of life and overall ability of pediatric stroke patients to function within their environments.[3] In order to address the psychosocial needs of the patients and their families, it is important to focus on prevention and management of the patient with persistent limitations and disabilities. Professionals providing care to children and their families following a stroke should help the parent and child adjust to the ways their lives have changed since the stroke. This includes helping them acquire the care and support they need and educating them about advocacy and resources, both financial and health benefits, that are available for children with stroke and that the patients and their families will need to manage lifelong impairments and disabilities.[4,6,7]

THE ROLE OF ADVOCACY IN THE CARE OF CHILDREN WHO HAVE SUFFERED A PEDIATRIC STROKE

When professionals work with children and their parents following a stroke, it is important to remember that the entire family is affected by the diagnosis and resulting disabilities that can change the dynamic of the family environment. Professionals can help parents and caregivers become advocates for their child and family, and they can help them recognize that needs will change over time.[7] The environment that the child and family will need to function and navigate in following the stroke will be dynamic and multifaceted. With the major change in the environment due the diagnosis of stroke, parents will need to learn to be

Box 13-1. Health Care Professionals

MEDICAL PROFESSIONALS	
Cardiologists	Cardiologists treat diseases and abnormalities of the heart and circulatory system. They are more likely to treat congenital diseases and defects that can be the underlying cause of the stroke in addressing related cardiac and circulatory issues. Cardiologists are typically involved in the care of the child with a hemorrhagic stroke, which is often caused by ruptured or weakened, or malformed arteries known as *arteriovenous malformations*. The risk of hemorrhage is higher with certain illnesses such as hemophilia. Cardiologists may also be involved in the care of the child with an ischemic stroke, which occurs when a blood clot forms in the heart and travels to the brain. Ischemic stroke can be caused by congenital heart problems such as abnormal valves, infections, or sickle cell disease.
Developmental Pediatrician	Developmental pediatricians manage the physical, mental, and emotional well-being of patients from birth to age 21 in every stage of development and in good health or in illness. Developmental pediatricians are trained to work with children who may have developmental, learning, or behavioral problems. Their assessments and treatments focus on the medical and psychosocial aspects of children's and adolescents' developmental and behavioral problems. In the case of a child diagnosed with a stroke, a developmental pediatrician is most likely to care for the child's overall health and wellness, including immunizations, and track the child's development. The pediatrician will work with the medical team, specifically the neurologist, and provide follow-up care based on the child's specific medical issues and as indicated by the specialist.
Hematologists	Hematologists specialize in the treatment of children diagnosed with cancer and hematologic disorders, including diseases of the blood, spleen, and lymph glands. The hematologist is a blood specialist who cares for patients with blood clotting disorders or occasional rare causes of stroke in children, such as anemia, clotting disorders, sickle cell disease, hemophilia, leukemia, and lymphoma, which may be an underlying cause of a pediatric stroke.
Neurologists	Neurologists are physicians who specialize in neurology and diagnosing and treating disorders that affect the brain, spinal cord, and peripheral nerves. In early treatment, they focus on protecting the brain and keeping blood vessels open to prevent more strokes. As children with stroke require specialized imaging and treatment, neurologists usually provide care in a children's hospital, which has all the facilities necessary to treat children and their specific pathologies and where the neurologist coordinates care and follows the patient for any complications related to the stroke. The focus of care for the neurologist changes with the age of the child. In infants and children age 0 to 5 years, neurologists focus on managing any underlying medical issues related to the stroke as well as preventing further strokes. As the children grow older, the neurologist focuses on the neurological deficits that children experience in physical, developmental, and psychosocial impairments. As the child becomes neurologically stable, the neurologist will follow the child yearly until he or she transitions to adulthood.
Neurosurgeons	Neurosurgeons provide neurosurgical care for infants and children concentrating on the special surgical problems of children involving the brain such as underlying causes of a stroke. They can be involved in the care of infants, children, and adolescents, and they also counsel parents expecting a baby who may have been diagnosed before birth with a neurosurgical problem or a neurological event such as a stroke that may have occurred prenatally.

(continued)

BOX 13-1 (CONTINUED). HEALTH CARE PROFESSIONALS

Physiatrists	Physiatrists are physicians who specialize in the diagnosis and nonsurgical treatment of diseases and injuries of the bones, muscles, and nervous system. They specialize in treating stroke, brain injury, spinal cord injury, and musculoskeletal conditions with a focus on rehabilitation. Physiatrists collaborate with other health care professionals to help direct the child's treatment, resulting in a rehabilitation program tailored to the needs of the child following a stroke while helping each patient reach the highest possible level of functioning and quality of life.
REHABILITATION SPECIALISTS	
Neuropsychologists	Neuropsychologists are professionals who study, assess, and aim to understand and treat behaviors directly related to brain functioning. They specialize in understanding the relationship between the brain, which is extremely complex, and behavior and disorders within the brain or nervous system that can alter behavior and cognitive function. A neuropsychological assessment focuses on the learning and educational needs of the child following a stroke. Neuropsychological services also include screening for school readiness among typical 4- to 5-year-olds and formal neuropsychology evaluation, if indicated, and in children suffering a pediatric stroke. Neuropsychologists are an essential part of the rehabilitation team for children after stroke, working closely with physicians, including neurologists.
Occupational Therapists	Occupational therapists focus on interventions that help the child adapt to different environments and modify tasks to meet his or her abilities. In particular, occupational therapists help children with hemiplegia, a common impairment after a stroke, improve their ability to perform tasks in their daily living. Occupational therapists may help children with hemiplegia improve their hand function and eating skills and strengthen their hand, shoulder, and trunk. They provide skills training and education in order to increase patient participation in and performance of daily activities, particularly those that are meaningful to the client. Occupational therapists help children succeed in their occupation of learning, playing, and growing. When skill and strength cannot be developed or improved, occupational therapy offers creative solutions and resources to help children carry out their daily activities.
Orthotists	Orthotists are specifically educated and trained to design, fabricate, and fit custom-made orthopedic braces, or orthoses, and to fit prefabricated devices and provide related patient care to address their patients' needs. Orthotic practitioners blend patient care with design and fabrication of devices. Their unique expertise in patient assessment, design, and materials offers patients increased mobility and independence. They may work with patients following a stroke to design orthoses that serve as adjuncts to rehabilitation care.
Physical Therapists	Physical therapists are rehabilitation specialists who focus on the impairment aspect of the ICF-CY, specifically the remediation of impairments and disabilities and the promotion of mobility, functional ability, quality of life, and movement potential, through examination, evaluation, diagnosis, and physical intervention. The physical therapy rehabilitation will focus on helping the child reach developmental milestones like sitting, rolling, crawling, standing, walking and running. Physical therapists work on balance, stretching, strengthening, coordination, and motor planning as well as focus on gross motor skills that are involved in activities like walking and running.

(continued)

BOX 13-1 (CONTINUED). HEALTH CARE PROFESSIONALS	
Social Workers	Social workers are also essential to the coordination of care for a pediatric patient following a stroke. Social workers seek to improve the quality of life and the well-being of an individual, group, or community by intervening through research, policy, crisis intervention, community organizing, direct practice, and teaching on behalf of individuals afflicted with poverty or any real or perceived social injustices and violations of civil liberties and human rights. Social workers help individuals, families, and groups restore or enhance their capacity for social functioning and work to create societal conditions that support communities in need.
Speech-Language Pathology Therapists	Speech-Language Pathologists specialize in communication and swallowing disorders that may result from a pediatric stroke. Speech-language pathologists are the primary care providers of speech-language pathology services and use professional judgment to determine if individuals with communication and/or swallowing disorders would benefit from their services. Speech-language pathologists assess and address speech or language challenges using a multimodality approach, including visual, auditory, and tactile modalities when working with children following a stroke.

advocates in that environment in order to address the ongoing needs of the pediatric stroke patient, as well as the needs of their other children and spouse.

Parents as Advocates for Children With Stroke

An advocate is someone who supports another person by obtaining what the individual needs, as well as by seeking policy and laws that support the individual in achieving his or her goals in life.[8,9] The parents or caregiver of a child who has suffered a stroke who will require ongoing poststroke care will need to become an advocate for their child and family. The parent/advocate will need to learn all of the systems that will support the child's recovery, ranging from the medical and rehabilitation care, educational services, and community resources, to public laws and policies. Although parents will need to navigate many systems and services, they must keep in mind that the child should always be the central focus of every decision. Professionals can use many theories and models to understand how to help parents keep the child as the central focus of the care. The child who has suffered a stroke still goes through a developmental process, although altered due to the stroke, in the environment of the family and community.

Bronfenbrenner's Ecological Systems Theory

Professionals can look to developmental theories that focus on the child and his or her environment. One well-known developmental theory that addresses overall development and the environment is Bronfenbrenner's ecological systems theory, which focuses on development and the influence of a multilevel system within the child's environment,

with the child at the center.[10-12] The Brofenbrenner ecological systems theory is composed of 5 socially organized subsystems that are theorized to support and guide human development: the microsystem, mesosystem, exosystem, macrosystem, and chronosystem.[10-12] The systems work in a bidirectional manner that implies that relationships have impact in 2 directions, both away from the individual and toward the individual.[10-12] In the ecological system of development at the microsystem, the child after a stroke will have the majority of the relationships and interactions with the immediate family and other caregivers, such as school and daycare environments.[10-12] The resulting disabilities after the stroke will affect the relationship and interaction the child has in this system. The parent can be an advocate for the child in this system by seeking support from the extended family, school, and immediate community. The ecological systems theory holds that as children develop, they encounter different environments throughout their lifespan that may influence their behavior in varying degrees.[10-12]

The remaining systems in Brofenbrenner's ecological developmental theory include the mesosystem, which is the connection between 2 systems such as the child's teacher and his or her parents or between his or her church and his or her neighborhood.[11,12] The ecosystem is the larger social system in which the child may not directly function but the parents would be the main people to interact with the structures in this layer. This may include the parent's workplace schedules or community-based family resources. The child may not be directly involved at this system, but he or she does feel the positive or negative force involved with the interaction with his or her own system.[10] The main exosystems that indirectly influence youth through their family include school and peers, parents' workplace, family social networks and neighborhood community contexts, local politics, and industry.[11,12] Each level of the ecological system in which the child and family live influences them differently, and they behave and interact with the environment differently depending on the system and the needs of the individual. The macrosysytem is the larger community, which is composed of cultural values, customs, and laws, which is the society as a whole. This is the outermost layer of the child's environment and the most difficult layer for the parent and child to navigate. The chronosystem encompasses the dimension of time as it relates to a child's environment. Elements within this system can be either external, such as the timing of a parent's death, or internal, such as the physiological changes that occur with the aging of a child or the medical event of a pediatric stroke. Bronfenbrenner suggests that, in many cases, families respond to different stressors within the societal parameters existent in their lives, and their success depends on how well they navigate the systems and advocate for their child.[10-12] At each layer or level of the ecological system, the parent must to learn to advocate for the child and family. In looking at the different systems and varying influences in the child's life, advocating for the child offers many challenges. Brofenbrenner's ecological theory of development fits with the environmental and personal components of the ICF-CY, which clearly provides challenges and opportunities to support the child and family as they address the impairments and disabilities resulting from the stroke.[3,12] Parents will have many different roles, including caregiver, team member, decision maker, and advocate for the community and school resources, peer relationships, and needs of the siblings. In communicating with others about the stroke, the parent will play these many roles while trying to have the child and rest of the family function as ordinary people. Parents will learn that advocacy can be a dynamic process that pushes them to be flexible and nimble in their interactions with professionals and the community as a whole. A parent/advocate's role may differ from the time of the diagnosis, which might be at birth, and continually changes as the child grows and changes over time.

Parents may need to advocate in the macrosystem, including the legal system, educational system, and social support service system, with the parent helping the child to start to develop skills needed to be a self-advocate.[8,12] The ultimate role of the parent/advocate is to do what is necessary to meet the child and family needs. Professionals can be the initial advocate for the child and parents and then transition to being the parents' ally as the parents move into the role of advocate. Both the parent and professional advocates can help not only to improve the system for their child or patient, but also to improve it for other children as well.[7,9]

Combining the knowledge of Brofenbrenner's ecological system and the role of the advocate is important so the parents can help their child be functional within his or her environment. Professionals can help parents work to understand the needs of the child while they learn to advocate for their child. In learning to be a parent/advocate, the parent must do the following[7-9]:

- Learn about the child's diagnosis of pediatric stroke and his or her special needs.

- Develop effective communication with health care professionals, the educational system, and social support systems. Learn what they want and why.

- Become a member of the health care team and an equal partner.

- Maintain records and information about the child's medical and educational records and individualized education program.

- Know their rights and responsibilities in relationship to the child's diagnosis and ongoing needs.

- Be familiar with the local, state, and federal laws, as well as public laws and policies such as the Individuals with Disabilities Education Act (IDEA).

- Be familiar with the child's health and social benefits such as Supplemental Security Income and Medicaid.

- Develop a portfolio of resources for the child and family.

- Develop strategies for problem solving.

Team-Based Advocacy for Children With Stroke

Professionals can support the parent by promoting a collaborative relationship of trust between the professional team and the parent.[13] When professionals are working as part of a health care team, it is important for them to facilitate open communication, listen attentively, and encourage the family to ask questions. The team should also create an atmosphere of respect for the family's cultural values and beliefs. Professionals can help parents become an important part of the care team and help them function as a coach and advocate for their child as they grow older to ensure that the child gets what he or she needs. The professional and parent can also start to help children learn to advocate for themselves. Advocating for children, simply stated, means actively supporting the needs of the child. This should be the team's approach as they provide care and services for the child and create mutually beneficial partnerships between the family, the child, medical professionals, education professionals, and the community. The driving goal is to give each child the support that he or she needs in order to utilize available resources to reach his or her full potential.

HELPFUL HINTS FOR PARENT/ADVOCATES

How to Support the Needs of Their Child

1. Perinatal, the last 18 weeks of gestation through the first 30 days after birth

    a. Understand the diagnosis of pediatric stroke and related medical management and impairments

    b. Perinatal stroke is often delayed or misdiagnosed for months, even years

2. Childhood, ages 1 month to 18 years old

    a. Recognize signs and symptoms of stroke in babies and children.

    b. Symptoms may not appear until 4 to 8 months of age.

    c. Seizures can be one of the first signs of stroke.

    d. Early recognition and treatment during the first hours after a stroke is critical in optimizing long-term functional outcomes and minimizing recurrence risk.

    e. Stroke symptoms in children can be missed by parents/caregivers as well as by emergency department medical specialists.

    f. Many children with stroke symptoms are misdiagnosed with common conditions that mimic stroke, such as migraines, epilepsy, and viral illnesses.

    g. Early hand preference (before 1 year of age) should be investigated.

    h. Investigate developmental delays with medical specialists.

3. Birth to 5 years of age

    a. Work with your pediatrician or family physician to create a team of specialists to support your child's needs. Health care professionals to consult may include a neurologist, physiatrist, developmental pediatrician, physical, speech, or occupational therapist, orthopedist, and ophthalmologist.

    b. Each state in the United States must provide early intervention evaluations to families who have children with disabilities per IDEA. The child is evalu-

ated to determine what services may be needed, and services are provided in a natural environment, typically in the child's home.

    c. For birth up to the third birthday, these services are provided through IDEA Part C. For ages 3 to 21, the program is provided through IDEA Part B www.parentcenterhub.org/).[13]

    d. Work with your child at home, using the stretches, exercises, and recommendations the medical specialists/therapists provide. Starting a daily routine at an early age can help with adhering to the program as the child ages.

    e. Activities, classes, and group sessions specifically designed for children with physical disabilities may not be available in your area. However, many park districts and community programs may accommodate your child into their programs for the general population. Minor modifications may need to be made, so work with the administrators of these programs to help your child participate in classes, sports, and activities.

4. Age 6 to 14 years

    a. Continue the partnership and team approach with your child's health care professionals and education personnel. It is especially important during this period of development to keep up with medical evaluations due to growth spurts and puberty. Peer pressure and wanting to fit in can also play a role in the child's compliance with wearing orthotics, going to therapy, etc.

    b. In addition to the health care professionals listed for ages birth to 5 years, consider adding a neuropsychologist to the team in the early school years. This evaluation could expose potential learning or educational concerns.

    c. IDEA Part B may still be utilized if the evaluations indicate educational-based needs for the child. Services will be provided through the public school education system. See Chapter 12 for more information.

    d. If your child doesn't qualify for IDEA, you may be able to get accommodations for your child under Section 504 of the Rehabilitation Act of 1973 (Section 504) and Title II of the Americans with Disabilities Act (ADA). See Chapter 12 for more information.

    e. Utilize health care insurance whenever possible for additional therapies, medical services, and treatment as necessary.

    f. Look for programs that incorporate therapy/exercises into an activity or sport, such as karate, swimming, yoga, or adaptive sports programs. These may need to be modified to fit the needs of the child, so working in partnership with the administrators/instructors/teachers will be important.

5. Age 15 years to young adulthood

a. Continue the partnership and team approach with your child's health care professionals and education personnel as suggested in the earlier ages.

b. IDEA Part B may still be utilized if the evaluations indicate educational-based needs for the child. Section 504 accommodations through the ADA may also be utilized. Services will be provided through the public school education system. See Chapter 12 for more information.

c. Utilize health care insurance whenever possible for additional therapies, medical services, and treatment as necessary.

d. Driving laws and ages vary from state to state. Check with your Department of Motor Vehicles to find the age and what will be required to start the driving process for your child. Some states may require extra testing for cognitive issues, spatial abilities, response time, extra vision screening, and auto adaption devices.

e. Steering knobs are useful for drivers with hemiplegia. The knob allows for steering with one hand. The knob can be placed on either side of the steering wheel, and it is easily removed when not in use.

f. Adaptive foot pedals can be installed in cars for drivers with right hemiplegia. The pedal can be removed when not in use, but the car does have to be fitted with a permanent plate.

g. Panoramic or wide-angle rear and side view mirrors can be helpful for drivers with impaired peripheral vision.

h. To locate any of these devices, special testing, or disability driving instructors, contact a local rehabilitation center; search on the Internet for "adaptive driving equipment" + "your local area"; or go to the Association for Driver Rehabilitation Specialists (ADED) website to search by state for members of the ADED.

LIST OF RESOURCES ORGANIZATIONS, COMMUNITY RESOURCES, AND SUPPORT GROUPS

There are a number of organizations, support groups, government programs, and community resources for pediatric stroke survivors and their families. The following is a list of some of these.

American Heart Association (www.heart.org/HEARTORG)

The AHA is the nation's oldest and largest voluntary organization devoted to fighting cardiovascular diseases and stroke.

American Heart Association/American Stroke Association Support Network for Pediatric Stroke (www.strokeassociation.org)

The AHA/ASA Support Network offers a dedicated pediatric stroke discussion board where you can connect with other stroke patients and their caregivers, share your stroke experiences, and give and get emotional support and encouragement. This website provides useful information about stroke, including pediatric stroke.

American Stroke Association (http://www.strokeassociation.org/STROKEORG/AboutStroke/StrokeInChildren/Stroke-In-Children_UCM_308543_SubHomePage.jsp)

The ASA is the division of the AHA that's solely focused on reducing disability and death from stroke through research, education, fundraising, and advocacy.

Brain Injury Association of America (http://www.biausa.org)

The Brain Injury Association of America is the country's oldest and largest nationwide brain injury advocacy organization.

Brain Injury Association of Pennsylvania (BIAPA) (http://www.biapa.org)

BIAPA provides a listing of support groups for regions across the state, a resource line, and pre-enrollment assistance information.

Brain Injury Association of the United States (www.biapa.org)

Each state has a statewide brain injury association. Many of the groups have yearly conferences in which the parents and child can participate and get involved.

Children's Hemiplegia and Stroke Association: CHASA (www.chasa.org)

CHASA provides information and support to families of children who have hemiplegia, hemiparesis, or hemiplegic cerebral palsy. CHASA exists to help children who have survived an early brain injury that results in hemiplegia or hemiparesis (weakness on one side of the body). They also help adults who have been living with a diagnosis of hemiplegia since childhood. This organization has online support groups for both parents and children. CHASA members in certain regional areas have organized activities for child pediatric stroke survivors and their parents.

Children's Hemiplegia and Stroke Association—Pediatric Stroke Awareness (www.chasa.org/you-can-help/pediatric-stroke-awareness)

This site provides information on infant and childhood stroke, including diagnosing stroke in an infant or child; causes of pediatric stroke; childhood stroke facts; how you can help increase awareness of pediatric stroke; and updates on the latest in utero, infant, and childhood stroke research. You'll also find a list of pediatric stroke researchers and a list of infant and childhood stroke clinical trials and studies that need participants.

HemiHelp (www.hemihelp.org.uk)

HemiHelp is a website in Great Britain formed by a group of parents in 1990 to offer information and support to children and young people with hemiplegia, to their families or caregivers, and to the professionals who work with them to increase general awareness of the condition.

Hemi-kids (www.hemikids.org)

This site provides an email discussion group where parents of infants and children who have mild to moderate hemiplegia or hemiplegic cerebral palsy share information. This site provides an online support group of over 900 families of children who have hemiplegia or hemiplegic cerebral palsy.

International Alliance for Pediatric Stroke (IAPS) (www.iapediatricstroke.org/home.aspx)

The IAPS is an organization founded by doctors and parent advocates in 2013 to provide ease of access to resources and information about pediatric stroke to families, caregivers, researchers, medical specialists, and anyone else involved with these children. Included on this website is a list of pediatric stroke organizations worldwide that are making a difference in the lives of this pediatric population. IAPS was created to unite pediatric stroke communities around the world. IAPS provides knowledge, hope, resources and the connection between families, medical specialists, researchers, health care providers and anyone affected by pediatric stroke. Their mission is supported by leading pediatric neurologists and all of their information is approved by the physicians on their board.

The Internet Stroke Center (www.strokecenter.org)

The Internet Stroke Center is an independent educational service provided by the Washington University School of Medicine. It aims to provide current, professional, and unbiased information about stroke.

National Institute of Neurological Disorders and Stroke (NINDS) (www.ninds.nih.gov/disorders/stroke/stroke.htm)

This is the nation's leading supporter of biomedical research on disorders of the brain and nervous system. The mission of NINDS is to seek fundamental knowledge about the brain and nervous system and to use that knowledge to reduce the burden of neurological disease.

National Stroke Association (www.stroke.org)

The National Stroke Association provides information and resources to the public and health professionals with the aim of reducing the incidence and impact of stroke.

National Stroke Foundation (http://strokefoundation.com.au/)

This site provides a PDF booklet with helpful information about childhood stroke, stroke assessment, stroke recovery, personal stories, and more.

Pediatric Stroke Infographic (http://www.iapediatricstroke.org/infographic.pdf)

Pediatric stroke can happen in infants, children, and even before birth. This infographic created by the ASA offers facts about perinatal and childhood stroke.

The information is also available in Spanish (http://www.iapediatricstroke.org/Spanish.pdf) and Portugese (http://www.iapediatricstroke.org/Portuguese.pdf).

Pediatric Stroke Program at The Children's Hospital of Philadelphia (http://www.chop.edu/centers-programs/pediatric-stroke-program)

The Pediatric Stroke Program at The Children's Hospital of Philadelphia provides comprehensive assessment and treatment for children and infants who suffer from strokes. We provide inpatient and outpatient consultation and coordination of care and recovery services, including family education and support.

The Pediatric Stroke Network (www.pediatricstrokenetwork.com/)

The Pediatric Stroke Network is a family support organization. Their website offers general medical information, practical suggestions for living with stroke, and links to numerous other sources of information and support.

Reaching for the Stars (www.reachingforthestars.org)

A foundation of hope for children with cerebral palsy. Launched in late 2005 by 2 mothers in Atlanta, Georgia, Reaching for the Stars has grown into the largest pediatric cerebral palsy nonprofit foundation in the world led by parents, with a focus on the prevention, treatment, and cure of cerebral palsy. They are committed to serving the needs of children with cerebral palsy, their families, and the caregivers involved in their care.

SUPPORT GROUPS

New support groups are set up and organized frequently. Parents or professionals may want to form new support groups in areas where groups do not yet exist. Existing support groups can be found in hospital and clinic settings where the child and family receive care for the stroke.

Sibshops for siblings (www.siblingsupport.org)

This organization provides support for brothers and sisters of a person with special needs. Many hospitals and rehabilitation facilities have ongoing sibshops.

Neonatal and Pediatric Stroke Programs/Clinics at Large Children's Hospitals With Support Groups

- Children's Hospital of Philadelphia, Pennsylvania
- Boston Children's Hospital, Massachusetts
- University of California—San Francisco Pediatric Stroke and Cerebrovascular Disease Center
- Pediatric Stroke Program at Johns Hopkins All Children's Hospital in St. Petersburg, Florida
- Denver Pediatric Stroke Clinic at University of Colorado—Hemophilia and Thrombosis Center

Neuro-Rehab Parent Support Group

The Neuro-Rehab Parent Support Group is open to parents and caregivers of children with acquired brain injury (including traumatic brain injury and stroke).

Teen Neuro-Rehab Support Group

The Teen Neuro-Rehab Support Group provides support to teens and young adults (ages 13 to 21) with acquired brain injuries (including traumatic brain injury and stroke).

VIDEO

Pediatric Stroke Awareness Video: A Stroke Can Happen at Any Age (www.youtube.com/watch?v=pvyocL0njPg)

The International Alliance for Pediatric Stroke, in partnership with the AHA/ASA, created a video about pediatric stroke to help raise awareness that a stroke can happen to infants, children, and even before birth.

TOOLS FOR SUCCESS AT SCHOOL

Special Education After Stroke

Find tips for children returning to school after a stroke and information about special education for children who have suffered a stroke.

Stroke Therapy Services in the School Environment

Learn about the difference between in-school and outpatient therapy for stroke recovery and how each can help your child meet his or her academic goals.

Tips for a Successful Transition to College After Stroke

Many young adults choose to pursue a college degree after a stroke. Whether you are considering attending a local community college or attending a university away from home, here are a few quick tips on how to have a successful transition to college.

- Work with your health care and educational teams for support as you transition.
- Contact a social worker who can assist you during the transition to college.
- Contact the Office of Disabilities as you are researching colleges.

COMMUNITY PROGRAMS

- Park and recreational programs
- Paralympic sports programs
- YMCA classes/sports, etc
- Social media (Facebook)

ACKNOWLEDGMENTS

Thank you to Julie A. Neitzke, RN, BSN for her contribution to this chapter. Her perspective and knowledge as a nurse working with children in a pediatric stroke clinic was essential and invaluable to this chapter

REFERENCES

1. deVeber G, Roach E, Riela A, Wiznitzer M. Stroke in children: recognition, treatment, and future directions. *Seminars in Pediatric Neurology.* 2000;7(4):309-317.

2. Tsze D, Valente J. Pediatric stroke: a review. *Emergency Medicine International.* 2011; 2-10. doi:10.1155/2011/734506.

3. ICF-CY, International Classification Of Functioning, Disability, And Health. Geneva, Switzerland: World Health Organization; 2007.

4. Lo W, Zamel K, Ponnappa K, et al. The Cost of pediatric stroke care and rehabilitation. *Stroke.* 2008;39:161-165.

5. FACTS Knowing No Bounds: Stroke in Infants, Children, and Youth. American Heart Association/American Stroke Association. http://www.strokeassociation.org/idc/groups/heart-public/@wcm/@adv/documents/downloadable/ucm_302255.pdf. Published 2013. Accessed March 14, 2016.

6. Paediatric Stroke Working Group. *Stroke In Childhood Clinical Guidelines For Diagnosis, Management And Rehabilitation.* London, United Kingdom: Royal College of Physicians of London; 2004.

7. A Family Guide To Pediatric Stroke. http://www.heartandstroke.com/atf/cf/%7B99452d8b-e7f1-4bd6-a57d-b136ce6c95bf%7D/A-FAMILY-GUIDE-TO-PEDIATRIC-STROKE-ENG.PDF. Published 2015. Accessed March 14, 2016.

8. Alper S, Schloss P, Schloss C. Families of children with disabilities in elementary and middle school: advocacy models and strategies. *Exceptional Children.* 1995;62(3):261-270.

9. Institute for Patient- and Family-Centered Care. Patient Safety Toolkit. http://www.ipfcc.org/tools/Patient-Safety-Toolkit-04.pdf. Accessed March 14, 2016.

10. Advocating for Your Child with Special Needs. http://www.directionservice.org/cadre/parent/artifacts/Matrix-1%20advocating.packet.6.11.pdf. Accessed March 14, 2016.

11. Darling N. Ecological systems theory: the person in the center of the circles. *Research In Human Development.* 2007;4(3-4):203-217.

12. Bronfenbrenner U. *The Ecology Of Human Development: Experiments By Nature And Design.* Cambridge, MA: Harvard University Press; 1979.

13. Bronfenbrenner U. The Bioecological Theory Of Human Development. In: Smelser NJ & Baltes PB, eds. *International Encyclopedia Of The Social And Behavioral Sciences.* New York, NY: Elsevier; 2001:6963–6970.

14. Maternal and Child Health Bureau. Definition of family-centered care. http://www.familyvoices.org/admin/work_family_centered/files/FCCare.pdf. Accessed March 14, 2016. 15.

15. Center for Parent Information and Resources. http://www.parentcenterhub.org/. Accessed March 15, 2016.

Financial Disclosures

Dr. Heather L. Atkinson has no financial or proprietary interest in the materials presented herein.

Mary Kay Ballasiotes has no financial or proprietary interest in the materials presented herein.

Dr. Juliana Bloom has no financial or proprietary interest in the materials presented herein.

Dr. Danielle Bosenbark has no financial or proprietary interest in the materials presented herein.

Dr. Phillip R. Bryant has no financial or proprietary interest in the materials presented herein.

Amy Colin has no financial or proprietary interest in the materials presented herein.

Anna Cooper has no financial or proprietary interest in the materials presented herein.

Dr. Susan V. Duff has no financial or proprietary interest in the materials presented herein.

Dr. Amanda Fuentes has no financial or proprietary interest in the materials presented herein.

Dr. Anne Gordon has no financial or proprietary interest in the materials presented herein.

Dr. Mardee Greenham has no financial or proprietary interest in the materials presented herein.

Dr. Gregory G. Heuer has no financial or proprietary interest in the materials presented herein.

Dr. Rebecca Ichord has no financial or proprietary interest in the materials presented herein.

Dr. Adam Kirton has no financial or proprietary interest in the materials presented herein.

Dr. Lauren Krivitzky has no financial or proprietary interest in the materials presented herein.

Dr. Shih-Shan Lang has no financial or proprietary interest in the materials presented herein.

Dr. Kim Nixon-Cave has no financial or proprietary interest in the materials presented herein.

Elisa Olson D'Achille has no financial or proprietary interest in the materials presented herein.

Dr. Mubeen F. Rafay has no financial or proprietary interest in the materials presented herein.

Dr. Lois J. Robbins has no financial or proprietary interest in the materials presented herein.

Dr. Sabrina E. Smith has no financial or proprietary interest in the materials presented herein.

Dr. Robyn Westmacott has no financial or proprietary interest in the materials presented herein.

Elizabeth Yeh has no financial or proprietary interest in the materials presented herein.

Index

activated protein C resistance, 45
activity measures, 94–98
    activities of daily living, 95–96
    balance, 96
    cardiopulmonary screen, 97–98
    coordination, 96
    functional mobility, 94
    gait analysis, 94–95
    gross motor skills, 96
    physical activity levels, 94
    prehension, 96–97
acute care rehabilitation therapists, role of, 72–73
acute care setting, 70
acute cerebellar ataxia, 6
acute disseminated encephalomyelitis, 6
adaptive aids, 127–128
Adaptive Behavior Assessment System, 174
admissions coordinator, role of, 73
advocacy, 248–253
    team-based, 252–253
allergies, 78–79, 91
American Heart Association, 17, 46, 247, 254
American Heart Association/American Stroke Association
    Support Network for Pediatric Stroke, 254
American Stroke Association, 247, 254
American Stroke Association Support Network for Pediatric
    Stroke, 254
anemia, 11, 45
antiphospholipid antibodies presence, 45
antithrombin III deficiency, 8, 22, 45–46
anxiety, 192–194, 214
    prevention, 82
    psychotherapy, 195–196
    treatments, 195–196
apathy, depression, 195
Apgar score, 22, 30
aphasia, 136–137
    expressive language deficits, 140–141
    global, 142–143
    receptive language deficits, 141–142
    symptoms, 138–143
    word finding, 138–140

apraxia of speech, 143–144
arterial ischemic stroke, 7–11, 21–30
    childhood, 3–20
    perinatal, 21–32
aspiration precautions, 72, 79
attention deficit hyperactivity disorder, 188–192
    behavior management, 191
    education, 191
    educational supports, 192
    identification, 188
    medication, 191–192, 196
    parent training, 191
    school support, 192
    symptoms, 188–190
    treatments, 190–192

Beery-Buktenica Developmental Test of Visual-Motor
    Integration, 174
behavioral conferences, 78–79
behavioral functioning, 185–203
    biopsychosocial model, 206–210
        family-centered care, 208–210
    giving up, 185
    scope of problem, 186–188
behavioral status, 79, 82
Behcet's disease, 9, 45
belief system, 218–219
BIAPA. *See* Brain Injury Association of Pennsylvania
Boston Naming Test, 137
boundary ambiguity, 216
Brain Injury Association of America, 254
Brain Injury Association of Pennsylvania, 254
Brain Injury Association of United States, 254
breastfeeding, swallowing, 150
Broca's area, 26, 136, 140, 143
Bronfenbrenner's ecological systems theory, 251–252

California Verbal Learning Test, Children's Version, 164,
    170, 174
cancer, 45, 61, 67, 98, 102, 195, 212, 249
cardiopulmonary screen, 97–98
caregiver burden, 217

case manager, role of, 73
cerebellar ataxia, 6
cerebral sinovenous thrombosis, 35–57
    Behcet's disease, 45
    diagnosis, 46–47
        antithrombotic therapy, 51–53
        supportive therapy, 51
    dural venous system
        anatomy, 35–36
        pathophysiology, 35–36
    etiologies, 38–46
    imaging, 46–47
    incidence, 36–37
    infectious, 38–45
    maternal, 46
    noninfectious, 45–46
    perinatal, 46
    rehabilitation, 53
    risk factors, 38–46
        maternal, 46
        noninfectious, 45–46
        perinatal, 46
channelopathies, 6
CHASA. *See* Children's Hemiplegia and Stroke Association
childhood arterial ischemic stroke, 3–20
    chronic management, 12–15
    clinical presentation, 5
    diagnosis, 5–7
    differential diagnosis, 6
    epidemiology, 3
    hematological disorders, 11
    neuroimaging, 5–7
    outcomes, 12–15
    pathophysiology, 4–5
        arterial circulation, 4
        brain injury, 4–5
        thromboembolism, 4
    prothrombotic disorders, 11
    risk factors, 7–11
        arteriopathies, 7–10
        cardiac, 10–11
    treatment, 11–12
Children's Category Test, 174
Children's Hemiplegia and Stroke Association, 203, 254–255
The Children's Hospital of Philadelphia, 255
chin down swallowing, 152
chorioamnionitis, 22, 30
circumlocution, 138
Clinical Evaluation of Language Fundamentals, 137
cognition, social, 168–169
cognitive ability, 161–163
cognitive changes, 161–183
    cognitive outcomes, 161–172
    neuropsychological assessment, 173
    rehabilitation strategies, 173–175

communication, 135–159
communication handoff, 76–78
community, 205–257
    evaluation, 105
    programs, 256
compensatory strategies, 128
complication prevention, 81–83
    anxiety, 82
    subluxation prevention, 82
conferences
    behavioral, 78–79
    family, 79
    interprofessional team, 78
congenital heart disease, 8, 10–13, 22, 45, 248
Conners' Continuous Performance Test, 174
Conners' Rating Scales, 174
contact precautions, 79
continuum of care, 1–88
contractures, 83–84
coordination of care, 103
coping strategies, 219–220
cortical reorganization
    in animals, 116–117
    in humans, 117
culture, impact of, 218–219
CVLT-C. *See* California Verbal Learning Test, Children's Version

day hospital rehabilitation, 80
decreased attention, 235–236
deep venous thrombosis prophylaxis, 79
dehydration, 41, 43, 45–46, 51–52
Delis-Kaplan Executive Function System, 174
depression, 82
    apathy, distinguished, 195
Developmental NEuroPSYcological Assessment, 174
developmental pediatrician, 249, 253
diabetes, 9, 11, 22, 46, 98, 195, 248
dietician, role of, 72
discharge planning, 103–109
disseminated encephalomyelitis, 6
dural venous system anatomy, 35–36

education
    504 Plan, 228
    absences from school, 231
    accommodations, 234–244
    college, intervention to, 232–234
    educational services, 232–234
    elementary school, 233–234
    gradual school re-entry, 230
    high school, 233–234
    homebound instruction, 230
    individualized education program, 227–228
    legislation, educational, 227–228

medical needs, 232
medication at school, 232
private school, 230
school problems, 234–244
student health care plan sample, 244
therapy services, 231–232
transition back to school, 229–231
transportation, specialized, 231
effortful swallow, 152
emotional functioning, 185–203
biopsychosocial model, 206–210
employment, parental, 223
encephalitis, 6, 8–9, 38, 45
environment, 205–257
epilepsy, perinatal arterial ischemic stroke, 29
equipment, 105
executive function, 166–167, 240
exogenous hormones, 45
Expressive One Word Picture Vocabulary Test, 137
Expressive Vocabulary Test, 137
extracorporeal membrane oxygenation, 8, 22

factor V Leiden mutation, 45
falls, 79, 84–86
family, 205–257
conferences, 79
education, 105–106, 129
family-centered care, 208–210
feeding, 147–155
breastfeeding, 150
chin down, 152
chin tuck, 152
dysphagia management, 151–155
effortful swallow, 152
fiber-optic endoscopic evaluation, 151
head turn, 152–153
instrumental assessment, 150–151
oral feeding assessment, 148–149, 152
oral feeding considerations, 149–150
swallowing phases, 147–148
videofluoroscopic swallow study, 150–151
fetal heart rate abnormalities, 22
fiber-optic endoscopic evaluation, 151
financial issues, 223
finding words, 138–140
fine motor difficulties, 238–239
focal transient cerebral arteriopathy, 7–9
functional outcomes, 89–204

gait dysfunction, 83–84, 94–95
gait training, 123–124
gestational diabetes, 22
giving up, 185
global aphasia, 142–143
grief, stages of, 216
guardianship, 223

head turn, swallowing, 152–153
Hemi-kids, 255
HemiHelp, 255
hemiplegic migraine, 6
hemorrhage, intracerebral, 59–68
congenital bleeding disorders, 60–61
elevated intracerebral hemorrhage, 63
elevated intracranial pressure, 63–64
epidemiology, 59
hemophilia, 60–61
idiopathic thrombocytopenia purpura, 60
initial evaluation, 61–62
malignancy, 61
management, 61–62
neonatal intracerebral hemorrhage, 61
neuroimaging, 62–63
newborn intracerebral hemorrhage, 61
risk factors, 60–61
sickle cell disease, 61
special populations, 60–61
heparin-induced thrombocytopenia, 45
high school, 233–234
home
evaluation, 105
modifications, 222
program, 80
homebound instruction, 230
hyperactivity, 188–192. *See also* attention deficit
hyperactivity disorder
hyperhomocysteinemia, 8, 45–46
hypertensive encephalopathy, 6
hypoglycemia, 6, 22

IAPS. *See* International Alliance for Pediatric Stroke
identity, change in, 217
impairment measures, 91–94
cognition, 94
movement analysis, 92
physical function, 91–92
posture, 92–93
sensibility, 93
visual function, 93–94
visual-motor function, 94
visual-perceptual function, 94
inborn errors of metabolism, 6
individualized education program, 227–228
infection, 4–7, 9, 11, 22, 37–38, 41, 43, 45–46, 51–52
infertility, 22, 30
inflammatory bowel disease, 8, 45, 55, 195
inpatient admission criteria, 73–76
inpatient rehabilitation, 70–72
insurance, 224
intellectual functioning, 161–163
International Alliance for Pediatric Stroke, 255–256
International Classification of Functioning, Disability and Health-Children and Youth, 207–210

Internet Stroke Center, 255
interprofessional conferences, 78
intracerebral hemorrhage, 59–68. *See also* Hemorrhage,
     intracerebral
intrauterine growth restriction, 22
iron-deficiency anemia, 11, 45

joint contractures, prevention of, 81–82
Judgment of Line Orientation, 174

L-asparaginase, 45
lactic acidosis, 6
language, 135–136. *See also* aphasia
learning difficulties, 14, 65, 119, 145, 147, 164–165, 177,
     199, 230, 236–238
legal issues, 223
legislation, educational, 227–228
liaison, role of, 73
locomotor training, 123–124
lower extremity orthoses, 125–127
lupus, 8–9, 45
lupus anticoagulant presence, 45

malignancy, 45, 61
maternal fever, 22, 46
medical management, 1–88
medication at school, 232
memory, 164–165, 167–168, 236–238
meningitis, 8–9, 14, 22, 38, 41, 43, 45–46
mental processing speed, 240–241
methylene tetrahydrofolate reductase gene mutation, 45
migraine, 5–6, 9, 11, 13
mirror therapy, 125
mitochondrial encephalomyopathy, 6
mobility difficulties, 239
modifications, home, 222
Modified Ashworth Scale, 92
Modified Tardieu Scale, 93
mood disorders, 194–195
     psychotherapy, 195–196
     treatments, 195–196
motor imagery, 124–125
motor skills, 113–134
     adaptive techniques, 125–129
     child education, 129
     cortical reorganization, 116–117
     family education, 129
     interprofessional team, 129–130
     neuroplasticity, 117–120
     therapeutic strategies, 122–125
moyamoya, childhood arterial ischemic stroke, 10
multiple sclerosis, 6

National Institute of Neurological Disorders and Stroke, 255
National Stroke Association, 255
National Stroke Foundation, 255

neologisms, 138, 141, 144
nephrotic syndrome, 45
networks of support, 222–223
Neuro-Rehab Parent Support Group, 256
neuroimaging, childhood arterial ischemic stroke, 5–7
neuromotor evaluation, 91–112
     activity measures, 94–98
     communication, 103
     coordination of care, 103
     diagnosis, 98–99
     discharge planning, 103–109
     equipment, 105
     examination, 91–98
     general appearance, 91
     goals, 100–101
     history, 91
     impairment measures, 91–94
     interview, 91
     Modified Ashworth Scale, 92
     Modified Tardieu Scale, 93
     orthoses, 105
     participation measures, 98
     plan of care, 100–101
     presentation, 91
     prognosis, 99–100
     re-evaluation, 101–103
     splints, 105
neuromuscular re-education, 122–123
neuroplasticity, 83, 116–120
     age at diagnosis, 118
     behavior, 119–120
     brain reserve, 119
     cognition, 119–120
     language, 119–120
     location of lesion, 118
     motivation, 120
     premorbid abilities, 119
     size of lesion, 118
     time since injury, 119
nurses, rehabilitation, 72
nursing care at school, 232
nutritional restrictions, 79

orthoses, 105
orthotists, 250
outpatient rehabilitation therapies, 80
ovarian stimulation, 22

pacing, 150–151
panic, 214
paraphasias, 138, 141–144
parental employment, 223
parents as advocates, 251
paroxysmal nocturnal hemoglobinuria, 45
participation measures, 98
pediatric rehabilitation physician specialist, role of, 72

pediatric stroke
   advocacy, 247–257
   behavioral functioning, 185–203
   cerebral sinovenous thrombosis, 35–57
   cognitive changes, 161–183
   communication, 135–159
   educational needs, 227–245
   emotional functioning, 185–203
   environment, 211–225
   family, 211–225
   feeding, 135–159
   intracerebral hemorrhage, 59–68
   motor skills, 113–134
   neuromotor evaluation, 91–112
   rehabilitation, 69–88, 247–257
   resources, 247–257
Pediatric Stroke Network, 255
Pediatric Test of Brain Injury, 137
perinatal arterial ischemic stroke, 21–32
   behavioral deficits, 27–29
   clinical presentation, 21–22
   cognitive deficits, 27–29
   cost, 29–30
   diagnosis, 23–25
   epilepsy, 29
   health status, 29–30
   motor deficits, 26–27
   outcome, 26–30
   quality of life, 29–30
   risk factors, 22–23
   sensory deficits, 26–27
perseverations, 138
phases of swallowing, 147–148
phonological treatments, 139
physician, communication with, 79
placental abnormalities, 22
plan of care, 100–101
polycythemia, 9, 22, 45
postdischarge, 79–80
posterior reversible encephalopathy syndrome, 6
poststroke surveillance, 81
posture, 92–93
preeclampsia, 22
prehension, 96–97
pressure sores, prevention of, 82
primary physician, communication with, 79
private school, 230
procoagulant drugs, 45
prolonged rupture of membranes, 22
protein C deficiency, 45–46
protein S deficiency, 8, 22, 45–46
prothrombin 20210A mutation, 45
prothrombotic disorders, 11, 26, 45
psychotherapy, for anxiety, 195–196

range-of-motion restrictions, 79, 126

re-entering community, 222
Reaching for Stars, 256
recreation, 223
Rehabilitation Act, 228, 253
rehabilitation nurses, role of, 72
religion, impact of, 218–219
resiliency of family, 220–222
resource organizations, 254–256
Rey-Osterrieth Complex Figure Test, 174
robotic support, treadmill training, 123–124

safety issues, 222
sarcoidosis, 45
school. *See also* education
   environment, stroke therapy services, 256
   evaluation, 105
   recommendations, 105
   rehabilitation, 80
seizures, 5–6, 14, 23, 29–33, 38, 51, 72, 78–79, 81, 83, 85,
   148, 155, 171–172, 228
sensory impairments, 174, 241–242
septicemia, 38, 45
shoulder pain, 82
siblings, 218
Sibshops for Siblings, 256
sidelying, 150–151
sinovenous thrombosis, cerebral, 35–57
   Behcet's disease, 45
   diagnosis, 46–47, 51–53
   dural venous system, anatomy, 35–36
   etiologies, 38–46
   incidence, 36–37
   infectious, 38–45
   rehabilitation, 53
   risk factors, 38–46
social cognition, 168–169
social workers, 73, 196, 206, 248, 251
spasticity, management of, 82–83
specialized transportation, 231
speech-language pathology therapists, 251
speech motor disorders, 143–144
   apraxia of speech, 143–144
   dysarthria of speech, 143
spirituality, impact of, 218–219
splints, 105
split belt, treadmill training, 124
stages of grief, 216
Stanford Binet Intelligence Scales, 174
steroids, 12, 14, 45, 177
strength training, 123
student health care plan sample, 244
support groups, 256
surveillance poststroke, 81
swallowing, 147–155
   breastfeeding, 150
   chin down, 152

chin tuck, 152
dysphagia management, 151–155
effortful swallow, 152
fiber-optic endoscopic evaluation, 151
head turn, 152–153
instrumental assessment, 150–151
oral feeding assessment, 148–149, 152
oral feeding considerations, 149–150
phases, 147–148
videofluoroscopic swallow study, 150–151
systemic emboli prophylaxis, 79
systemic lupus erythematosus, 8–9, 45

Teacher Report Form, 174
team-based advocacy, 252–253
Teen Neuro-Rehab Support Group, 256
Test of Auditory Processing Skills, 137
The Test of Everyday Attention for Children, 174
Test of Narrative Language, 137
Test of Reading Comprehension, 137
Test of Visual Perceptual Skills, 174
Test of Word Finding, 137
Test of Written Language, 137
thrombocythemia, 45
thrombocytopenia, 12, 45, 60, 62, 78
thromboembolism, childhood arterial ischemic stroke, 4
thrombophilia, 10, 12, 22, 25, 46
thrombotic thrombocytopenic purpura, 9, 45
thyroid disorders, 45

transportation, specialized, 231
treadmill training, 123–124
trusts, special needs, 223
twin-twin transfusion syndrome, 22

upper extremity orthoses, 127

vestibulopathy, 6
videofluoroscopic swallow study, 150–151
Vineland Adaptive Behavior Scale, 174
virtual reality devices, 124
visual function, 93–94
visual-perceptual function, 94
visuospatial processing, 163–164

Wechsler Adult Intelligence Scale, 174
Wechsler Intelligence Scale for Children, 174
Wechsler Preschool and Primary Scale of Intelligence, 94, 174
weight-bearing limitations, 79
Wide Range Assessment of Memory and Learning, 174
Wisconsin Card Sorting Test, 174
word finding, 138–140. *See also* aphasia
work force, preparing to enter, 224
working memory, 167–168
Working Memory Test Battery for Children, 174
wound care, 72, 79

Youth Self-Report, 174

Printed in the United States
by Baker & Taylor Publisher Services